ORGAN TRANSPLANTATION RESEARCH HORIZONS

KIDNEY TRANSPLANTATION

DENERVATION, REINNERVATION, ISCHEMIA, HYPOTHERMIA

ORGAN TRANSPLANTATION RESEARCH HORIZONS

Additional books in this series can be found on Nova's website
under the Series tab.

Additional e-books in this series can be found on Nova's website
under the E-books tab.

ORGAN TRANSPLANTATION RESEARCH HORIZONS

KIDNEY TRANSPLANTATION

DENERVATION, REINNERVATION, ISCHEMIA, HYPOTHERMIA

TAMAZ J. SHIOSHVILI

Nova Science Publishers, Inc.

New York

For permission to use material from this book please contact us:
Telephone 631-231-7269; Fax 631-231-8175
Web Site: http://www.novapublishers.com

LIBRARY OF CONGRESS CATALOGING-IN-PUBLICATION DATA

Shioshvili, Tamaz J.
Kidney transplantation : denervation, reinnervation, ischemia, hypothermia / Tamaz J. Shioshvili.
p. ; cm.
Includes bibliographical references and index.
ISBN 978-1-60692-487-7 (hardcover)
1. Kidneys--Transplantation--Complications. 2. Kidneys--Innervation. 3. Ischemia. I. Title.
[DNLM: 1. Kidney Transplantation. 2. Denervation. 3. Graft Survival. 4. Hypothermia, Induced. 5. Ischemia--therapy. 6. Kidney--innervation. WJ 368 S556k 2009]
RD575.S485 2009
617.4'610592--dc22

2008055748

Published by Nova Science Publishers, Inc. † New York

CONTENTS

PREFACE

The kidney transplantation is a versatile problem which includes very important specific (immune) as well as nonspecific aspects (the denervation and ischemia of the kidney, surgical complexity, infection, initially complicated somatic condition of patients and so on). The neglect or underestimation even of one of them inevitably leads to the failure of the whole intervention.

In the last twenty years an especially great progress in the transplantation immunology is observed. Very effective immunosuppressive substances were elaborated which to a marked degree extended the survival of the kidney transplant and patient. But at the same time a more attention has to be paid to other, nonspecific sides, particularly the denervation and ischemia of the transplant. Exactly they were the subject of the given work.

The god has nothing created aimlessly, including the kidney nervous apparatus. It is very rich structurally and loaded functionally. By the transplantation it occurs the total rupture of the kidney with the organism and with full sharpness arise the questions: how much harmless is the kidney denervation, is it needed its artificial reinnervation, which is the most effective method for that?

In the given work are described the existing data about the consequences of denervation of the kidney in situ and in connection with its autotransplantation in dogs. It was convincingly demonstrated that the mentioned interventions in 1-2 years caused the functional depression, atrophy and sclerosis of considerable part of the kidney parenchyma in spite of the absence of an immune rejection.

On the other hand, the comparison of results of the auto- and allotransplantations of the kidney and revealing some common signs (various degree of dystrophy, atrophy, local and diffusive sclerosis, lymphoid infiltration, circulatory disorders) testify that they could be caused not only by an immune rejection but also by the cessation of the trophic influence of the nervous system on the kidney.

Therefore proceeding from clinical interests, more persistently arise the questions: to leave the nervous apparatus of the kidney to the mercy of fate or to make an active artificial surgical reinnervation of the kidney transplant? The first attempts undertaken in this field showed the principle feasibility of surgical reinnervation of the transplanted kidney and its beneficial influence on the organ. But existing methods did not require utterly to the necessary demands because the used sources of reinnervation were not physiological enough.

It was obvious that the decisive criteria for the optimal decision in this respect should be the following: 1. The source of reinnervation should be natural for the kidney, providing its adequate supply with adrenergic and cholinergic mediators; 2. The surgical technique should insure the germination of nervous fibers up to the terminal level of the kidney nervous apparatus. 3. The method of reinnervation should be technically simple accessible for an ordinary transplantologist.

In this respect the I.D. Kirpatovsky-s method [189] seems as very promising and perspective. It consists in the connection of perivascular fascial shreds of anastomosed blood vessels of the transplant and recipient. This method used by the intestinal autotransplantation [205,237] showed a high efficacy. Because there were not any data about its action by the kidney transplantation with longterm following observation, I took the I.D. Kirpatovsky-s method as a basis of the given investigation. Of course, it should be an autotransplantation model in order to avoid at this time undesirable immune problems.

As far the objective examination of the finest changes related to the neural trophic was impossible on the background of normothermic ischemia, the second direction of this study was the minimization of ischemic injury of the transplanted kidney.

There is a very rich literature about the ischemised kidney hypothermic protection. But hypothermia has as positive as well as negative sides. Therefore it has to be emphasized, that it doesn`t exist any universal optimal level of hypothermia suitable for every duration ischemia. It is obvious that the longer is the ischemia of an organ the lower should be its temperature. In this respect the ischemia duration of two hours has its firm position in the experimental and clinical transplantology. This area includes: auto-and allotransplantation of the organs in experiments, clinical autotransplantation of the kidney, its allotransplantation from a leaving donor in the clinic, nephrolithotomy and partial resection of a kidney with the temporarily blockaded blood flow. The literary data concerning the optimal level of hypothermia for two hour ischemia are very controversial and contradictious as far various authors use the hypothermia in wide range from +32 C to +2 C. The special apparatus for the realization of hypothermia by above mentioned operations require also the further optimization. It concerns especially to the techniques for the maintaining of renal hypothermia during the blood vessels anastomosing of the transplanting kidney. Thus, the aims of the present work were following:

- evaluation of the kidney denervation in situ and in the autotransplantation model in dogs using modern high sensitive morpho-functional test-methods;
- examination of the most possible level of spontaneous reinnervation of the transplanted kidney;
- the trial of feasibility of I.D. Kirpatovsky-s method of surgical reinnervation by the kidney autotransplantation in the iliac fossa.
- investigation of the regeneration process in the nervous apparatus of the autotransplanted kidney after its surgical reinnervation in the long term following observation;
- determination of an optimal regime of hypothermic protection of the kidney by its two-hour long ischemia;
- perfection of the techniques for the local renal hypothermia.

Aproximately 100 000 kidney transplantations are carried out in the whole world every year. Many aspects of this intervention are elaborated in details and became routine. On the one hand, it is a positive phenomenon making available this operation for the more amount of surgeons and patients. But on the other hand, the routine means the stoppage of the progress.

The present work is an attempt to demonstrate that there are still some unused essential reserves for the improvement of general results in the transplantology. Particularly, the artificial surgical reinnervation and proper hypothermic protection of the transplanted kidney from ischemia can increase its morpho-functional potential for 30-40%. It means that the sclerosis and functional depression of the kidney observed after its allotransplantation and considered as a result of an immune (acute or chronic) rejection, actually are determined in a marked degree by the organ denervation and ischemia.

How much convincing looks this general conclusion, every reader can decide for himself after described impartial objective data. But, in my opinion, absolutely doubtless is that denervaton and ischemic injuries should not be underestimated and deserve more attention of the wide range of experimental and clinical transplantologists, scientists and scholars not only in respect of the kidney, but also of other transplanting organs. I would be very happy if I could activate this aspiration.

Taking an opportunity I express the highest gratitude to my consultants: Prof. Igor Kirpatovsky, Head of department of surgical anatomy at Moscow Peoples Friendship University, Prof. Vadim Shvalev, Head of department of neurohistology at Moscow Scientific Center of Cardiology, Prof. George Nasarishvili, Head of department of pathophysiology at Georgian National Center of Urology and all my colleagues in urologic department of Georgian State Medical Academy for the support and assistance in preparing this work.

I am very thankful to Mrs. Maya Columbus, Editor of Nova-Science- Publishers Inc. for the opportunity to publish the present material.

Chapter I

SURVEY OF THE LITERATURE

1.1. CONSEQUENCES OF KIDNEY DENERVATION IN SITU

1.1.1. The Methods of Kidney Denervation

The evaluation of kidney denervation still remains disputable in spite of countless works in that field. This contradiction is mainly determined by the variety of methods for kidney denervation, the insufficient sensitivity of tests that are used, and the short duration of follow-up observations.

There are a few methods for kidney denervation used in acute and chronic experiments. The partial denervation (the removal of ganglions of the spinal brain on various levels, or those of sympathetic border trunks, the cutting of hypogastric nerves, vagotomy, the cutting of pelvic nerves, the removal of the pelvic nervous plexus, the decapsulation of the kidney) are used mainly for the detection of sources of kidney innervation.

More complete denervation of the kidney in situ is achieved by means of cutting all visible nervous fibers in the kidney pelvic area along the renal artery, vein and ureter; their cultivation with neurolytic solutions and decapsulation of the kidney. In this case, all that remains untouched are the nerve fibers located in the middle layer of renal blood vessels.

Full denervation of the kidney occurs by transplantation. Simultaneously the kidney is affected by many other factors related to transplantation such as the mechanical trauma, temporary ischemia, circulatory disorders, cutting of lymphatic vessels, and immune factors, infection, which distort the real results of the kidney denervation.

Therefore, for objective evaluation of the kidney denervation, the type and volume of denervation has to be taken into account..

1.1.2. The Functional State of the Kidney after Denervation in Situ

The results of acute experiments in kidney denervation are, on the whole, monotonous.

Still, Clod Bernard (1859) [38] established that the cut of n. splanchnicus caused an increase of diuresis on the same side. This phenomenon was confirmed many times by other scientists especially after the wide use of separate ureterostomy in the experimental physiology. [267,279,280].

The cut of n. splanchnicus caused, in 1-2 days, a polyuria and an increase of chloride excretion. One week later the diuresis of the denervated and intact kidneys became equal, but by water loading the denervated kidney secreted less urine than the intact one. [220,221].

In analogous experiments, the denervation of one kidney was accompanied by polyuria on both sides. But water loading also revealed a lag in diuresis of the denervated kidney. [41,117,288].

The increase of diuresis and secretion of Na-ions after the cut of n. splanchnicus had been observed by many other authors [36,42-44,111,178,179,201,274,286,333]. One group of them considered it to be a result of an intensification of the tubular transport of Na-ions without any changes in glomerular filtration or renal blood flow [35,42,44,179,201,333,345,394].

Another group of authors, after unilateral sympathectomy in acute experiments on dogs, observed an increase in renal blood flow. They considered this fact to be a result of the increase of water and Na-ion secretion. By analogy, the positive influence of the kidney decapsulation in the case of glomerulonephritic anuria was considered to be a result of the removal of the neural control of the kidney and consequent intensification of renal blood circulation [172,206,346,380].

Other results were observed after the denervation of renal blood vessels, their cultivation with 5%-fenol and decapsulation of the kidney. The indices of filtration, reabsorption functions and blood flow in this kidney did not differ from physiologic individual fluctuations. Therefore, the authors concluded that efferent innervation does not have any influence on renal function [285,364,365,366].

On the contrary, by the same volume of denervation, the reduction of the glomerular filtration of 50%, tubular secretion of 67%, and increase of reabsorption of 20% compared with the intact kidney were observed [246].

After the analogous unilateral denervation of the kidney, in the first five days an equal reduction of the diuresis on both sides was observed. Later, the diuresis of the denervated kidney as well as its blood flow continued to decrease with a simultaneous increase in diuresis of the intact kidney. The authors consider that the renal nerves take part in the regulation of blood flow, as well as secretion and reabsorption in the kidney. The denervation of the kidney reduces its adaptive properties [16,65,67,90,108,163,195,305,327,382,383].

The following investigations [231-234] also testify to coordinated and differentiated nervous regulation of the kidney's various functions. Electrostimulation of the adrenergic nervous fibers of the kidney intestified the water reabsorption and tubular transport of Na and K ions. Analogous irritation during adrenergic blockade with guanetidin or reserpin did not produce the same results. On the other hand, electrostimulation of a cholinergic wandering nerve (n. vagus) caused an increase of diuresis at the expense of the tubular reabsorption reduction. But the blockade of acetylcholin with hemicholin or triethilcholin utterly excluded the influence of n. vagus on diuresis.

The whole range of special works revealed disorders in the adaptation-regulation mechanism of the denervated kidney by functional loading and perversion of its reactions after the injection of various pharmacologic substances. [33,44,194,255,256,257,278,289, 291,293,312,323,329,350,367,375,382,383].

Also mentioned was the perversion of reactions of a denervated kidney towards adrenalin and insulin. [56,57].

The sensitivity of the vascular system of the kidney was also observed after the cutting of the renal nervous plexus. Injection of adrenalin caused a greater reduction of diuresis of the denervated kidney, compared to the intact kidney. [203].

In analogous experiments, after the injection of adrenalin, the denervated kidney reacted with a more expressed and longer reduction of filtration and blood flow than the intact one [199,341].

Confirming these data, other authors [39,40,65,90] explained this by the increase of a contractive influence of adrenalin on the efferent arterioles of the denervated kidney.

It was discovered that a denervated kidney adapted much worse to the water-saline loading in the hyperthermy condition. [326].

The excretory and concentration functions of the denervated kidney are also disordered by functional loading. [391].

Furthermore, the depressing influence of the kidney denervation on erythropoetic activity was revealed [252,253].

Thus, summarizing the results of physiologic experiments on denervation of the kidney with short follow-up observations (up to 2-4 weeks) it can be concluded that the majority of them performed with the use of sufficiently sensitive methods and tests permits one to conclude that the denervation of the kidney causes specific disorders in varied functions related to the blood circulation, filtration, reabsorption, and erythropoesis. As well as the perversion of reactions to various pharmacologic substances and the reduction of adaptation-regulation abilities of the kidney by functional loadings.

Results of chronic experiments devided the authors into two groups. The first (small) one considered that denervation doesn`t introduce any changes in the kidney function examinated under normal conditions [120-127,323].

Further, in the model of one-side kidney denervation, they studied the influence of adrenalin injection, artificial acidosis and of electric irritation of efferent renal nerves on the water and Na-ion excretion functions. The indices of both kidneys were almost identical. Therefore, authors consider that the humoral factors are more important in the regulation of renal functions, whilst the efferent nerves act on the kidney only in the form of a duplicate mechanism.

The majority of scientists have a contrary opinion. [279-283] Long-term chronic experiments concluded that the denervated kidney works on an intermediate level and such a kidney is not able to adapt to the changing demands of the organism fast enough and with correct concentration levels. Therefore the author introduced the concept of an adaptive-trophic influence of the nervous system on the kidney.

These data coincide with experimental results, which showed that the denervated organ became "fragile" towards traumatic factors [37,201].

It has to be mentioned that the next authors [264-266] distinguished three stages after kidney denervation. In the first 2-3 weeks they mentioned the polyuria, hyperchloruria, and reduction of urea excretion on the denervated side. By water- and saline-loading the lag of the denervated kidney was observed because of reduction of its concentration ability.

In the period from three weeks to 5 months, the diuresis and urea excretion returned to normal, but the functional loading revealed, as before, a depression of the denervated kidney as compared with the intact one.

After five months the following observations were made, oliguria, reduction of concentration ability on the denervated side, and an increase of the functional asymmetry between the kidneys by water loading, while at the same time morphologic investigations revealed atrophy and sclerosis of the denervated kidney parenchyma, reduction of the glomerulas quantity, and some obliteration. The author concluded that the disorder of nervous regulation of the kidney leads to its functional depression, development of neurodystrophic alterations, which are followed with atrophy and sclerosis of the mentioned organ.

Within numerous pathophysiological investigations the authors [80-84] stated that the renal nerves are the communication link between the central nervous system and the kidney. In response to multiple peripheral and central inputs, efferent renal sympathetic nerve activity is altered so as to convey information to the major structural and functional components of the kidney, the vessels, glomeruli, and tubules, each of which is innervated. At the level of each of these individual components, information transfer occurs via interaction of the neurotransmitter released at the sympathetic nerve terminal-neuroeffector junction with specific postjunctional receptors coupled with defined intracellular signaling and effector systems. In response to normal physiological stimuli, changes in efferent renal sympathetic nerve activity contribute importantly to homeostatic regulation of renal blood flow, glomerular filtration rate, renal tubular epithelial cell solute and water transport, and hormonal release. Afferent input from sensory receptors located in the kidney participates in this reflex control system via renorenal reflexes that enable total renal function to be self-regulated and balanced between the two kidneys. In pathophysiological conditions, abnormal regulation of efferent renal sympathetic nerve activity contributes significantly to the associated abnormalities of renal function which, in turn, are of importance in the pathogenesis of the disease.

1.1.3. The Morphologic State of the Kidney after the Denervation in Situ

Various models of the partial or full denervation of the kidney were performed by morphologists mainly for the investigation of sources of the kidney innervation and the architectonic structure of its neurous apparatus.

In this respect it has to be distinguished as the merit of the Kasanian (Russia) group of scientists which suggested an original method for the objective examination of internal organ innervation. It consisted in the cutting of peripheric nervous fibers of an organ from their trophic centers (neurons) and an evoking of a secondary so-called "Vallerish" degeneration in the nervous terminals [155].

So the cut of spinal brain ganglions was performed beginning from the upper neck vertebrae to the sacral vertebrae inclusive on dogs, cats, rabbits, rats and ducks [367-370]. After the cutting of the lower thoracal and upper lumbal spinal ganglions, the specific changes in nervous terminals of the glomerulas, tubules, pyelon, blood vessels and kidney capsula were observed. In the first two days, there were reactive alterations such as argentophyllia, swelling, intensified impregnation, and coursing. With the third day came the degenerative changes of nervous receptors with their disintegration, previously on the level of preterminals and terminals. Only a few of them remained intact.

As a result, on the one hand, it was established that the kidneys have cross afferent innervation. On the other hand, the conclusion was made that five pairs of lower thoracal and five pairs of lumbal spinal ganglions take part in the innervation of the kidneys. But the highest amount of afferent neurons related to the kidney was found in the three lower thoracal and two upper lumbal pairs of spinal ganglions.

These data were confirmed by the following works [153,154,167,304].

So after the removal of the lower thoracal and upper lumbal spinal ganglions, the specific changes in the kidney parenchyma were observed (stasys, vasodilatation, leukocyte infiltration, lipoid dystrophy [149,150,360-362].

The excision of THXI - LII spinal ganglia caused the disorders of the content of nuclear acides, glycogen and lipids in the nephron tubules [439].

The same volume of deafferentation ultrastructurally revealed a blood stagnation, vacuolization in glomerulas, the swelling of mitochondrias, accumulation of lipoid drops and a progressive decrease of succinat dehydrogenase and cytochromoxydase activity in the proximal and distal segments of nephron. In the Henle's loop there was additionally a widening of diameter, and exfoliation of the apical parts of epithelial cells. In the straight tubules the same picture was observed. [2, 440-442].

The same authors concluded that the nervous apparatus constitutes an essential part of the structural safety and proper regulation of cellular metabolism in the kidney.

As far as the removal of upper lumbal spinal ganglions causing the degeneration of a part of renal receptors, the conclusion was made that the urinary organs have at least two conductive paths in the efferent innervation in the form of splanchnic and pelvic nerves. [369].

The other anatomists also consider the splanchnic nerves as very essential for afferent and efferent innervation of abdominal organs inclusive of the kidneys and furthermore, they defined more precisely that the most intimate connections with the kidney have minor splanchnic nerves which are the conductors of an afferent innervation, at the same time the splanchnic nerves have a sympathetic nature [109,218,249,383].

The role of the wandering nerve in the renal innervation was disputed for a long time among physiologists and morphologists.

Some of physiologists consider its role in the afferent kidney innervation as vague [62,63].

The other authors considered the possibility of an efferent influence of the wandering nerve on the kidney [6,17,157,158,226-228].

There is an opinion that this influence can be realized through post ganglion nervous fibers after switching the impulses on the neurons of the renal plexus [369].

As for morphologic manifestation of the cutting of a wandering nerve, there are only a few works revealing the lipoid dystrophy and necrotic changes in the cortical layer of the kidney.

But the overwhelming majority of neurohistologists could not state any signs of degeneration in intrarenal nervous fibers after the vagotomy. Their data testifies that the wandering (parasympathetic, cholinergic) nerve plays a very inessential role in the kidney innervation [55,238,239,369].

On the contrary, there are many works confirming that the kidney has on the whole sympathetic (adrenergic) innervation. So the removal of ganglions of sympathetic frontier trunks caused the disappearance of the unmielynized nerve fibers accompanying the intrarenal blood vessels [14,15,32,64,109,185,186,218,270].

By the interpretation of morphologic investigations of a denervated kidney it has to be mentioned that some of them emphasized the state of the nervous apparatus of the kidney, but others highlighted the state of the renal parenchyma. Such a one-sided approach made their objective evaluation difficult.

In this respect we can distinguish the work of [369] who denervated the kidneys of dogs, cats and rats on the level of the pyelon and examined their parallel common morphologic and neurohistologic states over two years.

Beginning from the first days the urine analyses showed the picture of denervation nephritis. Miscroscopically in the renal parenchyma were revealed a stagnation in the blood vessels, nephritic changes in glomerulas, a leukocitary infiltration in the cortical layer and a turbid swelling of tubular epithelial cells. Simultaneously the signs of sharp reactive alterations in the afferent nerve fibers were observed such as the large inflations of neuroplasma in the place of its crossing with blood vessels and demyelinization. But among the nerve fibers with obvious signs of degeneration, there were some that were quite intact.

Five days later, together with leukocytary infiltration in the kidney parenchyma, the amount of fat cells increased along the connective tissue stratums and blood vessels. It testified to the expressed metabolic disorders in the kidney parenchyma.

The majority of nerve fibers suffered the degenerative changes and furthermore, an unevenness in the process of degeneration was observed. More were in the following period, the lesser was the amount of intact nerve fibers, but even by the 14th day there were some that were only reactive changed fibers without any signs of degeneration.

After 1.5–2 years the denervated kidney was atrophic, sclerosed, and trailed the intact kidney in weight. Microscopically one could observe the growth of connective tissue in the parenchyma and atrophic alterations in the nephrons. The intraorganic neurons on a whole were disintegrated to this state. The spontaneously regenerated nerve fibers were found only in the structure of connective tissue stratum and along the intrarenal blood vessels.

At the same time the intact kidneys of these animals were increased and hypertrophied not only as compared with denervated kidneys but also with kidneys of unoperated animals.

Thus, in one author`s [369] opinion, by short-term observation the denervation of the kidney is accompanied by a degeneration of the majority of intrarenal nerve fibers and disorder of albuminous, carbo-hydrative and lipoid metabolism.

A long-term experiment revealed the atrophy and sclerosis of denervated kidney with partial preservation of an innervation along the intrarenal blood vessels.

These phenomena were confirmed in the next works.

On the fifth day after the kidney denervation in the nervous trunks accompanying the big renal arteries, the typical process of "Vallerish degeneration" was detected. In the juxtamedullar zone of the kidney, mielynized nerve fibers were also disintegrated.

After three months signs of a spontaneous reinnervation along the big blood vessels on the level of pyelon were noted, but they were not revealed in the kidney parenchyma in the form of nervous terminals.

One year later the state of the renal nervous apparatus remained as they were previously. The kidney parenchyma was stated as the linear place of sclerosis and atrophy of tubular epithelium. [52].

[74,75] The age aspect was studied as far as the content of polysaccharides and lipids in the denervated kidney. The experiments were made on two groups of rats, two weeks of age and adults.

They showed that the denervation affected the kidney parenchyma and renal blood vessels quite destructively. They were interpreted as the disorders of carbo-hydrative, albuminous and lipid metabolism and what`s more, the kidneys of adult animals suffered more than young ones.

On the contrary, in other experiments the denervation of the kidney caused its atrophy in six-day old puppies earlier than in adults [120].

In experiments performed on newborn rabbits, the denervated kidneys also underwent a rapid atrophy. [31].

After the denervation of the kidney, the paralytic changes in muscular walls of renal blood vessels, big centers of leukocyte infiltration, and the diffusive swelling of the parenchyma were also detected. In the proximal segment of nephron, the additional accumulations of lipids in the distal segment, dystrophic changes and exfoliation of a part of cells in the tubular channel, and widening of diameter in the Henle`s loop and straight tubules were observed. After forty days the sclerosis of glomerulas was mentioned [361,362].

Other authors [382] also found the paralytic widening of renal blood vessels four days after kidney denervation. Two months later many centers of leukocyte infiltration and sclerosis in the cortical layer of the kidney were observed.

A morphologic study of the kidney was performed within three months after its denervation [360]. In the first days a sharp hyperemia was mentioned, after seven days perivascular infiltration and granular dystrophy were observed. 1–1.5 months later the vacuoles filled with fat, appearing in the cortical layer of the kidney. After three months, the kidney reduced in volume 1.5 times. Connective tissue developed on many glomerulas. After four months, many tubules were disintegrated, the apical parts of tubular epithelial cells were exfoliated and fell into the tubular channel.

The experiments [348] which investigated the influence of denervation on the development of amyloidosis in rabbit kidneys were interesting. After the kidney denervation, the author injected 4 ml 10%-Na-Kaseinat into the animals. The experiments continued from 13 to 130 days. Initially the author found hemostasis, granular dystrophy of tubules, and leukocytary infiltration in the denervated kidney stroma. At the end of the experiment, atrophy, sclerosis, amyloidosis and decrease of weight of the denervated kidney were observed. At the same time the intact kidney was free from amyloidosis.

In the experiments on dogs [190], during the first days after the kidney denervation, degeneration of intrarenal nerve fibers was observed, and even 1.5 years later the fragments of disintegrated nerve fibers could be seen. The partial regeneration of nerve fibers was observed in the kidney after three months. But after one year, atrophy of many nephrons was seen.

1.2. The Influence of a Transplantation Denervation on the Kidney

The experiments on the denervation of the kidney in situ were the foundation for the investigation of renal nervous regulation. But the influence of full denervation could be found only by kidney transplantation.

The best model for this was the kidney autotransplantation, which was free from the factors of immune incompatibility.

1.2.1. The Functional State of an Autotransplanted Kidney

By interpretation of corresponding results, it has to be distinguished whether or not the contralateral (intact) kidney was preserved. In the latter version the sole autotransplanted kidney underwent complex processes of compensatory hypertrophy which could distort the exact dynamics in renal functional changes. The parallel investigations of a transplanted and intact kidneys permitted one to evaluate each of them in more physiologic conditions, because in this case the functional loading between them was equal.

Some authors [157,387] examined the difference between the in situ, denervated or autotransplantated kidney compared with the intact kidney. They consider that denervation is probably responsible for observed posttransplant urinary sodium and bicarbonic loss and the associated metabolic problems.

Other authors observed that 1 week after the operation the transplanted kidney excreted less urine which contained less urea and phosphates but more chlorides than the intact kidney [97]. Furthermore, it was stated that in the early period the transplanted kidney excreted as much urine as the intact one. But three months later thei ratio became 1:3.

The diuretic function of a transplanted kidney compared with the intact kidney was more comprehensively examined in long-term experiments [363-365].

After transplantation of the kidney to the neck area three functional periods were stated. The period of unsteady diuresis which continued for 40-50 days. The urine volume of the transplanted kidney was less, more or the same as of the intact one. The next period of steady diuresis was observed from 50 days to 1.0–1.5 years after the operation. The transplanted kidney excreted, as a rule, less urine than the intact one. Its volume constituted 30% of common diuresis of the animal. In this period an essential difference had to be distinguished between the reactions of the transplanted and intact kidneys to functional loadings. The first was considerably backward compared with the second. The author explained this phenomenon so that the transplanted kidney was subordinated only to humoral factors, whilst the intact kidney had additional nervous regulation. In the third period (1.5–2 years after the operation) the function of the transplanted kidney progressively worsened. Its diuresis decreased further and the kidney underwent atrophy, whilst the function of the intact kidney was compensatively increased.

The next works [75,215,216,250,251,340,341] confirmed that the function of the kidney transplanted to the neck consisted of 40% of the common function , with the intact kidney handling 60% of the common function. But the removal of the intact kidney increased the functional ability of the sole transplanted kidney.

In the followed works [210-217] the condition of the transplanted kidney was evaluated by means of more differentiated methods, such as partial functions of the kidney.

The authors confirmed the existence of three functional periods after transplantation. In the first period, the functional data were inconclusive. In the second, a steady period (from 1.5–2 months to 6 months) of glomerular filtration, effective renal blood flow and maximal tubular secretion of the transplanted kidney achieved 70–80% of the intact kidney function. Reduction of water- and Na-ions reabsorption was observed as well.

In the third period (six months and later) a further decrease of partial functions of the transplanted kidney was observed, particularly its glomerular filtration.

Thus, the functions of the transplanted kidney during the steady period was essentially backward and then continued to decrease further.

The next works are in concordance with those mentioned above.

In the very first hours after the kidney transplantation, the reduction of their glomerular filtration and paraaminohyppur acide clearence were mentioned. The authors explained this fact on the one hand, by the kidney ischemia related to the transplantation and, on the other hand, by the vascular paralycic effect of denervation. [173,401].

The other authors [245,382] also confirmed the decrease of glomerulary filtration, tubulary excretion and blood flow after transplantation.

The summarized experimental data about the functional state of the transplanted kidney testify that it is able to work quite a long time at a decreased level as compared with an intact kidney, but after 1.5–2 years it underwent further progressive functional depression accompanied with compensative hypertrophy of the intact kidney [13,49,104].

A great interest is represented by experimental works for the investigation of a transplanted kidney by injection of various biologic active and pharmacologic substances. It is much more interesting that in the case of partial, orthotopic in situ denervation the reactions of the kidney were distorted. In this respect the full denervation of the kidney by transplantation could reveal more unknown phenomena.

On the other hand, such investigations are very important from a clinical point of view, because in every clinical case of kidney transplantation the surgeons have to take into account the possible perverse reactions related to denervation.

The results of such investigations can be interpreted according to the main matter of the monograph "The increase of sensibility of denervated structures: The rule of denervation" [184]. It was stated that after the denervation of an organ its sensitivity occurs, and it has a specific character in respect to the nervous mediator. For example, if an organ has an adrenergic innervation, the denervation increased its sensibility to adrenalin, and in the case of cholinergic innervations, to acetylcholin.

According to this conformity the influence of the adrenalin was examined on the function of an autotransplanted kidney [366]. The intravenous injection of adrenalin caused an anuria of both kidneys, and what`s more, on the side of the transplanted kidney the anuria came earlier and lasted longer than on the opposite side.

In analogous experiments [212,213] the quantitative evaluation of partial functions of the transplanted kidney was made. The intravenous injection of adrenalin caused a greater reduction of glomerular filtration, renal bloodflow, reabsorption of glycose, secretion of phenolrot and a greater increase of water reabsorption than in the intact kidney. The author explained these facts by a sharp contraction of intrarenal blood vessels of transplanted kidney sensitized towards adrenalin.

The above-mentioned data are very important and essential in the point of view that they testify to the mainly adrenergic nature of the kidney innervation.

The examination of the filtration-reabsorption function of autotransplanted kidney after injection of acetylcholine [217] did not reveal an essential difference between it and an intact kidney. Reduction of filtration and increase of water reabsorption were observed in both cases, and what`s more, these changes could be explained, in the author`s opinion, mainly by the influence of acetylcholine on the other organs rather than by the direct action of acetylcholine on the various reactive systems of the nephron.

Acetylcholine caused a decrease in blood pressure and stimulation of antidiuretic hormone secretion, which consequently increased the water reabsorption in the nephron tubules. As for the main aim of the experiments, the author concluded that the transplanted kidney with deprivated innervation did not become more sensitive to acetylcholine as compared with the intact kidney.

The author [217] could not reveal any sensitivity of the transplanted kidney towards pituitrin as well. This preparation equally increased the water reabsorption in nephron tubules of both (transplanted as well as intact) kidneys.

The obtained data testifies to the inessential role of cholinergic nervous structures in kidney innervation, which coincided with results of other scientists [86,87,369].

A more distinct difference in reactions of transplanted and intact kidneys was traced by the injection of diuretics and functional loading.

So the diuretics (Salin solution, mercusal, coffein) stimulated the diuresis of both kidneys but in all cases the transplanted kidney excreted less volume of urine, it was backwards in glomerulary filtration and tubular water reabsorption from the intact kidney [352,353].

The functional loading by means of increasing doses of a water-milk mixture [364] also revealed the difference between the kidneys in favor of the intact one which, in the author`s opinion, was associated with the transplantation denervation.

The defect of the transplanted kidney was observed in other works [79,208,209]. By the electrolytless regime of nutrition, the transplanted kidney excreted more chlorides than the intact kidney. After the intravenous injection of saline solution, on the contrary, the transplanted kidney excreted less chlorides than the intact one.

It is interesting to mention that the function of the transplanted kidney was also changed under the influence of a range of pharmacologic preparations. Soporific drugs (luminal, chlorahydrate) caused a decrease of diuresis at the expense of depression of filtration and increase of water reabsorption, and what`s more, the decrease of diuresis was more expressed on the side of an intact kidney [342].

The same result was observed under the influence of morphine [91,363] and histamine [366]. Taking into account that the mentioned substances, at least for morphine, stimulate the secretion of antidiuretic hormone in the hypophysis, and the corresponding reaction of the denervated transplant. It is obvious that it happened by a solely humoral mechanism. It is very important to emphasize that the more expressed reduction of diuresis in the intact kidney was evidently determined at the expense of a duplication of an antidiuretic influence of the mentioned soporific drugs through efferent nerves on the intact kidney.

Summarizing the results of functional studies of autotransplanted and intact kidneys after the use of biologic active and pharmacologic preparations, the author [217] concluded that, on the one hand, the functional changes in both cases were one-sided, on the other hand, in the reactions of the transplanted and intact kidneys it was possible to find only quantitative but not qualitative differences. In the author`s opinion, this quantitative difference evidently could be determined: 1) by the sensitivity of denervated organ to adrenalin, 2) by the absence of active efferent innervation in the transplanted kidney, and 3) by the insufficient function of the transplanted kidney as a result of the operation and accompanying factors.

From the practical and theoretical points of view, also very interesting was the investigation of reflex regulation of the transplanted kidney, because the kidney carries out a vitally important role ensuring very complex and diverse functions and maintenance of stable homeostasis in an organism. Therefore, it was necessary to have a clear notion about the nature, possibilities and limits of this regulation.

Some authors [210,211] examined the opportunity of conditional reflex changes of diuresis after kidney autotransplantation. They accompanied the conditional irritation (an electric bell) with the feeding of the water-milk mixture. After 70 combinations they achieved the desired reflex of the electric bell causing an increase in diuresis.

The possibility of conditional-reflex stimulation in diuresis of the transplanted kidney in response to an electric or sound signal was confirmed by other authors [151].

As far as the increase of the urine volume accompanied by reduction of its density and concentration of creatinin and chlorides, the author explained this fact by a weakening of secretion of hypophis antidiuretic hormone [217].

At the same time, the attempts of other authors to reproduce the analogous effect were unsuccessful, even after 200 combinations of the conditional signal and milk feeding [119].

On the contrary, the next group of authors [330] achieved a conditional reflex for the depression of diuresis of the kidney transplant. They used an electric irritation. In these experiments the concentration of creatinin in the urine was increased, which the authors considered a result of stimulation of secretion of the hypophis antidiuretic hormone.

Thus, by the interpretation of the above-mentioned works, it can be concluded that the opportunity of a conditional reflex change of diuresis on the side of the autotransplanted kidney appears quite real and feasible. It has to be distinguished only that the obligatory link for this reflex is the antidiuretic hormone of hypophysis, which to a marked degree can compensate for the absence of efferent innervation in the kidney transplant. But the following works showed that this humoral compensation was not quite perfect.

So, the irritation of mechanoreceptors of the stomach caused the reflectory decrease of filtration and an increase of water reabsorption in autotransplanted as well as in intact kidneys. But for such an effect, the autotransplanted kidney required stronger irritation [117].

It is interesting to mention that in the case of initial introduction of chloralhydrate (the latter depressed the nervous regulation of the intact kidney) the strong irritation of gastric receptors caused one-type (equal) decrease of diuresis both in the intact and transplanted kidneys.

By experimental colic of the intact kidney, caused by temporary occlusion of its ureter, the diuresis of an opposite autotransplanted kidney decreased considerably less than in experiments on animals with both intact kidneys [11].

The difference between the functional possibilities of autotransplanted and intact kidneys was observed in such extreme conditions as artificial nitroglycerin collapse, massive blood loss, and when the organism presents the special, abnormally high demands for the maintenance of steady homeostasis.

It is known that the volume of circulating blood in the organism is regulated by kidneys as a result of cooperation of two reflexes, antinatriuretic and antidiuretic. This way, on the one hand, Na-ions are kept in the organism and, on the other hand, water [46].

In serious hemodynamic disorders, in the overwhelming majority of experiments, the increase of water reabsorption in the autotransplanted kidney was expressed less than in the intact kidney [217]. Therefore, he considered that in extreme vital circumstances, the functional reserves of the kidney transplant for the steady inner equilibrium in the organism were limited.

An important role of efferent nerves of the kidney which supplement the action of humoral factors was confirmed by other authors as well [124]. But the next works convincingly demonstrated that the duplicate mechanism of the influence of efferent renal nerves was not formal but played a very essential role in the adequate regulation of renal function, and a loss of efferent innervation made the kidney functionally insufficient. [213,217].

Not less interesting is the question of restoration of the afferent innervation of a transplanted kidney. The temporary occlusion of the ureter of the autotransplanted kidney or the introduction of liquid into the ureter up to a pressure of 220 mm Hg pole did not reveal any reaction in the animal, whilst the same irritation of the intact kidney caused distinct reflex reactions, such as an increase in moving anxiety and the respiration becoming more frequent.

The other forms of irritation of supposed interoceptors of the transplanted kidney as an electric influence on the parenchyma or irrigation of the pyelon with electrolytes also remained without any answer, while the same irritation of the intact kidney caused the typical reflex reactions [217].

In the following experiments on intact animals [76] the electrostimulation of one kidney parenchyma caused the specific reno-renal reflex, which was the increase of its diuresis and the simultaneous decrease of diuresis in the opposite kidney.

In an attempt of reproduction of the same experiments on dogs with autotransplanted kidney, its electrical irritation did not cause any changes of diuresis in the opposite (intact) kidney.

The performed experiments with autotransplantation of the kidney demonstrated that in the case of some degree of spontaneous regeneration of afferent nerves, their physiologic role in the conduction of afferent impulses up to the central neural system was very inessential.

But it did not at all mean that the transplanted kidney was an alien organ which did not affect the organism.

In this respect we must pay attention to the experiments related to the participation of an autotransplanted kidney in the regulation of blood pressure. Reportedly, if the dog had an artificial hypertonia beforehand (evoked by the removal of carotid globules or occlusion of the renal artery) the kidney autotransplantation caused a decrease of the hypertonia level. The removal of the intact kidney led to a further decrease of blood pressure [75].

Based of her experiments, this author concluded that in an autotransplanted kidney, because of its denervation, the incretory function participating in blood pressure regulation was distorted. The intact kidney made the pressure higher, while the transplanted kidney made it lower.

In other experiments in this field [106], electric irritation of the transplanted kidney parenchyma did not cause any changes of the filtration—reabsorption functions, but led to a statistically reliable decrease in blood pressure (in average, 10 mm Hg pole) in the first 10-20 minutes after the irritation.

As for the interpretation of the hypotensive influence of an autotransplanted kidney, there is no common opinion. One author [317] considered it to be a result of a decrease of renin production in the denervated kidney.

Other authors [75,106] proposed the possibility of secretion of a hypotensive substance by the autotransplanted kidney. In these authors' opinion, it could be prostaglandin E which contains the medullar layer of the kidney. [343,344].

But in all the interpretations of the mechanism of the hypotensive influence of the autotransplanted kidney, it is doubtless that this influence was realized not through the efferent nerves (it means without the central nervous system) but mainly by a humoral mechanism. In spite of the seeming favorable (hypotensive) influence of an autotransplanted (denervated) kidney on the experimental hypertonia, proceeding from everyday various clinical situations, it is obvious that the secession of an afferent innervation and subordination of a complex mechanism of blood pressure regulation to the phylogenetically more primitive humoral mechanisms and the distortion of an incretory function of denervated transplant (the production of hypotensive substance instead of hypertensive one) are not always adequate and correspond to the real demands of the organism. Thus, after the autotransplantation of one kidney and preservation of the opposite (intact) organ, the first could function satisfactorily at certain times with reduced indices as compared with the intact kidney, but 1.5-2 years later came the progressive functional depression of the transplanted kidney and parallel compensative hypertrophy of the opposite (intact) kidney.

The removal of an intact kidney created for the autotransplanted kidney an extreme situation, because, on the one hand, it was affected by various injurious factors related to denervation (ischemia, trauma) and on the other hand, it should fulfill an increased functional loading. Although these factors impeded the objective functional evaluation of the autotransplanted kidney, this model provided important information about its reserves and vitality.

The experiments with the sole autotransplanted kidney showed that it was able to ensure the survival of the animal for a long time—6 years [59,60], 3 years 2 months [259,260], and 2 years 8 months [76], and what`s more, the animals died not because of a loss of the kidney vitality, but in light of finishing of the experiment.

In experiments on dogs with an autotransplanted kidney, from the initial hours after the removal of the intact kidney the diuresis of the remaining sole transplanted kidney increased and continued on this high level for two months [366].

The followed works showed that the function of the sole autotransplanted kidney exceeded 50% of common functions of two healthy kidneys.

So in experiments of [259,260] the glomerular filtration, the sole autotransplanted kidney consisted of 76-78% of the initial common functions of both kidneys before the operation.

But for the objective evaluation of the functional abilities of the sole autotransplanted kidney, it seems to be more expedient and justified to compare this kidney with the sole intact kidney.

In such experiments [362,363], two months after the autotransplantation and simultaneous contralateral nephrectomy, in the period of the steady diuresis, the diuresis of the sole autotransplanted kidney did not differ from that of the sole intact kidney. But other functional indices were considerably reduced: the glomerular filtration consisted 80.3%, renal blood flow was 83.1%, water reabsorption was 77.9% of the corresponding indices of the sole intact kidney.

The radio-renographic examinations, with J131 hippuran made periodically within one year after the kidney autotransplantation and contralateral nephrectomy, showed a lengthening of secretion and excretion phases of its renograms as compared with the sole intact kidney.

These data coincided with the clinical results of the kidney transplantation between the monozygote twins. This model can be considered as a clinical parallel of an experimental autotransplantation. So, before the transplantation the glomerular filtration of both kidneys of the donor was equal at 147ml/min, and the plasma flow was 477ml/min. Eight months after the mentioned operation, the indices of the transplanted kidney became 84ml/min and 420ml/min respectively [48,242,243].

Analogous observations on twins were made by other authors [128,376]. They did not mention the rough disorders of the transplanted kidney. Unfortunately the authors did not describe the comparison between the pre- and post-operative indices of the transplanted kidney, or between the transplanted kidney and the sole kidney retained by the donor. But even in this case the changes of the water-saline regime were accompanied by the decreased natriuretic function of the transplanted kidney.

Thus, the cited data testifies to the high plasticity of the kidney tissue and its ability to carry out compensative hypertrophy in response to increased loading. The function of the sole autotransplanted kidney could exceed half of the common function of two healthy kidneys and maintain the life of experimental animals for several years. But this kidney was considerably backward as compared with the sole intact kidney after the functional indices, as well as after the reserve abilities.

1.2.2. The Morphologic State of the Autotransplanted Kidney

The morphologic state of a kidney autotransplanted to the neck area also differed from the norm. Many authors [60,61,76,78,190,197,236,382] in various terms after the operation from one to fifty months revealed atrophy, local and diffusive scleros in the cortical and medullar layers, the hyalinosis and sclerosis of glomerulas, periglomerulary lymphoid infiltration, various forms of dystrophy (parenchimatous, lipoid, hyaline-drop) in the tubular epithelium, perivascular and intimal sclerosis of intrarenal arteriols, and the thickening of the renal capsule. At the same time, parts of glomerulas and tubules were well preserved.

In reference to the morphological state of the kidney transplanted in the iliac fossa, there are only a few works which testify that, in the latter case, the changes were expressed less than by the transplantation to the neck.

Some authors [260], 28 and 38 months after the transplantation of the sole kidney in the iliac fossa, revealed irregular thickening of the Bowman capsule, and by morphometric measures, the 30% increase of glomerulas dimensions was stated. The sizes of the transplant on the whole also increased by 60%. The structure of epithelial cells, basal membranes and intrarenal arterial walls were relatively intact.

The same changes observed in other works [72,177] were considered a manifestation of a compensative hypertrophy.

Some authors [382], regarding the dystrophic alterations found out in the tubules of a sole autotransplanted kidney, explained them as being a result of the ischemia.

The comprehensive morphologic, neurohistologic, histoensymatic and ultrastructural examination of the autologous kidney transplanted into the iliac fossa were performed by [52,53,190]. Alterations observed in the first ten days, in the authors' opinion, could be considered as a reaction to the general operative trauma. They were the interstitial swelling of renal cortical and medullar substances, the stagnation of blood in glomerulas, the dystrophy of tubular cells in proximal and distal segments of the nephron, and local necroses.

Fourteen to thirty days later, like everything else, dystrophic changes in the tubular epithelium and the blood stagnation, and the beginning of sclerotic alterations were found. They consisted of the thickening of the basal membrane of glomerulas and tubules, a great number of sclerotic trips stretched radially at full length of the parenchyma from the capsule to the medullar substance, perivascular and periglomerular sclerosis, and diffusive lymphoid infiltration.

After two to five months of the local subcapsular sclerosis, single periglomerular lymphoid infiltration were mentioned, in some cases the structure of the kidney was usual.

Between six to eight months, single periglomerular lymphoid infiltrations and a thickening of tubular basal membranes were found.

One to one-and-a-half years later, local and diffusive sclerosis in the parenchyma were observed. They were presented by linear strips stretched through the whole parenchyma and accompanied by a more or less expressed lymphoid infiltration. Furthermore, there was a thickening of glomerular capillary membranes and sclerosis of arterioles.

By the histoensimatic study (succinat-, lactate-, malat-, alcohol-dehydrogenase and glucose-6-phosphatase) up to one year after the operation, the distribution of ferments in various segments of the nephron and their activity did not differ from the norm. Only one year later could a decrease of activity of the mentioned ferments, except for malat-dehydrogenase and glucose-6-phosphatase, be mentioned.

For comparison, twenty days after the allotransplantation of the kidney in the case of prolongation of its survival, atrophy of tubules, interstitial fibrosis, perivascular infiltration, fibrous thickening of some big arteries, and sometimes the obliteration of peritubular capillaries and arterioles were also found [164,165,171].

The ultrastructural changes revealed [248] that after two to six months, dystrophy in the autotransplanted kidneys could be assessed. The glomerular capillaries were widened, endothelium became thinner with wide pores, the podocytes were flat, and their cytoplasma vacuolized; mitochondrias were swelled. The glomerular basal membrane was thickened. In the tubular epithelium swelling and vacuolized mitochondrias were found, with local sclerosis in some areas.

It has to be mentioned for comparison that after an experimental allotransplantation in the kidney signs of artero-arteriolopathy, sclerosis and lipoid dystrophy of elastic membrane of renal blood vessels were found [112].

A few neurohistologic investigations of an autotransplanted kidney gave contradictory results.

One group of authors [8,49,139,260,274-276,387-389] did not find any signs of regeneration of adrenergic nerve fibers even in the location of renal vascular anastomoses.

At the same time, other authors [346] observed the maintenance of parts of nervous fibers in the transplanted kidney.

Some authors [72,119] even mentioned an opportunity of the germination of nerves into the kidney and what`s more, it happened six months after the transplantation.

The detailed neurohistologic examination of kidney autotransplants was performed from two days up to one-and-a-half-years [369,372,373].

Two days after the operation, obviously expressed reactive alterations of intrarenal nerve fibers were found. Many of them, especially thick myelinized fibers located in the juxstamedullar zone and between the blood vessels, showed a sharp argentophylia, varicosis and the creation of small growths of neuroplasma. There were a very wide range of changes. Just as the unmyalinized nerve fibers seemed intact, the myelinized fibers located in the same nerve fibers were damaged up to the initial form of degeneration.

Two weeks later the structure of the renal nervous apparatus was essentially changed. In the parenchyma, only single preserved nerve fibers were found. The rest, an overwhelming majority, of them were desintegrated, and their axial cylinders absorbed. Between three and four monhs after the operation, a few germinating nerve fibers were seen, mainly along the big blood vessels. Their disposition was atypical, particularly, the usual succession was absent. Parts of the nerves reached the pyelon. The regenerated nerve fibers were distinguished by round growths at the ends.

One to one-and-a-half-years after the kidney autotransplantation, the regenerated nerve fibers were found between the cortical and medullar substances. Some of them reached the tubules and pyelon walls. But in the author`s opinion, the neurohistologic structure of an autologous kidney transplanted into the iliac fossa is distinguished by a lack of nerve terminals and plexus. The author concluded that the spontaneous reinnervation of the autotransplanted kidney did happen, but it was only partial and insufficient.

Subsequent investigations revealed a distinct dissociation between the regeneration of adrenergic and cholinergic nerve fibers. Just as 48 hours after the kidney transplantation the intrarenal adrenergic structures had completely lost the specific fluorescence [102], the cholinergic activity was preserved, although in a weakened form [275,276,384].

The partial maintenance of cholinergic autonomous innervation was explained by the authors by the preservation of pyrenofores of cholinergic nerve fibers. They were located in the renal gate area along the plexus renalis and had not been separated from them during the kidney transplantation.

At the same time, the ggl. ggl. splanchnicum and aoticorenale that were mainly connected with renal adrenergic nerve fibers were usually cut during the transplantation. This resulted in a firm adrenergic denervation of the kidney, cessation of catecholamins output and serious upset in tissue metabolism [10,219].

Thus, the cited morphologic works showed the gradual degeneration of intraorganic neural structures beginning from the second day after the kidney transplantation. First of all, the afferent nerve fibers and their terminals were degenerated. The disintegration of unmyelinized fibers proceeded slowly. At the end of the first month there remained in the kidney only single nervous fibers related to intraorganic neurons. Three to four months later there were a few growing nervous fibers along the big blood vessels. But these fibers reached the tubules and pyelon walls only rarely and mainly ended in the connective tissue. Even one-and-a-half-years after the autotransplantation the renal nervous apparatus was represented poorly and existing nervous structures did not reach the mediatoric phase, which meant they had firmly lost the ability to produce catecholamins.

Consequently, through analysis the above-mentioned morphologic investigations, it can be concluded that spontaneous reinnervation of an autotransplanted kidney was insufficient by volume, as well as by quality. Evidently it was the cause of a cessation of the trophic influence of the nervous system and consequently the atrophy, local and diffusive sclerosis of parenchyma and blood vessels, and various forms of dystrophy in the transplanted kidney.

The cited works convincingly showed an insolvency of the nervous apparatus of the transplanted kidney, which harmed the latter thoroughly. Therefore, the question: "Is it justified to demand perfect work from the transplanted kidney under the conditions of its imperfect reinnervation?" arose [190,369,374].

The comparison of auto- and allotransplantations of the kidney and revealing many common signs (atrophy, sclerosis, lymphoid infiltration, various forms of dystrophy in the parenchyma, artero-arteriolopathy) caused the next questions: "Is it justified to attribute them solely to the immune rejection? Maybe they are determined by the cessation of a nervous trophic influence on the kidney too?"

Therefore, many scientists and transplantologists are more and more persistently recommending making a directed artificial surgical reinnervation of the transplanted kidney [138,140,190-193,215-217,357,364-366,369,373,374,384,387]. But in spite of logical arguments of this opinion, only a few works have been performed in this field.

1.3. First Attempts of Surgical Reinnervation of the Kidney and other Inner Organs

Several methods of surgical reinnervation of various organs have been described: 1) the junction of big nerve fibers "end to end" [215-217,364,366]; 2) the sewing of a big nerve fiber to the wall of an organ (neuro-nephropexy); 3) the sewing of a nervous plexus ganglion to the wall of an organ [130-132]; 4) organopexy, which is the sewing of an organ to any other reachable innervated organ, for example, deserosed thin intestine [328]; 5) the inclusion of carefully separated ggl. ggl. splanchnicum and aorticorenale in the transplanted complex [138,139,189,387-389]; and 6) the junction of perivascular fascial shreds containing the nervous plexus [189].

Four of these methods were used for the reinnervation of a transplanted kidney: the direct junction of nerves, neuro-nephropexy, ileo-nephropexy, and the transplantation of a kidney in complex together with the ggl. ggl. splanchnicum and aorticorenale.

For the first time the influence of a surgical reinnervation of the autotransplanted kidney was investigated by [364,366]. For this he sewed the peripheric end of the wandering nerve to nerves of the kidney autotransplanted to the neck area.

Two to three months after the operation there was a distinct difference between the functional abilities of the reinnervated and unreinnervated kidneys. Just as the unreinnervated kidney secreted 40% and the intact kidney secreted 60% of the volume of urine, the reinnervated kidney transplant secreted 48% and the intact one secreted 52% of the common volume of urine. Also, in the latter case the correlation of the urine density and amount of excreted chlorides and nitrogen were equal.

A specific peculiarity of the autotransplanted kidney reinnervated with the wandering nerve was the cough reflex due to the increased diuresis after water loading. This fact was considered an irritation of the wandering nerve by the afferent nerves regenerated in the kidney after the transplantation. The author especially emphasized that by this model he never observed kidney atrophy. He did not consider the use of the wandering nerve as natural for the reinnervation of the kidney. But it principally deserved great attention, because it ensured more perfect functioning of the organ.

The experiments in this field were continued by [215-217] who examined the state of afferent and efferent innervation after kidney autotransplantation to the neck and innervation with the wandering nerve.

18 days after the operation, the mechanical irritation of the kidney caused a cough reflex. These reactions reached a maximum at four to five months and, furthermore, several successive cough pushes were finished with vomiting movements. The irritation of pyelon baroreceptors by means of temporary compression of the ureter, as well as the same action on

the opposite (intact) side, caused a moving excitement, and respiration became more frequent. The rapid increase in intrapyelon pressure by means of introduction of a liquid caused coughing and vomiting as well. The same vagus reflexes were observed by irritation of kidney chemoreceptors with various electrolytes as well as with electric irritation of the parenchyma.

If the anastomosed wandering nerve was cut, the above-mentioned irritations did not cause the same reactions.

The author considered the results of these investigations evidence of regeneration of afferent nerve fibers in the pyelon and parenchyma of the transplanted kidney.

In parallel experiments for the examination of efferent nervous structures of the transplanted and reinnervated kidney, six months after the operation, fluctuations in filtration and reabsorption were observed by direct as well as by central irritation of the wandering nerve. Specifically, they were accompanied by the depression of filtration and increase of reabsorption in the transplanted side. The excitement of the vomit center with parenteral introduction of morphine or apomorphine caused the same reaction, a reduction of diuresis at the expence of depression of filtration and activation of reabsorption. The cut of the anastomosed wandering nerve resulted in the cessation of this reflex.

Furthermore, the author convincingly showed that the reinnervation of a transplanted kidney with the wandering nerve an essentially reduced sensitivity of the kidney to an adrenalin injection, although it did not remove it fully.

Based on his neurophysiologic investigations the author [217] concluded that, in spite of the heterogenic nature of the wandering nerve for the kidney, the efferent nerve fibers were regenerated in the transplanted kidney with consequent specific reflexes.

The efficacy of afferent and efferent innervation and its favorable trophic influence on the transplanted kidney were confirmed by functional examinations. In the first one to two months after the operation, a period of unsteady diuresis was observed with a decrease of filtration and reabsorption functions compared to the contralateral (intact) kidney. From months two to eight the filtration and reabsorption functions of the transplanted and reinnervated kidney approached preoperative levels. This circumstance could be related to the regeneration of afferent and efferent nerves, and their favorable influence on the organ.

The above-described physiologic results [217] were confirmed by histologic investigation. 12 to 15 months after the autotransplantation and reinnervation with the wandering nerve in the cortical, medullar substances and pyelon, side by side with the empty (degenerated) Shwann nervous membranes, quite normal nerve fibers and their approximately equal correlation could be seen. At the same time in the autotransplanted but unreinnervated kidney, the nerve fibers were in overwhelming majority degenerated and represented by empty Shwann nerves.

The author considered his results as evidence non- complete but clear anatomic and functional regeneration of the wandering nerve in the parenchyma and pyelon of the transplanted kidney.

Another author [130,131] performed an analysis one month after reinnervation of the transplanted kidney with sewing of n. hypogastricus to the pyelon or renal artery, and found many nerve growths in the pyelon walls.

The next author [328] reinnervated the transplanted kidney by sewing its decapsulated surface with the deserosed area of the thin intestine. Seven days after the operation the beginning of nerve fiber regeneration was observed. Two to four months later some nerve fibers reached the kidney parenchyma. After 9–12 months the regenerated nerves were found in cortical as well as in medullar layers of the kidney. The examination of creatinin and residual nitrogen in the plasma did not show any changes.

By autotransplantation of the kidney together with carefully separated ggl. ggl. splanchnicum and aorticorenale [134,137-139] there was preservation of the autonomic nervous regulation of the organ. The intrarenal adrenergic nerve fibers continued to take part in the regulation of noradrenalin and to a marked degree prevented the sensitivity of the kidney to noradrenalin within the whole period of experiments (up to 2 years). The authors recommended preserving the autonomic renal nerve ganglions by kidney transplantation.

The positive influence of surgical reinnervation by autotransplantation was confirmed not only in respect of the kidney but also of other organs.

So, the spleen autotransplanted to the neck and reinnervated with the wandering nerve maintained during a year showed contractive ability in response to adrenalin injection, just as the unreinnervated spleen transplant soon lost the contractive ability [217].

Based on 300 lung autotransplantations in animals [175,176], was the statement that surgical reinnervation with the wandering nerve in 1.5–2 months led to a rapid and full recovery of partial spirographic data, just as the functional ability of an unreinnervated lung was much lower, even 45 and 58 months after the operation.

An essential lag of the unreinnervated lung transplant compared with the reinnervated organ was mentioned in reference to the specific Gering-Braier reflex and coefficient of oxygen utilization [94,292,310].

By the surgical reinnervation of an allotransplanted lung [176] the growth of the wandering nerve fibers through the anastomosis was revealed, but their regeneration proceeded with slower rates and did not give an efficiently functional effect. The distinct effect from the surgical reinnervation was observed only by the autotransplantation of the lung.

In the next works [205,237] a thin intestine was autotransplanted in dogs and reinnervated through a junction of perivascular fascial shreds along the anastomosed blood vessels and an additional junction of large nerve fibers located there.

The regenerated nerve fibers in the intestinal walls were found three months after the operation. Full normalization of the rectoenteral reflex, excretory, secretory, fermentative, and reabsorption functions of the transplanted intestine had taken place within 5–7 months.

In control experiments, without reinnervation of an intestinal autotransplant, no signs of nerve regeneration (in 24 months) nor recovery of functional indices of the intestine were found within 3 to 5 years after the operation.

In the case of reinnervation of a urinary bladder (in animal experiments) using n. hypogastricus and ganglion of the caudal plexus [132] as well as by the ileovesicopexy, [153,154] the growth of the functioning nerve fibers into the bladder wall was observed. The irritation of the bladder was accompanied by changes of blood pressure and breathing. On the other hand, breach of the junction between the bladder and thin intestine ceased the conduction of nervous impulses.

The obvious favorable influence of surgical reinnervation on the bladder in experiments stimulated the first attempts of its clinical application.

So, the ileovesicopexy was performed in 22 patients with neurogenic upsetting of the mixtion act. In 7 cases a full recovery occurred, in 2 cases the volume of residual urine reduced, in 9 cases it disappeared fully, arose the feeling of mixturishen, and the state of 4 patients remained unchanged. The author`s evaluation of this method on the whole was positive [334].

While the surgical reinnervation of inner organs is still mainly performed only in experiments and in the form of first clinical trials, it is very widespread and is an obligatory stage in traumatologic and plastic operations with an accompanying injury of innervation [45,147,148,168,182].

The experimental data and clinical experience showed that by damage of a nerve, the sewing of its ends was possible only in 71% of cases. In the rest of the cases, it was impossible because of the contraction of ends or deficiency of large nerve segments [341]. But even the careful junction of nerve fibers was not a reliable guarantee of success [428]. The worst recovered was n. ischiadicus. In 80% of cases an insufficient normalization of sensitivity had taken place. Not infrequently, the damage of n. ischiadicus was finished with partial extremity amputation because of trophic ulcers or osteomyelite [147,148]. But without a junction of nerve ends, the corresponding organ was condemned to sharp atrophy. Therefore if the direct junction of nerve endings was impossible, the plastic surgeons used various heterotopic or heterogenic substitution methods of reinnervation.

So, the plasty of facial nerves was made with the use of accesorial [7,50,386,438] sub-lingual or phrenical nerves [105,146,162,290]. The authors' work resulted in a good functional recovery of mimic muscles.

The plastic operations were also described with the junction of the sublinguale nerve with the wandering nerve, n. reccurence with the descending branch of the sublinguale nerve, also with good results [318].

The nerve regeneration was comprehensively described in the book of [182]. Based on neurophysiologic, experimental and clinical investigations, the author showed quite satisfactory functional and cosmetic results by the plasty of a facial nerve with a ventral branch of the 2nd neck nerve, with recovery of all facial expression and differentiated contractions.

Interesting are the experimental investigations of the author concerning reinnervation of the heart with the wandering nerve, of the recurrent laryngeal nerve with an intercostal nerve [114], and of ischiadic nerve with femoral, upper and lower gluteal nerves. The results were not always positive. For example, the junction of the sensitive nerve with the moving intercostal nerve was less effective than the junction of the sensitive recurrent nerve with a sensitive ventral branch of the 2nd or 3rd neck nerves. Nevertheless, the authors concluded that the direct junction, even of heterogenous nerve fibers, caused a certain rebuilding of the inner structure of the recipient nerve and its approach to the structure of the donor nerve. At the same time the functional recovery of the recipient nerve proceeded according to the function of the reinnervated peripheric organ.

1.4. Discussion of Information about Denervation and Reinnervation of the Kidney

A survey of literary data leads to the following conclusions. The decentralization of the kidney by its orthotopic denervation in situ or in connection with autotransplantation was accompanied by germination of only single nerve fibers along the renal blood vessels with a distinct dissociation in the regeneration dynamics of adrenergic and cholinergic nervous structures. Therefore the spontaneous reinnervation of the organ was obviously defective in quantitative as well as qualitative relations. This circumstance did not lead to the direct ruin of the kidney but caused considerable functional, metabolic and morphologic upsettings as in acute as well as in chronic experiments, with profound disorders of adaptive and trophic mechanisms in response to an increased functional loading. In long-term experiments it led to irreversible neurodystrophic alterations which were followed by atrophy and sclerose of the organ and its blood vessels.

Comparison of results in auto- and allotransplantations of the kidney and the discovery of many common changes mentioned above put scientists on to an idea that an important role in their origin was played not only by the immune rejection but also by the transplantative denervation of the organ.

By surgical reinnervation of the kidney autotransplanted to the neck and reinnervated with the wandering nerve, its germination occurred along the emptied Schwann membranes of degenerated renal nerves into the kidney parenchyma and pyelon. It resulted in the creation of a working nervous anastomose which determined a very satisfactory conduction as afferent as well as efferent impulses to the kidney. In spite of the heterogeneous character of this anastomose, it decreased to a marked degree the specific sensitivity of the transplanted kidney to various biologically active preparations and rendered a favorable adaptive-trophic influence on the kidney autotransplant insuring its long-term satisfactory capacity for work.

The positive action of surgical reinnervation in long-term prospects was confirmed not only by kidney transplantation but also by the transplantation of the spleen, lung, and intestine by surgical treatment of neurogenic diseases of the urinary bladder as well as by various neuroplastic operations.

Nevertheless, in spite of the obvious positive influence of the wandering nerve on the kidney autotransplanted to the neck [217,364,366], such a model can not be transferred in the clinic, because, on the one hand, the method of transplantation of the kidney into the iliac fossa used at present in clinics is more physiologic and on the other hand, the reinnervation of the kidney with a wandering nerve in this area would be technically impossible and genetically not optimal. This is because the wandering nerve renders a cholinergic innervation whilst the kidney requires mainly an agrenergic one.

Less useful for the clinic is the reinnervation of the transplant in the form of ileonephropexy [328], because it is connected with an unjustified complication from the operation as well as with a danger of intestinal problems. The method of kidney reinnervation with n. splanchnicus sewed to the renal gate or renal artery [132] represents a certain interest, but the cut of this nerve can cause denervative changes of inner organs innervated before (intestine, bladder), and the technical complexity related with finding and separating this nerve has to be taken into account.

The preservation of autonomous innervation of the kidney by its transplantation together with ggl. ggl. splanchnicum and aorticorenale [134-139,387-390] also deserves some attention. But it means only the preservation of an autonomous postganglionic innervation of the kidney which loses its central (preganglionic) nervous regulation. There is no remote evidence in the literature of how perfect its functional ability is.

Taking into account the considerations mentioned above, professor I.D. Kirpatovsky [189] suggested a method of surgical reinnervation of transplanted inner organs by a nervous plexus located above the fascial shreds along the anastomosed large blood vessels of the recipient and transplant.

This method seems very expedient for reinnervation of the kidney, because along the iliacal blood vessels there is a dense accumulation of nerves which are the branches of the aortic plexus. It is well known that the latter takes part in natural conditions in the kidney innervations, providing it with the corresponding adrenergic innervation [247]. The method`s technical simplicity has to be distinguished too. In spite of theoretically logical grounds and the practical feasibility of I. Kirpatovsky`s method for transplanted kidney surgical reinnervation, in accessible literature there was not any experimental or clinical trials in this field with long-term prospects.

Therefore, it was considered expedient to carry out an experimental investigation which would be able to answer the following questions:

1. Does the sewing of perivascular fascial shreds constitute the conditions for germination of nerve fibers up to the functional and morphologic terminal units of the autotransplanted kidney?
2. Under what terms does it happen?
3. Is there any dissociation in the dynamics of regeneraton of adrenergic, cholinergic, afferent and efferent nervous structures and does it reflect on the state of the autotransplanted kidney?
4. Does it ensure the germinated nerve fibers of the innervation are adequate for the kidney?
5. How perfect is the surgical reinnervation of the autotransplanted kidney by I. Kirpatovsky in connection with remote functional and morphologic results?
6. Is it expedient to use the surgical reinnervation in the clinical kidney autotransplantation?
7. Is the use of surgical reinnervation in the clinical kidney allotransplantation justified?

In my opinion, the investigations in this field would present a certain scientific as well as practical contribution in kidney transplantology.

Chapter II

MATERIAL AND METHODS

Proceeding from the fixed aim and chosen direction of investigations, the experiments were performed on 175 mongrel dogs of both sexes. All animals were divided into five groups and two subgroups (Table 1). In the first group (25 dogs) a left kidney orthotopic denervation in situ was made; in the second group (24 dogs) the denervated left kidney was surgically reinnervated by I. Kirpatovsky`s method; in the third group (51 dogs) the homolateral autotransplantation of the left kidney in the iliac fossa without surgical reinnervation was carried out; the animals of this group were divided into two subgroups: "a" (25 dogs) with preservation of contralateral (intact) kidney and "b" (26 dogs) with contralateral nephrectomy; in the fourth group (50 dogs) the homolaterally in the iliac fossa autotransplantated left kidney was surgically reinnervated; the animals of this group were also divided into two subgroups: "a" (25 dogs) with preservation and "b" (25 dogs) with nephrectomy of the opposite (intact) kidney; the fifth group (25 dogs) was a control in which only a right-side nephrectomy was made and the sole left kidney was kept intact.

The choice of the left kidney as an object of study was made in order to achieve the standard conditions of experiments, avoid the factors of physiologic functional asymmetry of kidneys and also in connection with convenience of manipulations on the longer vascular pedicle of the left kidney.

The surgical reinnervation of the autotransplanted kidney by I. Kirpatovsky [189] was fulfilled in the following way [Figure 1]. Under general anaesthesia Sol. Droperidoli 0.005% 1 ml intramuscularly, Sol. Phentanili 0.25% 1.0 and Sol. Hexenali 1% 5.0–10 ml/kg intravenously through a middle transabdominal approach the left iliacal blood vessels were found on the level of the crossing with the ureter. From the perivascular fascial tissue along a. iliaca int. a shred was carefully separated with a dimension of 1.0–1.5 cm which was fixed with a thread. The a. iliaca int. and v. iliaca ext. themselves were also separated and fixed with the threads. Then the left kidney was mobilized and before the nephrectomy the analogous perivascular fascial shred along the renal magistral blood vessels with the basis towards the kidney was separated and fixed as mentioned above. Directly after the nephrectomy the kidney was cooled from the external side by means of a special apparatus for local renal hypothermia (T.J. Shioshvili [354]) up to +20+25C in the cortical layer of the kidney. In such conditions of local hypothermia the kidney was transferred into the left iliac fossa turning the kidney poles 180 degrees (in order to avoid the crossing of renal and iliacal blood vessels0 and then the a. renalis was anastomosed with a. iliaca int, "end to end" but v. renalis with v. iliaca ext. "end to side'. After the junctioning of blood vessels which continued for 30–45 minutes and recovery of blood circulation in the kidney, the sewing of the above-mentioned perivascular fascial shreds was made by means of П-form catgut suture with tender tightening of the knot insuring the soft contact between the shreds only. with tender tightening of the knot insuring the soft contact between the shreds only.In the overwhelming majority of cases the perivascular fascial shreds contained 1-2-3 pairs of quite large nerve trunks which were sewed directly "end to end" by means of epineural sutures. The elementary microsurgical techniques and 4.5–6 times magnification was quite enough.

The ureter was left untouched in order to avoid additional problems related to the ureterocystoneostomy. Its superfluous part was placed only in the position which prevented the formation of occlusive fixed bends.

In the majority of cases (99) when the intact kidney was preserved, a two-chamber bladder was formed by G. Nasarishvili`s method [267] in order to study the partial functions of the kidney. Both halves of the bladder were led on the skin out.

In the rest (76) of the cases, accompanied by contralateral nephrectomy, the bladder was left untouched.

In the third group where the surgical reinnervation of the transplanted kidney was not foreseen, the usual stages of operation were fulfilled except of the junction of perivascular fascial shreds and the accompanying nerve trunks.

Table 1. Scheme of experiments in denervation and reinnervation of kidneys

Kinds of operations		Quantity of animals according to observation terms								In all
		3 days	10 days	1 month	2 months	4 months	6 months	1 year	2 years	
1st gr.	Denervation in situ	3	3	4	3	3	3	3	3	25
2nd gr.	Denervation, reinnervation in situ	3	3	3	3	3	3	3	3	24
3rd a gr.	Transplantation without reinnervation	3	3	3	4	3	3	3	3	25
3rd b gr.	Transplantation without reinnervation, contralateral nephrectomy	3	3	3	5	3	3	3	3	26
4th a gr.	Transplantation with reinnervation	3	3	3	4	3	3	3	3	25
4th b gr.	Transplantation with reinnervation, contralateral nephrectomy	3	3	4	3	3	3	3	3	25
5th gr.	Right side nephrectomy	3	3	4	3	3	3	3	3	25
										175

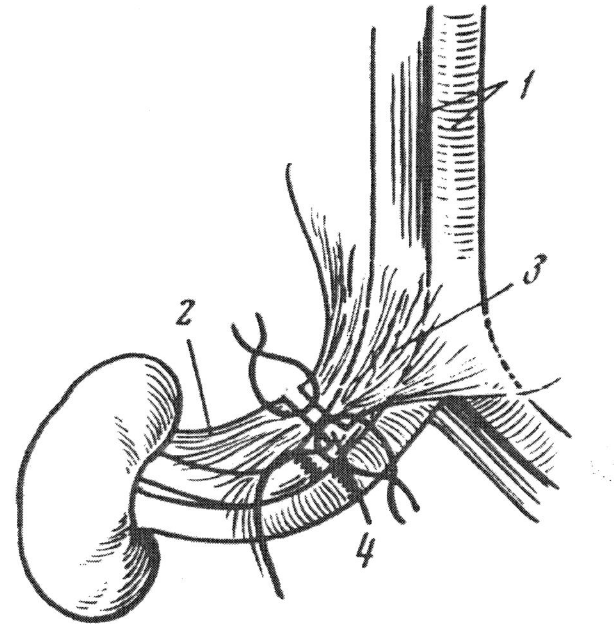

Figure 1. I. D. Kirpatovsky's method for surgical reinnervation of the kidney transplant.
1.$_1$ – magistral blood vessels;
1.$_2$ – fascial shred above the transplant vessels;
1.$_3$ – fascial shred above the recipient vessels;
1.$_4$ – sewing of fascial shreds.

The denervation of the kidney in situ was carried out by means of the cutting of all visible nerves along the renal artery, vein, pyeloureteral junction, their denudation and full decapsulation of the kidney. For ensuring equal conditions of experiments, the denervated in situ kidney also underwent 45-minute ischemia under local hypothermia +20+25 °C.

The surgical reinnervation of the kidney after its denervation in situ was made by means of sewing the perivascular fascial shreds and accompanying nerve trunks separated beforehand as mentioned above.

Thanks to autotransplantation of the kidney, homolaterally with turning of its poles 180 degrees and sewing of a. renalis to a. iliaca interna "end to end" and v. renalis to v. iliaca ext. "end to side" firstly, the animal underwent less trauma than by heterolateral autotransplantation; secondly, we avoided the crossing of renal and iliacal blood vessels and disorders in hemo- and urodynamics; and thirdly, we created favorable conditions for the forming of natural cortico-visceral relations and the corresponding representation of right and left kidneys in the central nervous system which was important for their normal function [351].

For the study of the kidneys, we used the modern functional and morphologic methods which were objective, exact and specific: radio-renography, reno-scintigraphy, excretory urography with X-ray cinematography, examination of partial and general secretory functions of kidney, biopotentials of the renal nerve, general morphologic methods (with impregnation by hematoxilin-eosin, Van-Gison and Mallory, general neurohistologic methods (with impregnation by Bilshovsky-Gros-Lavrentiev, Rasskasova) special neurohistologic methods (the study of cathecholamins through luminescence by Falck-Hillarp-Govyrin [100-102,142-144], Shvalev-Juchkova [379], of cholynestherase by Carnovsky-Roots [180], the dynamics of horse redish peroxidase transport through the nerve conductors by Mesulam[145,244]) and ultrastructural investigations of the kidney. The above-mentioned investigations were performed in the periods of three or ten days; one, two, or six months; one and two years after the operation.

The radio-renography was performed on animals fixed in belly recumbent position by means of intravenous injection of J^{131} Hippuran in the dose 0.5 mccjuri /1kg of animal weight, gamma-radiation was registered through radiographic device Gamma. These examinations were made under normal conditions and after the intravenous injection of adrenalin (0.3 ml of 0.1% solution). Results of radio-renography were evaluated quantitatively as well as qualitatively. With this aim we determined: 1) a percentage correlation of amplitudes of corresponding segments of renograms of operated and intact kidneys;

2) a definition of a universal renografic index RI by Hirakawa a. Corcoran [161] which was calculated by the formula:

$$K=\frac{(B-A)^2+(B-C)^2}{B^2}\times 100,\ \text{where}$$

A - amplitude of vascular segment,
B - amplitude of maximal secretion.
C - height of the curve 15 minutes after the isotope injection.

The quantitative indices of radiorenograms were analysed statistically by Student`s t-test and index of reliability p.

Usually a normal RI of a man according to various authors is 59±4, 52-70 [161]. In dogs it was 47-74 [352-355].

Renoscintigraphy was performed in fixed position as described above by means of intravenous injection of Neohydrin Hg^{203} or Hg^{197} in the summary dose 30-35 mccjuri.

The scanning was begun 30 minutes after injection on the device SCINTIKART. 624 radiorenographic and 168 radioscintigrafic investigations was made on the whole.

The excretory urography was fulfilled in the same position, 3, 7, 15 minutes after the intravenous injection of 20ml of 60% verographin (96 investigations). In 57 cases it was made using the cinematographic device SIMENS.

The kidney filtration and reabsorption were determined after endogenous creatinin, and its bloodflow after cardiotrast.

The renal absolute functional indexes fluctuated considerably in dependence on the weight and surface of the body, their percentage correlations between the operated and intact kidneys of the same animals were calculated.

The renal general secretory function by D. Murvanidze [262] was examined under normal conditions and after functional loading (50 ml/1kg water-milk mixture). The urine samples were collected over 3 hours. The diuresis and urine density were stated and then after D. Murvanidze`s table the index of general secretory function for each kidney was calculated. Later the percentage correlations between the operated and intact kidneys were determined.

The investigations of biopotentials of the renal nerve consisted of two parts. In the first was the examination of the background spontaneous impulsation of the renal nerve and afferent impulsation in response to intravenous injection of biologically active preparation of adrenalin and acetylcholine, and also by an increase of intrarenal pressure up to 200 mm Hg pole by means of retrograde introduction of Saline Solution.

In the second part the biopotentials of the renal nerve were investigated in response to an electric irritation.

In both cases they were performed in a screened and earthed room in conditions of general anaesthesia and manageable respiration of animals. Through the middle transabdominal approach the operated kidney and its anastomosed nerves were carefully separated. Very small nerve fibers of the plexus near the kidney were not suitable for the perfect recording of biopotentials, but it was possible, usually to separate 1-2 large nerves including the anastomosed section. One of these nerves was cut in 1–2 cm centrally away from the anastomose location, it means that on the aorta side, and the free end of the nerve was placed on the silver bipolar electrode with an interelectrode distance of 0.5 cm. A two-ray oscillographic device DISA with symmetric amplifier from electroencephalograph ALVAR was used for the biopotential recording. Its frequency characteristic was linear in the range of 10 to 1500 Hertz and sensitivity was 1 mcV for 1 mm deflexion of ray on the oscillograph screen. On one channel the biopotentials of the renal nerve and on the other an electrocardiogram and irritative electric impulses were registered. The picture from the screen was fixed on the film. In the moment of photography the respiration of the animal was stopped.

After the registration of the background spontaneous impulsation of the renal nerve, the adrenalin was injected intravenously in a concentration of 1:50000 with a velocity of 4 ml/min over 3-4 minutes. Then (after a 30-minute interval) the acetylcholine was injected in the same concentration and velocity. The registration of biopotentials as described above were performed periodically in a condition of ceased respiration (at 30 seconds each).

In the second part of these investigations, the renal nerve, distally away from the anastomose place, on the kidney side was irritated by electro-stimulator ESL-2. The excited biopotentials were led from this nerve proximally from the anastomose location by means of the same bipolar silver electrodes. The renal nerve between the irritative and register electrodes was earthed.

At first a threshold of excitement from the renal nerve was determined. Then the velocity of conduction of impulses through the nervous anastomose was calculated using the formula: $V=S/T$ - where V is the velocity of nervous impulse conduction, S is the distance between electrodes, T is the time between the moments of appearance of an artefact and ascendant phase of the biopotential.

After completion of functional investigations in the terms mentioned above the morphologic material was taken. The specimens for general morphologic and neurohistologic examinations with impregnation by hematoxilin and eosin, by Mallory, Van-Gison, Bilshovsky-Gros-Lavrentiev, Rasskasova were prepared using well-known methods.

The adrenergic nerve structures were revealed by Falck-Hillarp-Govyrin`s method. The pieces of kidney were frozen on the artificial ice directly after being taken, then the cuts were prepared by means of a cryostate. After the liophilization in the vacuum (10^{-4} atm) the cuts were placed in paraform steam at 80°C for one hour, embedded in the polystirole and examined in the luminescent microscope ML-2 or LUMAM I-1. The cuts were incubated in 2% solution of glyoxil-acid by Shvalev-Juchkova`s method [379].

Cholinergic nerve fibers were detected by Karnovsky-Root`s method [180]. The fresh pieces of kidney were frozen on artificial ice, the cuts were prepared by means of a cryostate and immersed in an incubative medium containing acethyl-thio-cholin-iodide, which gave a specific brown coloration in the location of cholinestherase activity.

The investigation of axonale transport in the horse, redish peroxidase was performed by Mesulam`s method [22,244,335,336]. 20-25 mg of trade-mark SIGMA-VI was injected into the kidney parenchyma of an animal which was under general anaesthesia. 48 hours later the ganglia of the spinal cord, brain and sympathetic trunk on the ThIX-LIII level were removed. If they were penetrated with the mentioned ferment the latter reacted with benzidin and created specific granules of blue color in ganglion cells.

For ultrastructural investigations, the 1 mm pieces of kidney were taken from animals which were under general anaesthesia. The pieces underwent a preliminary fixation in 2.5% glutaraldehyde mixed with 2% dimethylsulfoxide [77] and then were fixed in temperatures up to +4°C, with 1.3% buffered solution of 0s04 within 2 hours. A preliminary perfusion of the whole organ with fixation substance (by Maunsbuch, [235]) was performed in only 12 cases in 1, 2, 3a and 4a groups of animals 10 days, 2 and 6 months after the operation. The kidney material was taken for other morphologic and histoensymatic investigations as well (particularly for detection of adrenergic and cholinergic nervous structures) where the perfusion method of fixation was not acceptable.

After the dehydration in alcohol the cuts, prepared by means of ultramicrotom OmU2 (Reichert), were contrasted by Reinold`s method and observed in ultramicroscopes JEM-7 and JEM-100-B by accelerative voltage 80 kV.

In all cases, the intact kidneys were considered normal.

After removing the morphologic materials, the animals were brought out from the experiment under general anaesthesia by air embolia.

Chapter III

The Influence of Surgical Reinnervation on the Functional State of Denervated In Situ and Autotransplanted Kidneys

3.1. Radiologic Functional Examinations

The radio renograms of intact dog kidneys did not differ essentially from those of man. The renograms consisted of three segments: ascendant (vascular), secondary ascent secretion and the descending (excretion) segment. The amplitude of the vascular segment was 60% of the maximal secretion amplitude which was taken as 100% with the amplitude of the excretion segment 15 minutes after the J^{131} Hippuran injection was 40% of the maximal secretion. The correlation between the right and left kidneys of intact dogs was 98.2±1.1%; the duration of secretion was 3.2±0.3 min and of excretion – 5.6±1.5min, with a renographic index 47-74. The kidney scintigrams were represented by frequent touches which corresponded to the contour and dimensions of the kidneys.

On the excretion urogram and cinematogram the pyelon, as a rule, was intrarenal and was represented as a sickle form strip. Two or three segments were observed in the ureter, which were filled, not simultaneously, with the contrast medium.

In the first group, 3 days after the left kidney denervation in situ, the amplitudes of its vascular and secretion segments were decreased to 87.5±2.4% and 76.9±3.3% respectively, the excretion segment was represented by an ascendant curve instead of a descendant one (obturation type), which showed the residual radioactivity to 15 minutes 250.0±5.5% instead of 40% in the norm (Tables 2-4, Figure 2.1). Half the excretion period essentially exceeded 15 minutes. RI was sharply decreased (9.0±3.5, p<0.001, Table 5).

After the adrenalin injection the amplitude of the intact kidney vascular segment became 80.5±3.4% of the standard, but the corresponding amplitude of the denervated kidney decreased further and became 42.3±2.5% of the intact kidney. The amplitude of the secretory segment was 65.2±2.0% and residual activity was 128.5±3.0% of the intact kidney, p<0.001, Tables 6-8, Figure 2.9.

The semi-excretion period exceeded 15 minutes. RI became 8.4±2.5 (of the intact one – 45.6±2.5, p<0.001, Table 9).

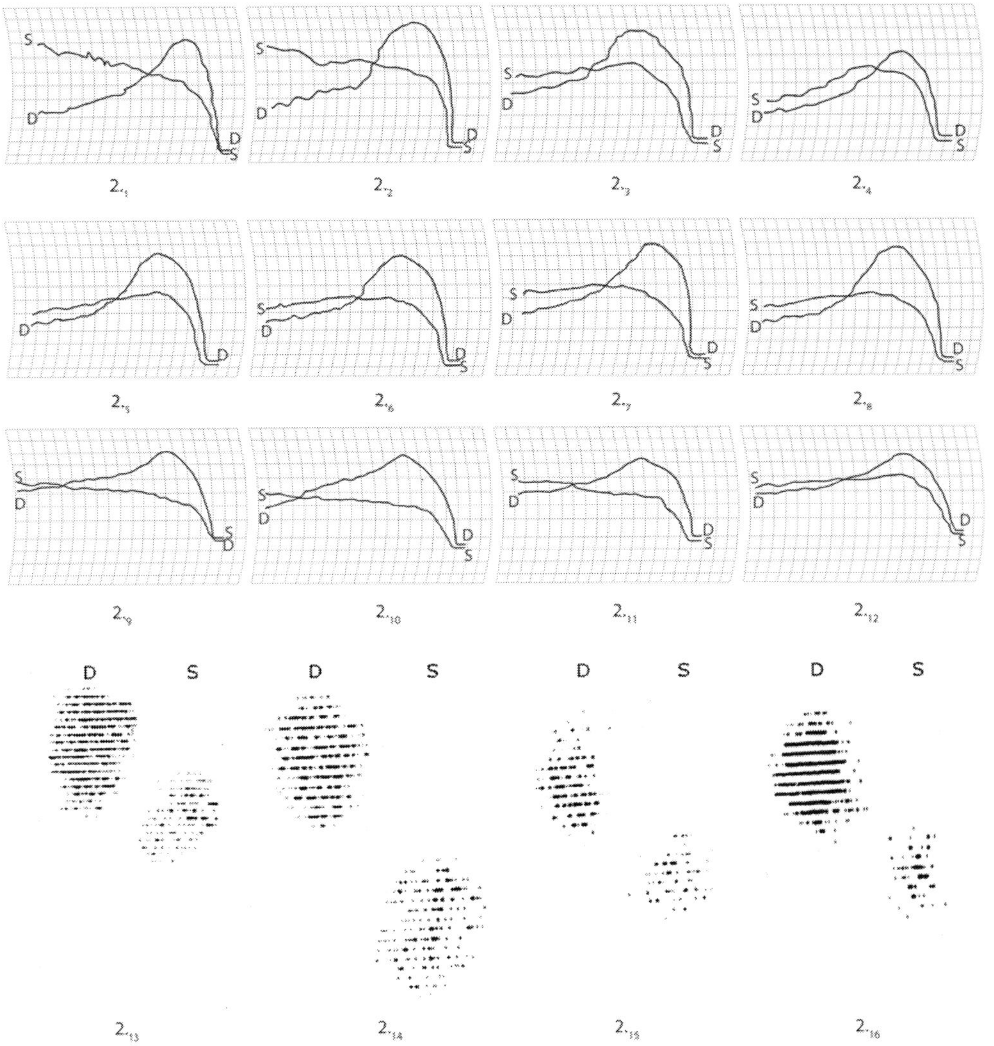

Figure 2. Denervation of the left kidney without surgical reinnervation.
Radiorenograms:
$2._1$ – 3 days after the operation; $2._2$ – after 10 days; $2._3$ – after 1 month; $2._4$ – after 2 months; $2._5$ = after 4 months; $2._5$ = after 4 months; $2._5$ = after 4 months; $2._6$ = after 6 months; $2._7$ = after 1 year; $2._8$ = after 2 years; Radiorenograms after intravenous injection of adrenalin; $2._9$ = 3 days after the operation; $2._{10}$ – 1 months lager; $2._{11}$ – 4 months later; $2._{12}$ – 2 years later,
Nephroscanograms:
$2._{13}$ – 10 days after the operation; $2._{14}$ – 1 month later; $2._{15}$ – 6 months later; $2._{16}$ – 2 years later.

The same state was maintained 10 days later as by usual radiorenography as well as after the adrenalin injection (Tables 2-9, Figure 2.2).

After a month, the excretion phase of the curve became descending but, as before, all the indices of the denervated kidney were backward as compared with the intact one, the amplitude of vascular segment was 85.7±3.8%, secretion segment – 76.0±2.4%, and residual activity – 150.0±9.8%. The period of half excretion exceeded 15 minutes. RI was 2.8±2.3, p<0.001 (Tables 2-5, Figure 2.3).

The adrenalin injection had influence over both the intact as well as the denervated kidneys, but nevertheless, the period of semi-excretion of the intact kidney did not exceed 15 minutes. At the same time the curve of the denervated kidney became an obturative type again; its vascular and secretion amplitudes were 52.8±3.6% and 60.3±1.8%, residual activity was 120.6±5.0% of the corresponding segments in the intact kidney.

RI decreased to 15.5±4.8 (p<0.001, Tables 6-9, Figure 2.10).

By two months the indices of the denervated kidney improved slightly. All three segments of the renogram became clearly differentiated. The amplitudes of vascular secretion and excretion segments reached 80.1±1.8%, 84.2±1.9%, 140.0±10.5% respectively, and RI increased to 34.6±6.4, p<0.01. Tables 1-4, Figure 2.4). But the adrenalin injection caused their depression again. The above-mentioned indices became 56.2±2.4%, 66.2±2.7% and 116.2±3.0 of the intact renogram, respectively, and RI became 20.4±6.0%, p<0.001 (Tables 6-9).

Beginning at four months a more expressed reduction of the main qualitative as well as quantitative renogram indices were observed. The amplitude of vascular and secretion segments decreased to 62.5±1.4%, 69.1±3.6%, respectively, and the amplitude of residual activity increased to 125.0±3.5%. RI became 23.4±3.6 (p<0.001, Tables 2-5, Figure 2.5).

The adrenalin injection caused the same depression of renographic indices of the denervated kidney as in previous terms (Tables 6-9, Figure 2.11).

In the more remote period (after six months, one and two years) the amplitudes of vascular and secretion segments of renograms remained on the same low level as before , but the residual activity gradually increased to 125.0±4.5%, 160.0±4.0% and 153.3±8.0%, respectively. After two years the RI reduced to 16.6±5.5 (p<0.001). (Tables 2-5, Figure 2.6-8).

In the same terms (6 months, 1, 2 years) the adrenalin injection did not cause essential worsening of renographic indices as compared with previous terms (Tables 6-9, Figure 2.12).

The renoscyntigrams of the denervated kidney within the first two months became distinguished with rare touches which testified to a low accumulation of the isotope in the kidney (Figures 2.13-14). From four months up to two years the renoscyntigrams showed a distinct reduction of functioning parenchyma of the denervated kidney and vicarious hypertrophy of the intact one (Figures 2.15-16).

By excretory urography within the first two months the contrast medium was excreted only on the late picture. Later (from four months to two years) the left ureter atony was observed (Figures 3.1,2).

The X-ray cinematograms in the same terms revealed the more rare and slack contractions of the ureter; its diameter was two times more than that of the intact one and was filled with the contrast medium in the whole space from the kidney up to the bladder, without a distinct differentiation of ureteral segments.

In the second group of experiments three days after the denervation and following surgical reinnervation of the kidney, the amplitudes of vascular and secretion segments decreased (80.0±4.3% and 85.7±4.8%) from the norm, respectively; the excretion phase of the curve was ascendant, and RI was reduced to 20.5+/-3.2, p<0.001 (Tables 2-5, Figure 4.1). Ten days later the curve of the renogram of the operated kidney became three-phase, although all its indices were depressed (Tables 2-5, Figure 4.2).

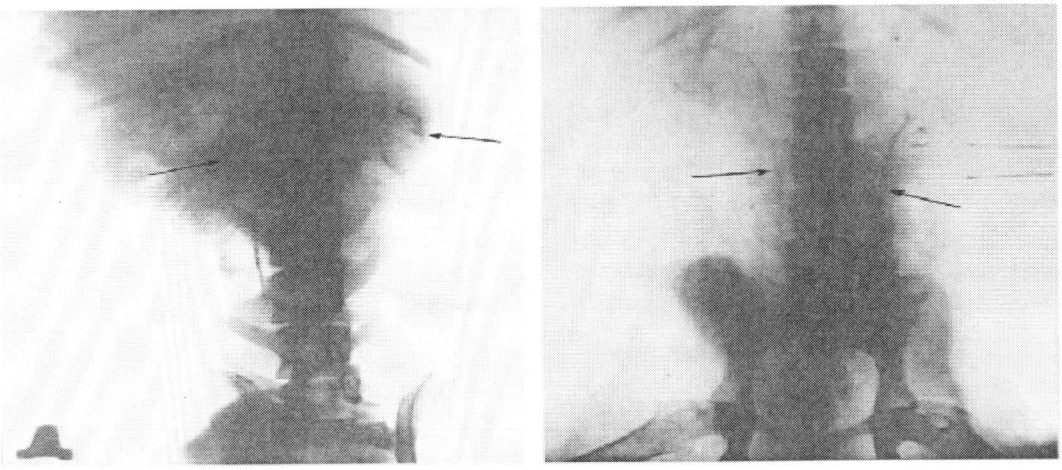

3.$_1$ 3.$_2$

Figure 3. Denervation of the left kidney without surgical reinnervation.
Excretory urograms:
3.$_1$ – 1 month after the operation;
3.$_2$ – 6 months after the operation. On the left side a more late excretion of contrast medium and an atony of ureter are observed.

After one month the amplitude of the vascular segment of this kidney reached the norm, but the secretion one was 86.8±3.6% of the norm; and RI increased as compared with the previous terms (32.2±4.4, $p<0.01$) (Tables 2-5, Figure 4.3).

Within one month of the operation, the adrenalin test caused a considerable reduction of renogram indices: the amplitude of the vascular segment decreased to 45.6±2.6%, 57.5±3.8%, 63.2±4.8%, the amplitude of the secreting one decreased to 62.0±2.2%, 63.4±1.8%, 63.2±1.0% and amplitude of residual activity decreased to 126.4±3.0, 128.2±3.4%, 130.8±4.7% of the corresponding indices of the intact kidney. RI decreased to 10.2±3.0; 12.5±2.0; 18.3±1.0 ($p<0.001$) (Tables 6-9, Figures 4.9,10).

After two months the indices of the reinnervated kidney improved considerably. Amplitudes of vascular and secretion segments (100.0±1.0%, 94.4±3.0%) as well as RI approached the lower limit of the norm (44.1±3.6, $p>0.05$) (Tables 2-5, Figure 4.4).

After four months and up to two years no asymmetry between the operated and intact kidneys was observed. The RI became stable at a level of 52.3±4.3; 62.8±5.2, ($p>0.05$) (Tables 2-5, Figures 4.5-8).

By four months the adrenalin test did not cause changes in the vascularization and secretion of the reinnervated kidney as compared with the intact one. Only the period of semi-excretion was prolonged (12.3±1.2 min, $p<0.01$) and RI was slightly reduced (to 36.4±4.1, $p>0.05$) (Tables 6-9, Figure 4.11).

At six months and up to the end of the experiments (two years) the mentioned indices did not differ from the corresponding indices of the intact kidney (Tables 2-9, Figures 4.6-8).

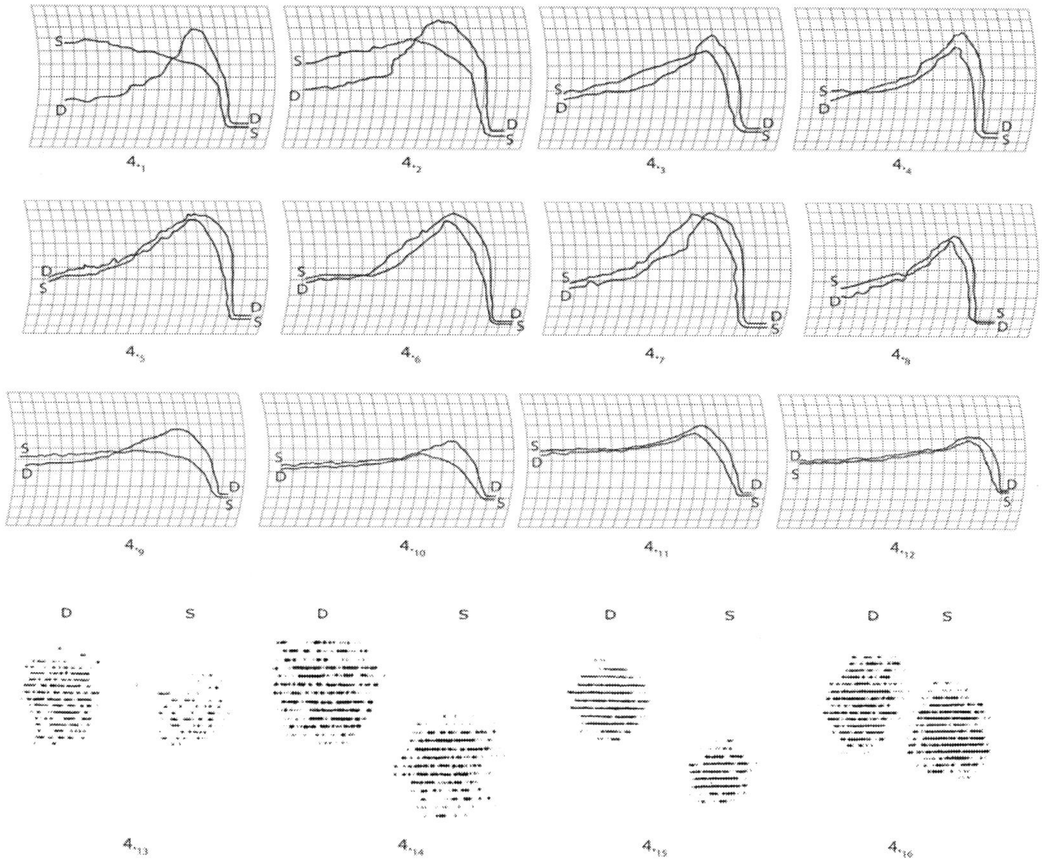

Figure 4. Denervation and surgical reinnervation of the left kidney.
Radiorenograms:
4.$_{1}$ – 3 days after the operation; 4.$_{2}$ – 10 days after; 4.$_{3}$ – 1 month after; 4.$_{4}$ – 2 months after; 4.$_{5}$ – 4 months after; 4.$_{6}$ – 6 months after; 4.$_{7}$ – 1 year after; 4.$_{8}$ – 2 years after, Radiorenograms after intravenous injection of adrenalin: 4.$_{9}$ – 3 days after the operation; 4.$_{10}$ – 1 month later; 4.$_{11}$ – 6 months later; 4.$_{12}$ – 2 years later.
nephroscanograms:
4.$_{13}$ – 10 days after the operation, 4.$_{14}$ – 1 month later; 4.$_{15}$ – 6 months later; 4.$_{16}$ – 2 years later.

Diffusive rare touches of renoscintigrams observed within the first two months after the operation, were replaced 4-6 months later with complete normalization of the picture (Figures 4.$_{13-16}$). Four months to two years after the operation the excretory urograms and x-ray cinematograms showed normal excretion of the contrast medium (Figures 5.$_{1,2}$).

In the third group ("a" subgroup) after the kidney autotransplantation in the iliac fossa without surgical reinnervation, within the first month, the renograms were two-phase, ascendant, with a low amplitude of the vascular segment, (90.0±4.2%; 83.3±3.3%; 75.1±1.8% of the intact side, $p<0.001$), low, prolonged secretion (76.1±3.8%; 76.0±4.2%; 85.2±4.6%, $p<0.01$) and absent excretion, and RI was decreased to (6.4±1.8; 11.7±3.0; 25.1±2.5, $p<0.001$, Tables 2-5, Figures 6.$_{1-3}$).

After two and four months the renograms became three phase, but their characteristics were considerably behind the corresponding indices of the intact kidney. So the amplitude of the vascular segment was 66.7±1.0%; 57.1±5.5%; the secretion segment was 71.7±3.8%; 63.6±4.2% and residual activity was 121.7±10.0%; 111.9±8.5% of the intact kidney, ($p<0.01$), and RI fluctuated between 29.4±2.5 and 36.7±1.8 ($p<0.01$) (Tables 2-5, Figures 6.$_{4,5}$).

Six months later and up to two years, the amplitude of the vascular and secretion segment were on a low level, as before (66.7±3.9%; 60.0±4.6%; 56.7±4.8% and 62.2±4.0%; 62.5±5.0%; 57.7±5.2% of the intact kidney, respectively, $p<.001$). The residual activity after 15 minutes was 130.0±4.5%; 150.0±8.5%; with 125.0±9.5% of the intact side. By two years the renogram curve was only slightly raised over the background line. RI, after six months and up to two years, was firmly decreased (18.7±2.1; 16.2±3.3; 13.9±2.1, $p<0.001$) (Tables 2-6, Figures 6.$_{6\text{-}8}$).

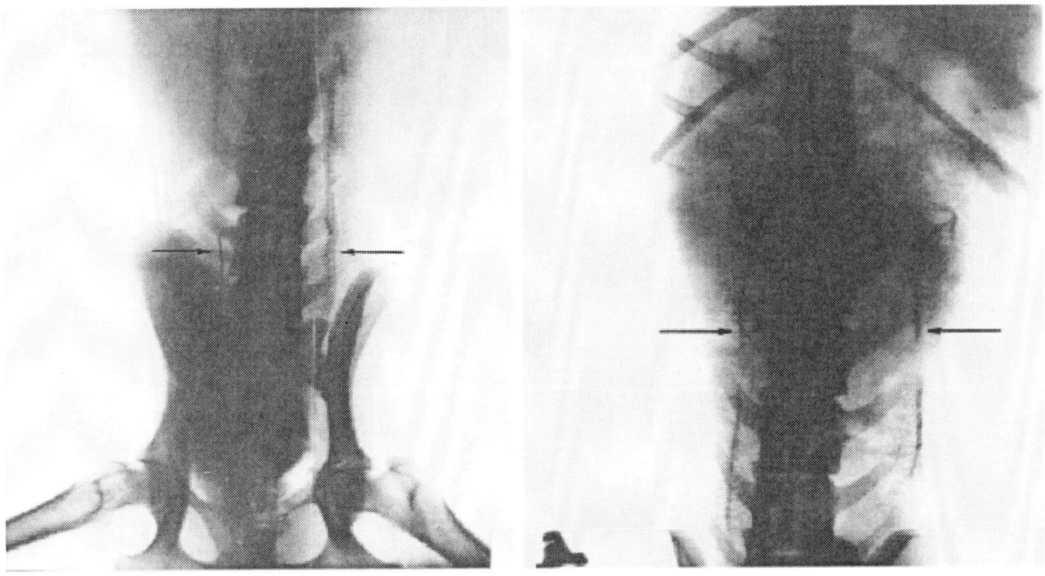

5.$_1$ 5.$_2$

Figure 5. Denervation and surgical reinnervation of the left kidney.
Excretory urograms:
5.$_1$ – 1 month after the operation, on the left side there is an atony of the ureter;
5.$_2$ – 6 months later, excretory and motor functions of the operated (left) kidney are normal.

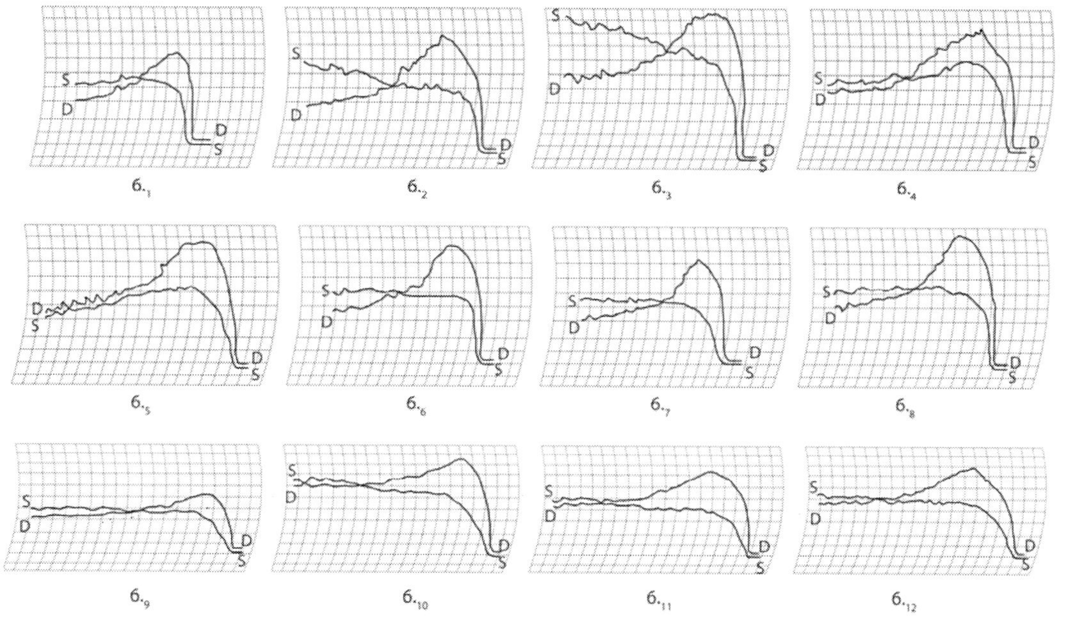

Figure 6. Autotransplantation of the left kidney in the iliac fossa without surgical reinnervation. Radiorenograms: $6._1$ – 3 days after operation; $6._2$ – 10 days after; $6._3$ – 1 month after; $6._4$ – 2 months after; $6._5$ – 4 months after; $6._6$ – 6 months after; $6._7$ – 1 year after; $6._8$ – 2 years after. Radiorenograms after the intravenous injection of adrenalin: $6._9$ – 3 days after the operation; $6._{10}$ – 2 months later; $6._{11}$ – 6 months later; $6._{12}$ – 2 years later.

The radiorenography after the intravenous adrenalin injection showed an additional firm decrease of amplitudes of vascular (40.2±2.5%; 54.3±2.5%) and secretion segments (52.2±1.2%; 53.5±2.2%), the residual activity was 135.6±3.5%, 128.5±3.6% of the intact kidney, and RI was greatly decreased (5.0±1.5; 10.5±2.2, $p<0.001$) (Tables 6-9, Figures $6._{9\text{-}12}$).

The renoscintigrams showed a weak accumulation of isotope in the kidney; after six months and up to two years the functioning parenchyma of the operated kidney decreased more with the vicarious hypertrophy of the intact kidney (Figures $7._{1\text{-}8}$).

One month after the operation the excretion urography showed only a track of contrast medium in the pyelon (Figure $8._1$). After six months it was revealed in the ureter only under remote possibilities and in lower concentration as compared with the intact kidney (Figure $8._2$). In the same terms the x-ray cinematograms showed the atony and slack contractions of the transplanted kidney ureter.

In the third group (subgroup b), three days after the autotransplantation of the left kidney without surgical reinnervation and contralateral nephrectomy, the renogram was two phase. RI reached 16.4±1.8 ($p<0.001$) (Table 5, Figure $9._1$).

After 10 days the renogram became three phase but all its indices were depressed. RI was 36.0±2.6, $p<0{,}01$. In the same periods the adrenalin test caused an additional decrease of RI (10.8±1.6; 22.6±1.5, $p<0{,}001$), (Table 5, Figure $9._9$).

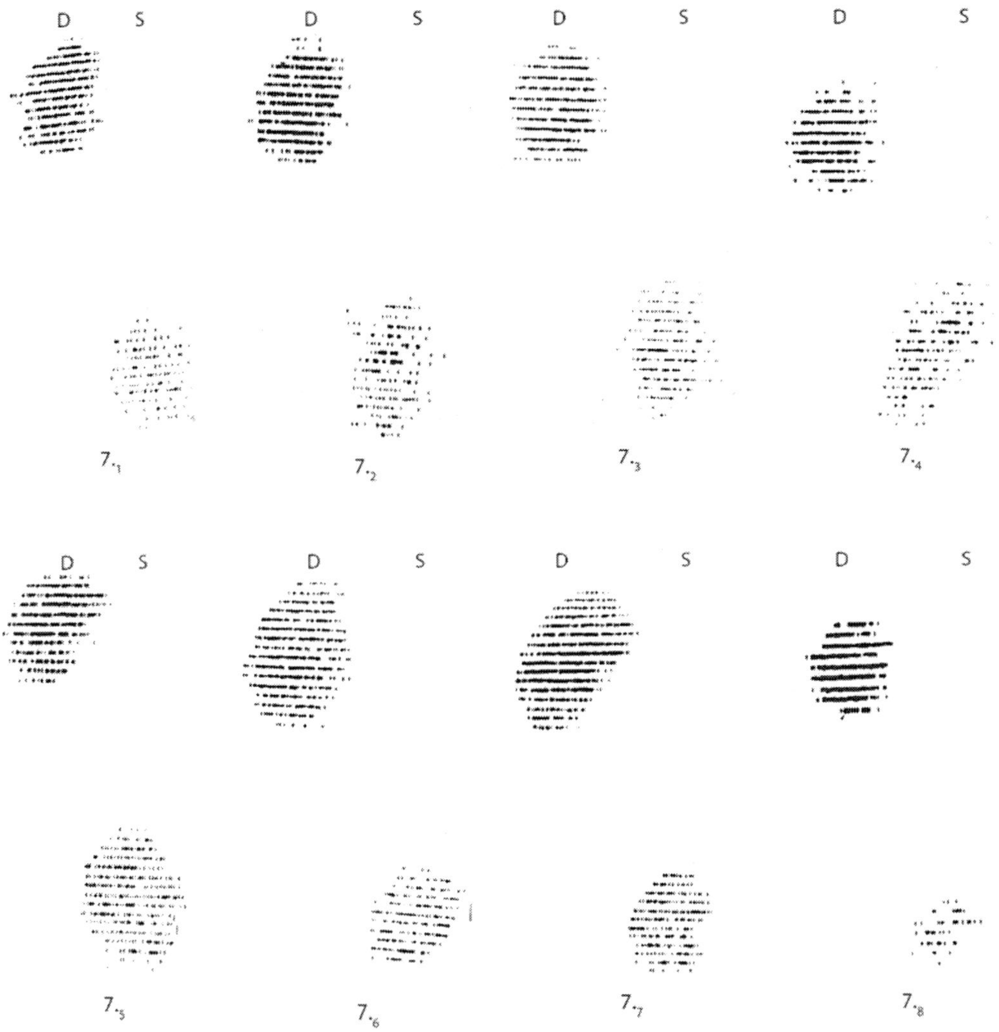

Figure 7. Autotransplantation of the left kidney in the iliac fossa without surgical reinnervation. Renoscintigrams:
$7._{1}$ – 3 days after the operation; $7._{2}$ – 10 days later; $7._{3}$ – 1 month later; $7._{4}$ – 2 months later; $7._{5}$ – 4 mohts later; $7._{6}$ – 6 monts later; $7._{7}$ – 1 year later; $7._{8}$ – 2 years later.

After one month the amplitudes of vascular and secretion segments increased gradually (Figure 9.3).

In the interval from two-to-six months after the operation the renogram indices approached the low limits of the norm (Figures 94-6). RI fluctuated between 43.8±8.7; 42.8±7.2; 44.4±5.5 ($p>0.05$, Table 5). But the adrenalin test revealed in the same terms a considerable decrease of RI (23.7±2.2; 28.7±2.4; 24.5±2.5) as compared with the preoperative level (41.5±0.8, $p<0.001$) (Table 9, Figure 9.11).

Further, even the usual renography (without adrenalin injection) showed a firm prolongation of excretion phase and decrease of RI (36.9±3.8; 36.4±5.0, $p<0.01$), (Table 5).

The adrenalin injection caused an additional reduction of RI (20.8±1.8; 25.8±2.2, $p<0.001$), (Table 9, Figure $9._{12}$).

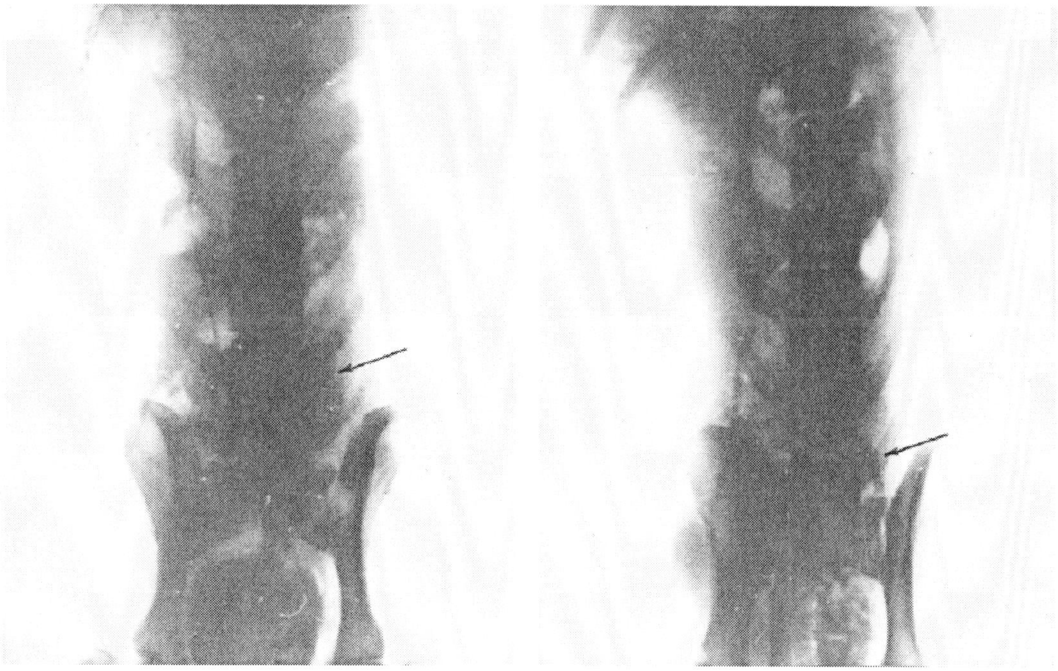

$8._1$ $8._2$

Figure 8. Autotransplantation of the left kidney in the pelvis without surgical reinnervation.
Excretory urograms:
$8._1$ – 1 month after the operation, left in the pelvis only nephrogram of the transplanted kidney is seen;
$8._2$ – 6 months later, an atony of the left ureter is observed.

The renoscintigrams within the first month were distinguished by a weak accumulation of the isotope (Figures $9._{13\text{-}14}$); later (after two months) the frequency of touches was normalized and by six months the vicarious hypertrophy of the sole transplanted kidney was revealed (Figures $9._{15\text{-}16}$).

The excretory urocinematograms after two months showed more late excretion of the contrast medium and rare contractions of the ureter as compared with the sole intact kidney (Figure 14).

In the fourth group (subgroup a) of the experiments, three and ten days after the autotransplantation and surgical reinnervation of the left kidney, the renograms were two-phase, with amplitude of the vascular segment of 86.7±3.3%; 86.0±2.4%, the secretion was 76.1±3.6%; 82.3±4.0%; residual activity was 114.5±10.8; 188.3±12.0% of the norm, and RI decreased (18.4±2.0; 12.6±2.2, $p<0.001$), (Tables 2-5), (Figures $10._{1,2}$).

After one month the renogram became three phase (Figure $10._3$).

Two months later the amplitude of the vascular segment approached normal (95.0±3.3%, $p>0.05$), but secretion was still behind the norm (87.1±4.4%), and the residual activity was 125.5±8.6%. RI increased to 39.5±2.4, $p<0.05$, (Tables 2-5, Figure $10._4$).

After four months the amplitude of the vascular segment was normal, as before (100.0±1.0%, p>0.05). At the same time the amplitude of secretion segment also reached the norm (100.0±1.0%). RI also increased and approached the norm (44.3±3.8%, p>0.05), (Tables 2-5, Figure 10.3).

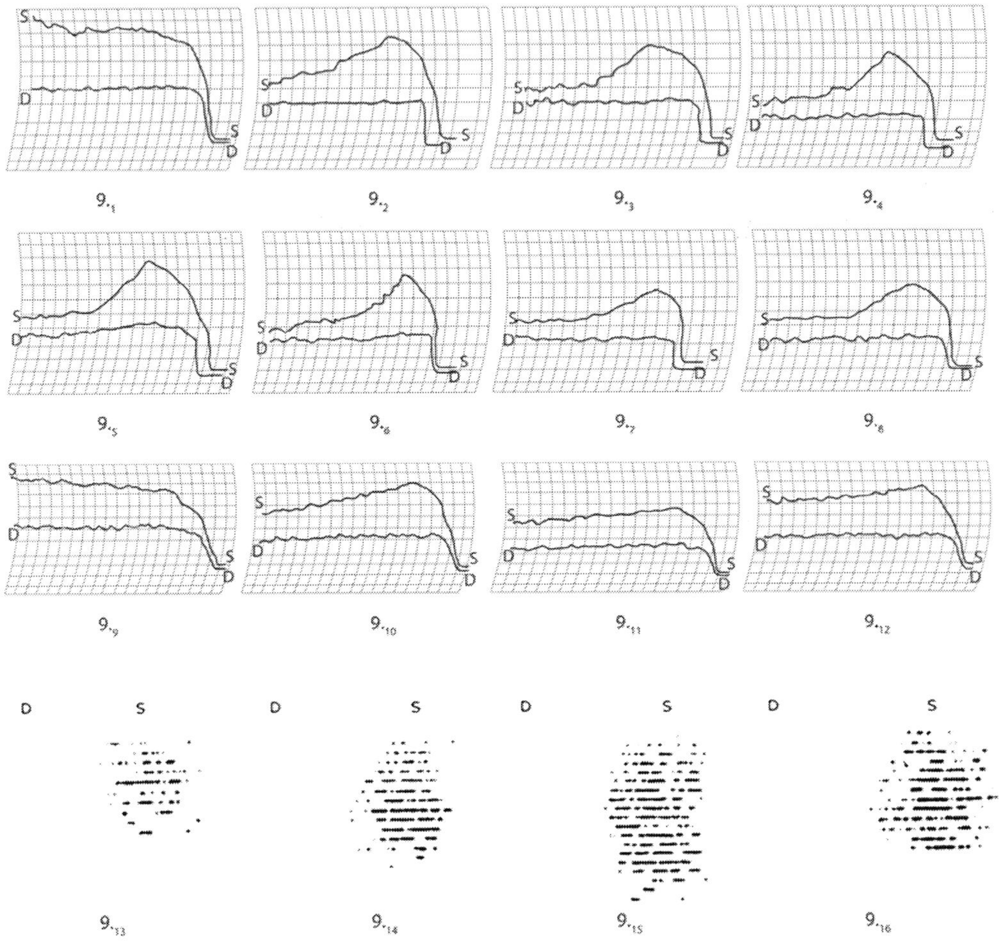

Figure 9. Autotransplantation of the left kidney in the iliac fossas without surgical reinnervation, contralateral nephrectomy.
Radiorenograms: $9._{1}$ – 3 days after the operation; $9._{2}$ – 10 days after; $9._{3}$ – 1 month after; $9._{4}$ – 2 months after; $9._{5}$ – 4 months after; $9._{6}$ – 6 months after; $9._{7}$ – 1 year after; $9._{8}$ – 2 years after. Raqdiorenograms after the intravenous injection of adrenalin; $9._{9}$ – 3 days after the operation; $9._{10}$ – 1 month later; $9._{11}$ – 4 months later; $9._{12}$ – 2 years later. Renoscintigrams: $9._{13}$ – 10 days after the operation; $9._{14}$ – 1 month later; $9._{15}$ – 6 months later; $9._{16}$ – 2 years later.

Six months after the operation, there was not quantitative or qualitative asymmetry between the operated and intact kidneys. Such a condition was maintained within the following period up to two years. RI was stabilized at a normal level (54.9±4.5; 48.6±3.6; 49.9±2.5, $p>0.05$), (Tables 2-5, Figures 10.$_{6-8}$).

In the same test-group within one month after the operation, the preliminary adrenalin injection caused an additional decrease of renogram indices. But after two months the reliable difference between the vascular segments disappeared, after four months between the secretion and after six months between the excretion segments of the operated and intact kidneys. By six months and later RI also reached the norm, as in the case of simple renography as well as adrenalin injection (Tables 6-9, Figures 10.$_{9-12}$).

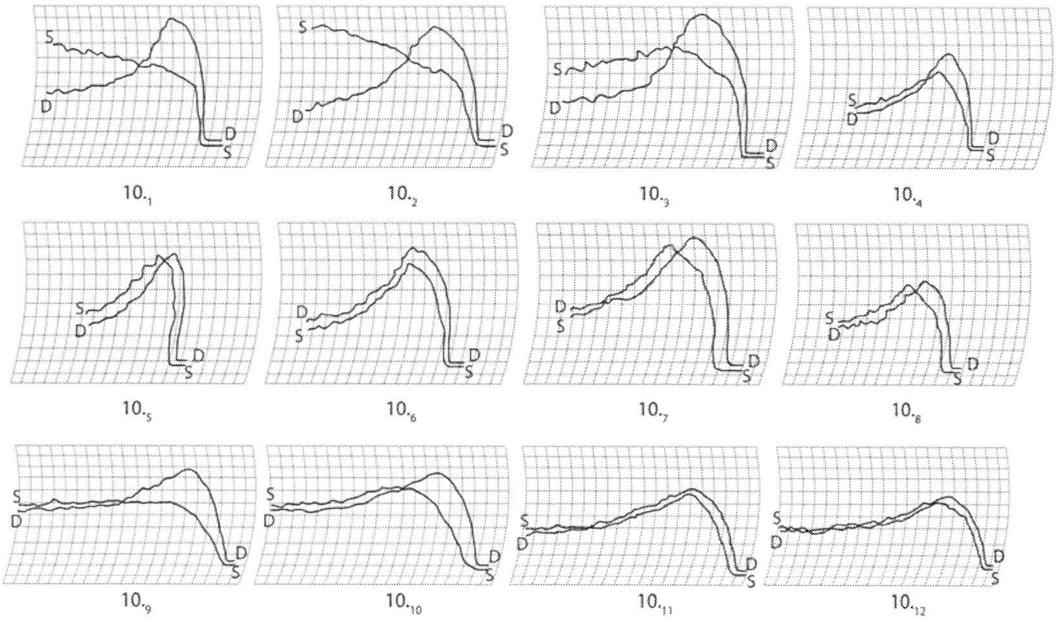

Figure 10. Autotransplantation of the left kidney in the iliac fossa with a surgical reinnervation. Radiorenograms: 10.$_1$ – 3 days after the operation; 10.$_2$ – 10 days after; 10.$_3$ – 1 month after; 10.$_4$ – 2 months after; 10.$_5$ – 4 months after; 10.$_6$ – 6 months after; 10.$_7$ – 1 year after; 10.$_8$ – 2 years after. Radiorenograms after the intravenous injection of adrenalin: 10.$_9$ – 3 days later; 10.$_{10}$ – 2 months later; 10.$_{11}$ – 6 months later; 10.$_{12}$ – 2 years later.

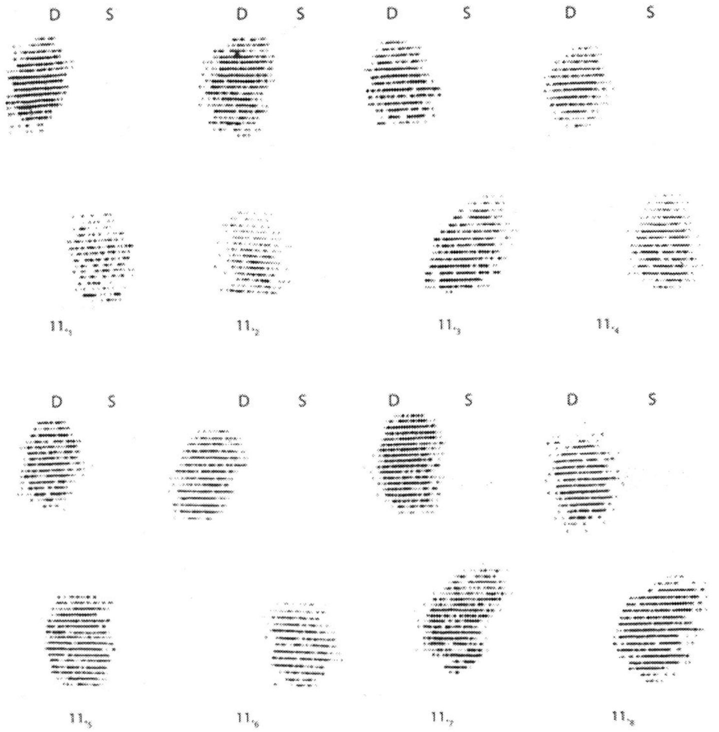

Figure 11. Autotransplantation of the left kidney in the iliac fossa with a surgical reinnervation. Renoscintigrams: 11.₁ – 3 days after the operation; 11.₂ – 10 days later; 11.₃ – 1 month later; 11.₄ – 2 months later; 11.₅ – 4 months later; 11.₆ – 6 months later; 11.₇ – 1 year later; 11.₈ – 2 years later.

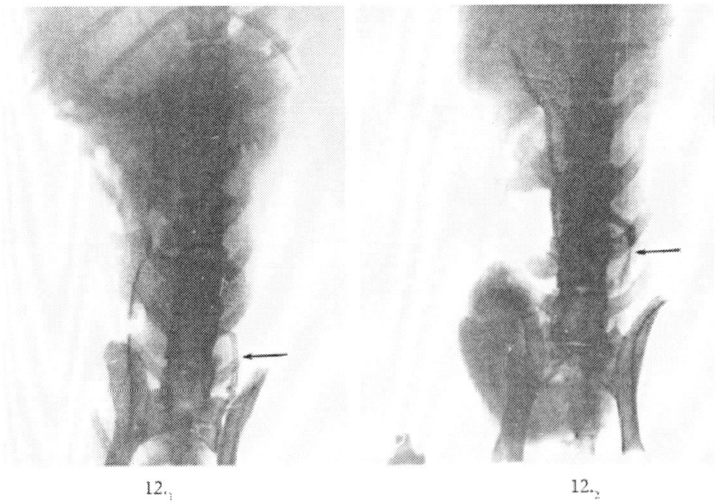

Figure 12. Autotransplantation of the left kidney in the iliac fossa with a surgical reinnervation. Excretory urograms: 12.₁ – 1 month after the operation, left there is a light atony of ureter; 12.₂ – 6 months later, the excretory function of the operated (left) kidney is normal.

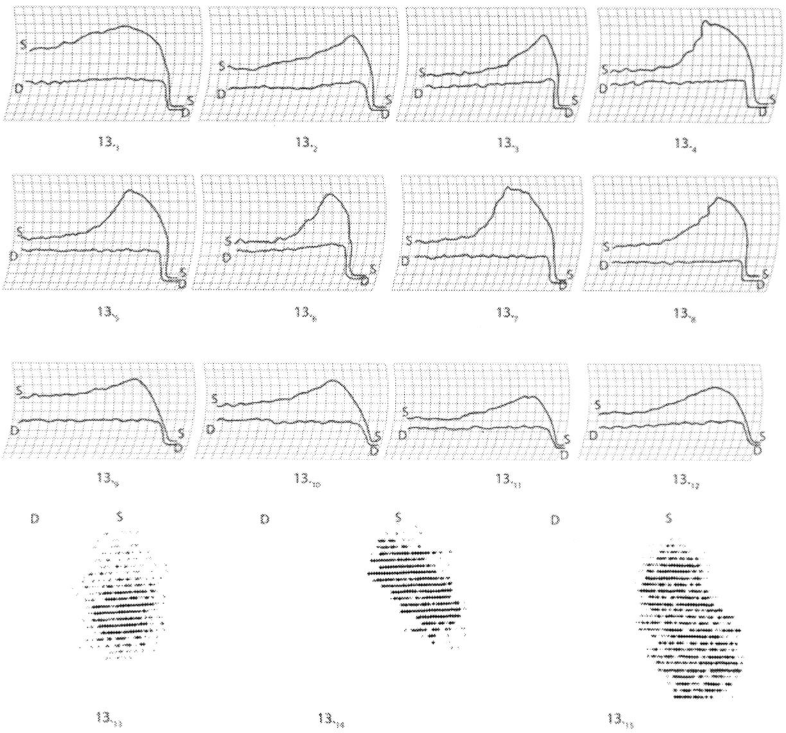

Figure 13. Autotransplantation of the left kidney in the iliac fossa with a surgical reinnervation, contralateral nephrectomy. Radiorenograms: $13._1$ – 3 days after the operation; $13._2$ – 10 days after; $13._3$ – 1 month after; $13._4$ – 2 months after; $13._5$ – 4 months after; $13._6$ – 6 months after; $13._7$ – 1 year after; $13._8$ – 2 years after. Radiorenograms after the intravenous injection of adrenalin: $13._9$ – 3 days as after the operation; $13._{10}$ – 2 months later; $13._{11}$ – 6 months later; $13._{12}$ – 2 years later. Renoscintigrams: $13._{13}$ – 10 days after the operation; 13.1_4 – 1 month later; $13._{15}$ – 2 years later.

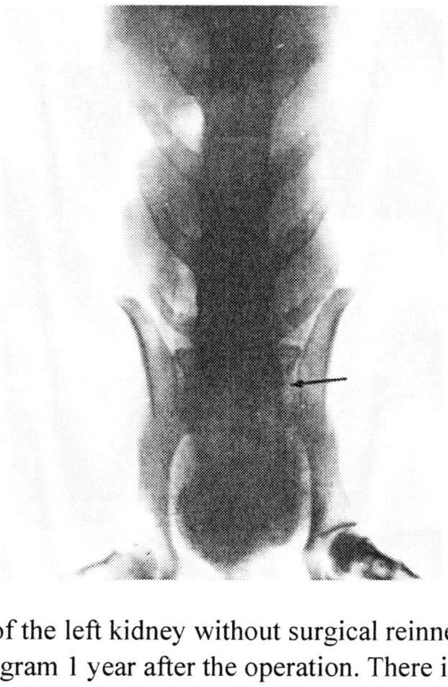

Figure 14. Autotransplantation of the left kidney without surgical reinnervation, contralateral nephrectomy. The excretory urogram 1 year after the operation. There is an atony of ureter.

The renoscinitigrams during the first ten days (Figures 11.1,2) were represented by rare diffusive touches. After two months the normal distribution of the isotope in the operated kidney was observed (Figures 11.4-8).

The excretory urograms and x-ray cinematograms after two months and later showed a normal function of the operated kidney (Figures 12.1,2).

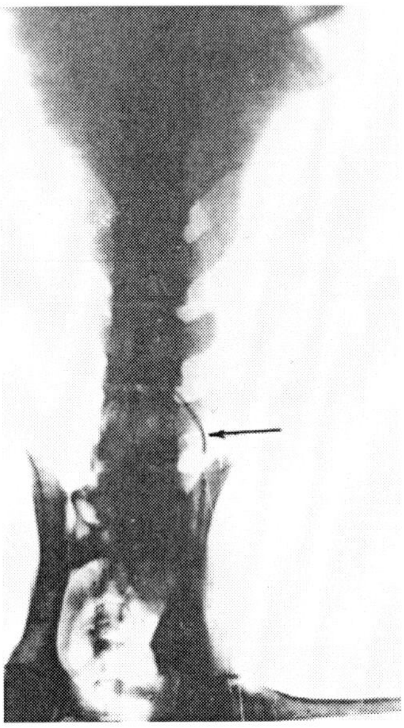

Figure 15. Autotransplantation of the left kidney with the surgical reinnervation, contralateral nephrectomy. The excretory urogram 1 year after the operation. The excretory and motor functions of the kidney is normal.

Table 2. Denervation in situ and autotransplantation of the kidneys without and with surgical reinnervation: Correlation of renogram vascular segment amplitudes of operated and intact kidneys

Kinds of operations			Terms of observations							
			3 days	10 days	1 month	2 months	4 months	6 months	1 year	2 years
1st gr.	Denervation in situ	M±m	87.5±2.4	87.5±3.2	85.7±3.8	80.1±1.8	62.5±1.4	71.4±2.2	66.7±5.7	66.7±3.9
		n	3	3	4	3	3	3	3	3
		p	<0,001	<0.001	<0.001	<0.001	<0.01	<0.001	<0.001	<0.001
2nd gr.	Denervation, reinnervation in situ	M±m	80.0±4.3	80.0±5.5	100.5±0.5	100.0±1.0	100.0±1.5	100.0±1.0	100.0±1.0	98.9±1.8
		n	3	3	3	3	3	3	3	3
		p	<0.001	<0.001	>0.05	>0.05	>0.05	>0.05	>0.05	>0.05
3rd a gr.	Transplantation without reinnervation	M±m	90.0±4.2	83.3±3.3	75.1±1.8	66.7±1.0	57.1±5.5	66.7±3.9	60.0±4.6	56.7±4.8
		n	3	3	3	4	3	3	3	3
		p	<0.01	<0.001	<0.001	<0.001	<0.001	<0.001	<0.001	<0.001
4th a gr.	Transplantation with reinnervation	M±m	86.7±3.3	86.0±2.4	83.3±3.8	95.0±3.3	100.0±1.0	100.0±0.5	100.0±1.0	100.0±1.0
		n	3	3	3	4	3	3	3	3
		p	<0.001	<0.001	<0.001	>0.05	>0.05	>0.05	>0.05	>0.05

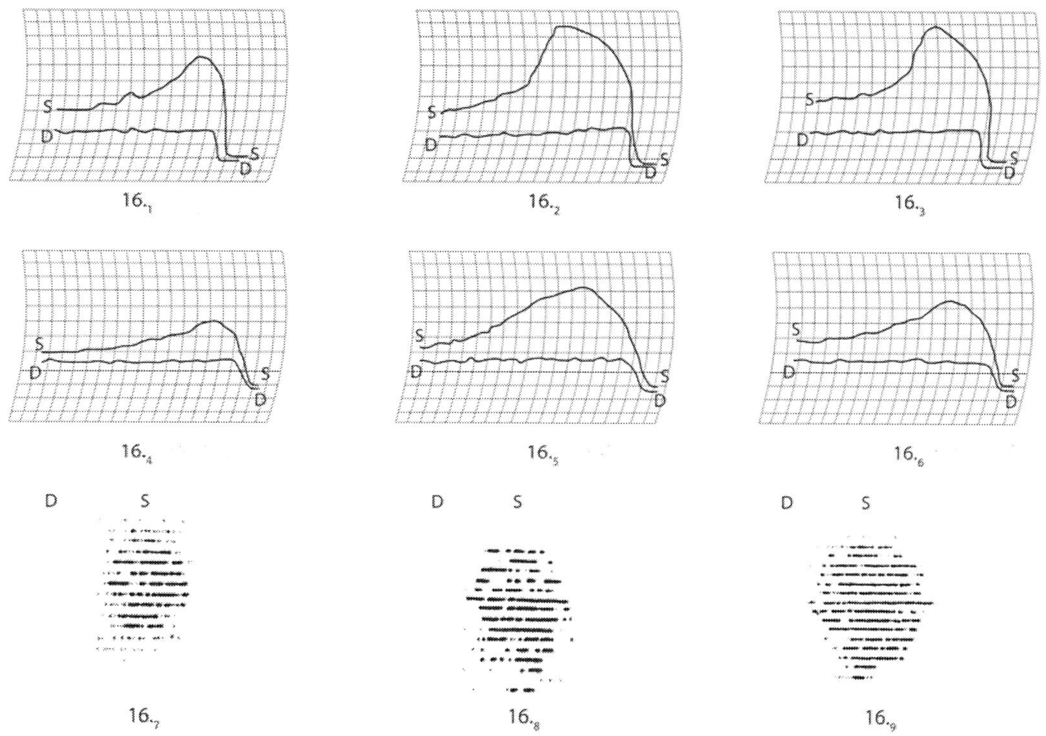

Figure 16. Right side nephrectomy (control test – group).
Radiorenograms: 16.1 – 3 days after the operation; 16.2 – 1 month later; 16.3 – 2 years later.
Renoscintigrams after the intravenous injection of adrenaline: 16.4 – 3 days after the operation; 16.5 – 1 month later; 16.6 – 2 years later.
Renoscintigrams: 16.7 – 3 days after the operation; 16.8 – 1 month later; 16.9 – 2 years later.

In the fourth group (subgroup b) three and ten days after the autotransplantation, surgical reinnervation of the left kidney and conralateral nephrectomy, the renograms maintained all three phases, although the amplitudes of vascular and secretion segments were behind the norm. RI was also reduced (22.2±1.0; 32.1±3.3, $p<0.01$), (Table 5, Figures 13.1,2).

One month later an improvement of the mentioned indices (especially of vascularization and secretion) was observed (Figure 13.3).

Two months later and within the whole period of experiment (up to two years) a firm normalization of renograms was observed in all indices. RI also reached the norm (47.1±3.2; 50.6±4.4; 52.3±6.0; 52.6±5.6; 59.9±3.8, $p>0.05$) (Table 5, Figures 13.5-8).

After six months the adrenalin injection did not reveal the reliable changes in the operated kidney as compared with its preoperative data and indices of the intact kidney made in parallel terms after the operation (Table 9, Figures 13.9-12).

Table 3. Denervation in situ and autotransplantation of the kidneys without and with surgical reinnervation: Correlation of renogram secretory segment amplitudes of operated and intact kidneys

Kinds of operations			Terms of observations							
			3 days	10 days	1 month	2 months	4 months	6 months	1 year	2 years
1st gr.	Denervation in situ	M±m	76,0±3,3	82,0±4,6	76,0±2,4	84,2±1,9	69,1±3,6	72,7±4,2	61,9±5,5	60,0±4,8
		n	3	3	4	3	3	3	3	3
		p	<0,001	<0,001	<0,001	<0,001	<0,001	<0,001	<0,001	<0,001
2nd gr.	Denervation, reinnervation in situ	M±m	85,7±4,8	84,0±3,2	86,8±3,6	94,4±3,0	93,3±2,8	93,8±2,7	102,2±1,0	97,2±1,6
		n	3	3	3	3	3	3	3	3
		p	<0,001	<0,001	<0,001	>0,05	>0,05	>0,05	>0,05	>0,05
3rd a gr.	Transplantatin without reinnervation	M±m	76,1±3,8	76,0±4,2	85,2±4,6	71,7±3,8	63,6±4,2	62,2±4,0	62,5±5,0	57,7±5,2
		n	3	3	3	4	3	3	3	3
		p	<0,001	<0,001	<0,01	<0,001	<0,001	<0,001	<0,001	<0,001
4th a gr.	Transplantatin with reinnervation	M±m	76,1±3,6	82,3±4,0	80,0±3,6	87,1±4,4	100,0±1,0	98,4±2,0	100,0±1,0	96,9±0,5
		n	3	3	3	4	3	3	3	3
		p	<0,001	<0,001	<0,01	<0,01	>0,05	>0,05	>0,05	>0,05

Table 4. Denervation in situ and autotransplantation of the kidneys without and with surgical reinnervation: Correlation of residual radioactivity in operated and intact kidneys

Kinds of operations			Terms of observations							
			3 days	10 days	1 month	2 months	4 months	6 months	1 year	2 years
1st gr.	Denervation in situ	M±m	250,0±5.0	270,0±5,0	150,0±9,8	140,0±10,5	125,0±3,5	125,0±4,5	160,0±4,6	153,3±8,0
		n	3	3	4	3	3	3	3	3
		p	<0,001	<0,001	<0,001	<0,001	<0,001	<0,001	<0,001	<0,001
2nd gr.	Denervation, reinnervation in situ	M±m	250,0±20,0	150,0±10,0	130,0±5,0	103,8±5,5	88,9±6,6	105,3±4,6	106,7±5,5	94,6±4,8
		n	3	3	3	3	3	3	3	3
		p	<0,001	<0,001	<0,01	>0,05	>0,05	>0,05	>0,05	>0,05
3rd a gr.	Transplantation without reinnervation	M±m	142,8±10,0	223,5±20,0	187,5±12,5	121,7±10,0	111,9±8,5	130,0±4,5	150,0±8,5	125,0±9,5
		n	3	3	3	4	3	3	3	3
		p	<0,001	<0,001	<0,001	<0,001	<0,01	<0,001	<0,001	<0,001
4th a gr.	Transplantation with reinnervation	M±m	114,5±10,8	188,3±12,0	150,0±8,5	125,5±8,6	108,5±4,3	96,5±3,5	95,0±5,5	104,3±3,5
		n	3	3	3	4	3	3	3	3
		p	<0,01	<0,001	<0,001	<0,001	<0,05	>0,05	>0,05	>0,05

Table 5. Denervation in situ and autotransplantation of the kidneys without and with surgical reinnervation: Changes of Hirakawa-Corcoran renographic index

Kinds of operations			Intact kidney	Terms of observations							
				3 days	10 days	1 month	2 months	4 months	6 months	1 year	2 years
1st gr.	Denervation in situ	M±m	53,5±3,5	9,0±3,5	13,2±5,4	25,8±2,3	34,6±6,4	23,4±3,6	28,1±9,3	15,9±6,8	16,6±5,5
		n	25	3	3	4	3	3	3	3	3
		p		<0,001	<0,001	<0,001	<0,01	<0,001	<0,001	<0,001	<0,001
2nd gr.	Denervation, reinnervation in situ	M±m	61,7±4,4	20,5±3,2	16,3±4,3	32,2±4,4	44,1±3,6	52,3±4,3	48,9±5,2	56,6±4,1	62,8±5,2
		n	24	3	3	3	3	3	3	3	3
		p		<0,001	<0,001	<0,01	>0,05	>0,05	>0,05	>0,05	>0,05
3rd a gr.	Transplantation without reinnervation	M±m	52,2±5,0	6,4±1,8	11,7±3,0	25,1±2,5	29,4±2,5	36,7±1,8	18,7±2,1	16,2±3,3	13,9±2,1
		n	25	3	3	3	4	3	3	3	3
		p		<0,001	<0,001	<0,001	<0,001	<0,01	<0,001	<0,001	<0,001
3rd b gr.	Transplantation without reinnervation, contralateral nephrectomy	M±m		16,4±1,8	36,0±2,6	32,9±5,1	43,8±8,7	42,8±7,2	44,4±5,5	36,9±3,8	36,4±5,0
		n		3	3	3	5	3	3	3	3
		p		<0,001	<0,01	<0,01	>0,05	>0,05	>0,05	<0,01	<0,01

4th a gr.	Transplantation with reinnervation	M±m	55,5±4,2	18,4±2,0	12,6±2,2	26,5±3,5	39,5±2,4	44,3±3,8	54,9±4,5	48,6±3,6	49,9±2,5
		n	25	3	3	3	4	3	3	3	3
		p		<0,001	<0,001	<0,001	<0,01	>0,05	>0,05	>0,05	>0,05
4th b gr.	Transplantation with reinnervation, contralateral nephrectomy	M±m		22,2±1,0	32,1±3,3	43,8±4,8	47,1±3,2	50,6±4,4	52,3±6,0	52,6±5,6	59,9±3,8
		n		3	3	4	3	3	3	3	3
		p		<0,001	<0,01	>0,05	>0,05	>0,05	>0,05	>0,05	>0,05
5th gr.	Right side nephrectomy	M±m		48,5±2,8	50,9±3,7	52,3±6,6	52,3±6,6	55,6±4,9	50,3±2,9	60,7±5,8	56,8±5,0
		n		3	3	4	4	3	3	3	3

Table 6. Denervation in situ and autotransplantation of the kidneys without and with surgical reinnervation: Correlation of intact (D) and operated (S) kidneys renogram vascular segment amplitudes after adrenalin intravenous injection (%)

Kinds of operations			Terms of observations								
			Before the operation	3 days after	10 days	1 month	2 months	4 months	6 months	1 year	2 years
1st gr.	Denervation in situ	M±m D	83,5±2,5	80,5±3,4	84,3±5,3	82,2±2,5	80,4±3,8	80,4±3,8	89,5±3,2	80,5±3,4	82,5±2,5
		S	84,1±1,5	42,3±2,5	51,6±3,2	52,8±3,6	56,2±2,4	56,2±2,4	62,6±3,6	63,5±2,7	62,4±3,4
		n	25	3	3	4	3	3	3	3	3
		p	>0,05	<0,001	<0,001	<0,001	<0,001	<0,001	<0,001	<0,001	<0,001
2nd gr.	Denervation, reinnervation in situ	M±m D	81,4±3,6	78,8±3,8	82,5±2,5	85,2±1,6	82,6±2,4	80,5±3,2	86,3±1,8	82,6±2,4	81,4±3,0
		S	82,5±2,5	45,6±2,6	57,5±3,8	63,6±4,8	72,5±5,0	75,3±3,0	80,1±1,2	76,0±1,2	78,3±1,0
		n	24	3	3	3	3	3	3	3	3
		p	>0,05	<0,001	<0,001	<0,001	<0,05	>0,05	>0,05	>0,05	>0,05
3rd a gr.	Transplantation without reinnervation	M±m D	84,3±2,1	85,2±2,5	80,5±3,0	83,3±1,8	79,8±1,5	81,2±3,0	86,0±1,6	80,1±2,4	82,5±1,0
		S	83,5±1,0	40,2±2,5	43,3±3,2	46,4±3,0	48,5±2,7	47,2±2,5	52,6±3,0	57,1±1,0	54,3±2,5
		n	25	3	3	3	3	3	3	3	3
		p	>0,05	<0,001	<0,001	<0,001	<0,001	<0,001	<0,001	<0,001	<0,001
4th a gr.	Transplantation with reinnervation	M±m D	83,4±1,2	82,4±2,0	84,1±2,1	85,5±3,0	80,3±3,5	82,2±1,0	81,0±1,2	88,5±2,5	85,7±2,7
		S	83,0±1,5	47,3±2,2	52,6±3,0	66,2±2,1	74,4±3,0	75,3±2,2	76,8±1,8	82,0±2,0	80,2±2,7
		n	3	3	3	3	4	3	3	3	3
		p	>0,05	<0,001	<0,001	<0,001	>0,05	>0,05	>0,05	>0,05	>0,05

Table 7. Denervation in situ and autotransplantation of the kidneys without and with surgical reinnervation: Correlation of intact (D) and operated (S) kidneys renogram secretory segment amplitudes after adrenalin intravenous injection (%)

Kinds of operations			Terms of observations								
			Before the operation	3 days after	10 days	1 month	2 months	4 months	6 months	1 year	2 years
1st gr.	Denervation in situ	M±m	75,2±1,2	80,2±2,5	79,5±1,2	82,4±1,8	83,1±0,5	75,0±1,9	77,7±2,2	74,8±1,0	73,3±2,5
		D	74,3±2,0	65,2±2,0	62,4±1,4	60,3±1,8	66,1±2,7	60,5±1,7	65,0±1,4	55,2±1,8	55,5±1,6
		S	25	3	3	4	3	3	3	3	3
		n	>0,05	<0,001	<0,001	<0,001	<0,001	<0,001	<0,001	<0,001	<0,001
		p									
2nd gr.	Denervation, reinnervation in situ	M±m	76,4±1,8	75,5±3,0	80,2±2,0	74,5±1,4	73,4±1,8	79,2±1,1	81,0±0,5	76,5±2,8	78,3±2,7
		D	74,2±1,0	62,0±2,2	63,4±1,8	63,2±1,0	70,3±2,0	75,2±1,6	77,4±2,0	74,3±1,0	76,0±1,2
		S	24	3	3	3	3	3	3	3	3
		n	>0,05	<0,001	<0,001	<0,01	>0,05	>0,05	>0,05	>0,05	>0,05
		p									

Table 7. (continued)

3rd a gr.	Transplantation without reinnervation	M±m	78,3±2,6	75,4±2,5	78,2±2,7	80,1±1,8	74,5±1,6	79,3±3,0	82,2±1,8	76,5±2,7	78,5±2,8
		D	76,4±0,5	52,2±1,2	53,4±1,4	50,5±2,7	55,3±0,5	60,2±1,0	54,5±1,5	57,7±2,0	53,5±2,2
		S	25	3	3	3	4	3	3	3	3
		n	>0,05	<0,001	<0,001	<0,001	<0,001	<0,001	<0,001	<0,001	<0,001
		p									
4th a gr.	Transplantation with reinnervation	M±m	80,5±1,0	81,0±1,0	78,2±2,7	75,5±1,6	82,3±2,5	84,2±0,5	80,1±1,0	76,5±2,5	79,8±2,7
		D	82,2±0,5	57,5±2,0	60,2±1,2	62,4±1,0	70,3±2,7	80,1±2,2	78,4±3,0	74,2±1,0	75,5±1,5
		S	25	3	3	3	4	3	3	3	3
		n	>0,05	<0,001	<0,001	<0,001	<0,05	>0,05	>0,05	>0,05	>0,05
		p									

In the same subgroup, the renoscintigrams were represented by relatively rare touches within only 10 days (Figures 13.13). After one month and later up to two years, the intensity of the isotope accumulation in the operated kidney was normal (Figures 13.14,15).

The excretory urograms and x-ray cinematograms performed in the same period testified about the normal function of this kidney (Figures 15).

In the fifth (control) group of experiments, after only a right-side nephrectomy, all the radiologic and x-ray data of the sole intact left kidney were normal (Table 5, Figures 16.1-3, 7-9). Although, the adrenalin injection caused a temporary reduction of RI to 38.6±1.0; 43.8±2.9; 39.0±2.0, p<0.05, (Table 9, Figures 16.4-6).

3.2. Partial and Common Excretion Renal Functions

The results of investigations of partial functions of the operated kidney mainly coincide with the radiologic and x-ray functional data mentioned above.

In the first group within four months after the kidney denervation in situ its glomerular filtration was 62.6±3.2%; 60.7±2.5%; 66.6±5.6%; 45.3±4.5%; 64.0±6.2% of the corresponding function of the contralateral intact kidney. From six months its further reduction was observed (56.9±4.8; 38.3±8.2%), and after two years was 53.3±3.8% of the intact kidney, p<0.01, (Table 10).

The correlation of reabsorption function of the denervated and intact kidneys during the first four months fluctuated between 85.5±6.5%; 85.4±4.4%; later it decreased gradually and after two years reached 75.2±4.2% (p<0.001, Table 11).

The correlation of renal blood flow in operated and intact kidneys in the first four months changed from 75.4±3.8; 68.8±4.2%; 81.2±3.8% to 78.3±5.1%, after six months it began to reduce (62.2±3.8%; 59.9±4.6%) and after two years was 56.6±5.5% (p<0.001, Table 12).

The common excretion function of the denervated kidney after D. Murvanidze`s table, three days after the operation, reduced to 80.4±3.5% of the norm; in the following terms (to two months) slightly increased (84.5±2.7%; 85.1±4.7%), but further decreased again and for up to two years was 63.3±4.0% of the corresponding index of the intact kidney (p<0.001, Table 13).

By water-milk loading the above dynamics of the common excretory functions were kept on the whole, but the denervated kidney was far behind the intact one. So, 3 days after the operation the common excretory function of the denervated kidney was 72.2±5.2%, after two months it was 80.4±4.2%, and after two years it was 58.5±5.5% of the corresponding function of the intact kidney ($p<0.001$, Table 14).

Table 8. Denervation in situ and autotransplantation of the kidneys without and with surgical reinnervation: Correlation of the residual radioactivity in the intact (D) and operated (S) kidneys after adrenalin intravenous injection (%)

Kinds of operations			Terms of observations								
			Before the operation	3 days after	10 days	1 month	2 months	4 months	6 months	1 year	2 years
1st gr.	Denervation in situ	M±m D S n p	111,5±2,5 105,8±3,0 25 >0,05	108,2±5,0 128,5±3,0 3 <0,01	116,2±2,4 124,4±2,5 3 <0,05	114,3±3,1 120,6±5,0 4 >0,05	110,5±3,2 116,2±3,0 3 >0,05	118,2±3,8 124,2±4,1 3 >0,05	110,5±5,1 128,6±3,0 3 <0,05	108,4±7,0 130,3±4,8 3 <0,001	108,1±2,0 125,5±2,0 3 <0,001
2nd gr.	Denervation, reinnervation in situ	M±m D S n p	116,6±3,8 110,6±4,6 24 >0,05	116,3±4,2 126,4±3,0 3 <0,05	112,8±2,0 128,2±3,4 3 <0,01	110,7±3,0 130,8±4,7 3 <0,01	114,5±3,6 120,0±5,2 3 >0,05	110,5±2,0 116,6±4,0 3 >0,05	118,2±3,8 120,0±5,7 3 >0,05	105,5±5,0 110,4±3,2 3 >0,05	120,0±5,5 116,6±3,5 3 >0,05
3rd a gr.	Transplantation without reinnervation	M±m D S n p	114,5±2,5 115,0±3,5 25 >0,05	112,1±2,0 135,6±3,5 3 <0,01	116,2±4,2 130,3±3,0 3 <0,01	118,4±2,8 125,5±3,1 3 <0,05	114,4±4,4 130,0±4,6 4 <0,01	110,8±2,6 126,2±4,0 3 <0,01	112,4±3,6 124,8±4,0 3 <0,01	114,4±2,8 130,0±3,2 3 <0,01	110,2±2,7 128,5±3,6 3 <0,01
4th a gr.	Transplantation with reinnervation	M±m D S n p	112,2±3,5 110,3±3,5 25 >0,05	110,7±3,8 120,5±3,2 3 <0,01	118,2±4,6 130,5±5,0 3 <0,01	120,2±3,5 130,0±3,2 3 <0,01	110,0±3,0 122,2±2,4 4 <0,01	104,1±3,1 116,0±4,6 3 <0,01	106,6±3,7 110,0±3,6 3 >0,05	116,3±2,8 114,2±2,7 3 >0,05	110,5±2,7 112,3±3,9 3 >0,05

In the second group, in the first ten days after the denervation and surgical reinnervation, the filtration function of the kidney was reduced (60.0±5.4%; 70.7±3.8%, $p<0.001$). After one and two months it increased considerably (93.1±4.2; 91.6±6.8%, $p>0.05$) and beginning at four months reached the norm (100.2±8.1%, 103.8±8.8%; 93.8±4.5% of the contralateral kidney filtration ($p>0.05$, Table 15).

Reabsorption function within the first month was 84.2±4.2%; 85.4±6.3% of the intact kidney ($p<0.01$), after two months we observed its increase (96.3±4.2%, $p>0.05$) and beginning from month four it reached 98.5±3.8%; 97.1±3.2%; 99.0±5.5%; 98.6±4.6% of reabsorption function of the intact kidney ($p>0.05$, Table 11).

The renal blood flow within the first ten days decreased (80.2±5.2%; 78.9±3.6%) as compared with the intact kidney ($p<0.001$), but from two months and further it stabilized at the normal level (98.2±6.2%; 99.6±5.6%; 100.6±5.0%, $p>0.05$, Table 12).

The common excretion function within one month was reduced (82.2±3.0%; 88.1±3.9%, $p<0.01$), then it increased gradually, and after four months did not differ from the common excretion function of the intact kidney (Tables 13,14). The same dynamics were observed during water-milk functional loading.

Table 9. Denervation in situ and autotransplantation of the kidneys without and with surgical reinnervation: Changes of Hirakawa-Corcoran`s renographic index after adrenalin intravenous injection

Kinds of operations			Terms of observations								
			Before the operation	3 days after	10 days	1 month	2 months	4 months	6 months	1 year	2 years
1st gr.	Denervation in situ	M±m	45,6±2,5	8,4±2,5	9,3±5,0	15,5±4,8	20,4±6,0	16,3±3,8	18,8±3,0	6,6±3,5	10,1±2,9
		n	25	3	3	4	3	3	3	3	3
		p		<0,001	<0,001	<0,001	<0,001	<0,001	<0,001	<0,001	<0,001
2nd gr.	Denervation, reinnervation in situ	M±m	48,4±2,0	10,2±3,0	12,5±2,0	18,3±1,0	22,4±3,0	36,4±4,1	38,3±3,6	40,5±2,5	42,6±1,8
		n	24	3	3	3	3	3	3	3	3
		p		<0,001	<0,001	<0,001	<0,001	>0,05	>0,05	>0,05	>0,05
3rd a gr.	Transplantation without reinnervation	M±m	42,3±2,5	5,0±1,5	9,2±1,8	12,6±3,0	15,5±3,2	18,8±1,8	22,4±2,8	14,6±2,7	10,5±2,2
		n	25	3	3	3	4	3	3	3	3
		p		<0,001	<0,001	<0,001	<0,001	<0,001	<0,001	<0,001	<0,001
3rd b gr.	Transplantation without reinnervation, contralateral nephrectomy	M±m	41,5±0,8	10,8±1,6	22,6±1,5	24,5±1,0	23,7±2,2	28,7±2,4	24,5±2,5	20,8±1,8	25,8±2,2
		n	26	3	3	3	5	3	3	3	3
		p		<0,001	<0,001	<0,001	<0,001	<0,001	<0,001	<0,001	<0,001
4th a gr.	Transplantation with reinnervation	M±m	46,1±1,0	12,6±2,7	10,6±1,9	16,4±1,0	22,2±1,5	30,5±2,0	42,0±1,8	44,8±1,2	45,4±2,0
		n	25	3	3	3	4	3	3	3	3
		p		<0,001	<0,001	<0,001	<0,001	<0,01	>0,05	>0,05	>0,05
4th b gr.	Transplantation with reinnervation, contralateral nephrectomy	M±m	45,3±0,6	16,4±1,4	20,5±1,5	24,8±1,8	35,6±2,0	40,0±2,8	41,5±2,7	43,3±2,5	42,6±2,0
		n	25	3	3	4	3	3	3	3	3
		p		<0,001	<0,001	<0,001	<0,05	>0,05	>0,05	>0,05	>0,05
5th gr.	Right side nephrectomy	M±m	40,8±1,1	38,6±1,0	32,5±0,5	39,2±1,0	42,5±2,7	43,8±2,9	38,6±2,2	44,5±3,3	39,0±2,0
		n	25	3	3	4	3	3	3	3	3

Tabel 10. Denervation in situ and autotransplantation of the kidney without and with surgical reinnervation: Correlation of their and intact kidneys filtration function (%)

Kinds of operations			Terms of observations							
			2-4 days	8-10 days	1 month	2 months	4 months	6 months	1 year	2 years
1st gr.	Denervation in situ	M±m	62,6±3,2	60,7±2,5	66,6±5,6	45,3±4,5	64,0±6,2	56,9±4,8	38,3±8,2	53,3±3,8
		n	3	4	3	3	3	3	3	3
		p	<0,001	<0,001	<0,001	<0,001	<0,001	<0,001	<0,001	<0,001
2nd gr.	Denervation, reinnervation in situ	M±m	60,0±5,4	70,7±3,8	93,1±4,2	91,6±6,8	100,2±8,1	97,6±5,6	103,8±8,8	93,8±4,5
		n	3	3	4	3	3	3	3	3
		p	<0,001	<0,001	>0,05	<0,05	>0,05	>0,05	>0,05	>0,05
3rd a gr.	Transplantation without reinnervation	M±m	64,9±5,5	46,2±4,2	73,8±3,6	51,9±4,6	57,7±6,5	49,7±5,9	50,0±7,5	49,7±5,7
		n	3	4	3	3	3	3	3	3
		p	<0,001	<0,001	<0,001	<0,001	<0,001	<0,001	<0,001	<0,001
3rd b gr.	Transplantation without reinnervation, contralateral nephrectomy	M±m	54,3±5,7	63,5±4,8	44,5±4,6	63,9±3,6	48,8±5,8	44,2±6,0	43,4±5,7	35,9±3,2
		n	3	3	4	3	3	3	3	3
		p	<0,001	<0,001	<0,001	<0,001	<0,001	<0,001	<0,001	<0,001
4th a gr.	Transplantation with reinnervation	M±m	52,7±6,8	62,6±3,9	66,6±6,9	90,2±8,2	97,7±8,9	94,8±7,7	93,1±8,6	100,8±8,2
		n	3	4	3	3	3	3	3	3
		p	<0,001	<0,001	<0,001	<0,05	>0,05	>0,05	>0,05	>0,05
4th b gr.	Transplantation with reinnervation,	M±m	66,2±4,2	83,3±6,2	98,4±7,8	97,2±6,2	94,1±8,5	94,5±6,8	101,2±7,5	94,3±5,9
		n	3	3	3	4	3	3	3	3
		p	<0,001	<0,01	>0,05	>0,05	>0,05	>0,05	>0,05	>0,05

	contralateral nephrectomy									
5th gr.	Right side nephrectomy	M±m n p	100 3	100 3	100 3	100 3	100 3	100 3	100 3	100 3

Table 11. Denervation in situ and autotransplantation of the kidney without and with surgical reinnervation: Correlation of their and intact kidneys reabsorption function (%)

Kinds of operations			Terms of observations							
			2-4 days	8-10 days	1 month	2 months	4 months	6 months	1 year	2 years
1st gr.	Denervation in situ	M±m n p	85,5±6,5 3 <0,001	68,2±6,8 4 <0,001	80,5±4,3 3 <0,001	69,6±5,2 3 <0,001	85,4±4,4 3 <0,01	80,1±7,6 3 <0,001	78,2±4,2 3 <0,001	75,2±4,2 3 <0,001
2nd gr.	Denervation, reinnervation in situ	M±m n p	84,2±4,2 3 <0,01	80,1±5,6 3 <0,001	85,4±6,3 4 <0,01	96,3±4,2 3 >0,05	98,5±3,8 3 >0,05	97,1±3,2 3 >0,05	99,0±5,5 3 >0,05	98,6±4,6 3 >0,05
3rd a gr.	Transplantation without reinnervation	M±m n p	80,3±5,1 3 <0,001	75,1±4,8 4 <0,001	85,0±5,3 3 <0,01	80,3±6,3 3 <0,001	76,6±4,0 3 <0,001	69,5±5,3 3 <0,001	70,8±3,6 3 <0,001	72,4±4,8 3 <0,001
3rd b gr.	Transplantation without reinnervation, contralateral nephrectomy	M±m n p	75,4±5,8 3 <0,001	80,5±4,6 3 <0,001	90,1±4,6 4 <0,05	91,4±3,7 3 <0,05	89,1±3,7 3 <0,05	92,2±3,9 3 <0,05	81,8±4,0 3 <0,001	76,6±3,0 3 <0,001
4th a gr.	Transplantation with reinnervation	M±m n p	82,2±4,0 3 <0,001	86,4±3,9 4 <0,01	89,1±4,1 3 <0,01	90,8±3,0 3 <0,05	94,6±4,1 3 >0,05	98,7±3,1 3 >0,05	99,0±3,6 3 >0,05	99,1±3,4 3 >0,05
4th b gr.	Transplantation with reinnervation, contralateral nephrectomy	M±m n p	86,4±3,9 3 <0,01	89,6±3,9 3 <0,01	92,1±2,4 3 <0,05	97,6±3,2 4 >0,05	99,0±4,0 3 >0,05	98,2±3,9 3 >0,05	99,1±4,4 3 >0,05	99,2±5,5 3 >0,05
5th gr.	Right side nephrectomy	 n	100 3	100 3	100 3	100 3	100 3	100 3	100 3	100 3

In the third group ("a" subgroup) within four months of the autotransplantation of the kidney in the iliac fossa without surgical reinnervation its glomerular filtration was considerably depressed (64.9±5.5%; 57.7±6.5%), from six months up to two years its further decrease was observed (49.7±5.9%; 49.7±5.7% of the filtration of the intact kidney, $p<0.001$, Table 10).

The same dynamics were observed in connection with the reabsorption function, within the first two months there was a moderate decrease (80.3±5.1%; 85.0±5.3%) then, up to two years later, a more expressed reduction of reabsorption as compared with the intact kidney (76.6±4.0%; 72.4±4.8%, $p<0.001$, Table 11).

The blood flow of the denervated kidney was also decreased and after two years became 59.8±5.9% of the intact kidney blood flow ($p<0.001$, Table 12).

The common excretion function of the denervated kidney within four months was moderately decreased by normal conditions as well as by functional loading (82.2±3.2%); it decreased further after six months (70.2±4.1%) and by two years became 60.5±5.7% of the intact kidney function ($p<0.001$, Tables 13, 14).

In the "b" subgroup of this third group the same dynamics of partial function changes was observed as in the "a" subgroup. By two years, the glomerular filtration, reabsorption and blood flow of the autotransplanted (without reinnervation) sole kidney was 35.9±3.2%,

76.6±3.0% and 60.6±5.9% of the corresponding indices of the sole intact kidney (p<0.001, Tables 10-12).

Table 12. Denervation in situ and autotransplantation of the kidney without and with surgical reinnervation: Correlation of their and intact kidneys blood flow (%)

Kinds of operations			Terms of observations							
			2-4 days	8-10 days	1 month	2 months	4 months	6 months	1 year	2 years
1st gr.	Denervation in situ	M±m	75,4±3,8	68,8±4,2	70,3±5,2	81,2±3,8	78,3±5,1	62,2±3,8	59,9±4,6	56,6±5,5
		n	3	4	3	3	3	3	3	3
		p	<0,001	<0,001	<0,001	<0,01	<0,001	<0,001	<0,001	<0,001
2nd gr.	Denervation, reinnervation in situ	M±m	80,2±5,2	78,9±3,6	87,3±5,1	98,2±6,2	98,2±5,5	99,6±5,6	99,1±4,0	100,6±5,0
		n	3	3	4	3	3	3	3	3
		p	<0,01	<0,001	<0,05	>0,05	>0,05	>0,05	>0,05	>0,05
3rd a gr.	Transplantation without reinnervation	M±m	70,2±4,5	69,5±5,7	65,2±4,8	70,1±4,8	62,1±3,6	67,2±4,8	60,2±5,8	59,8±5,9
		n	3	4	3	3	3	3	3	3
		p	<0,001	<0,001	<0,001	<0,001	<0,001	<0,001	<0,001	<0,001
3rd b gr.	Transplantation without reinnervation, contralateral nephrectomy	M±m	50,8±3,6	70,5±4,2	76,2±5,8	82,5±4,4	79,8±6,1	85,7±4,2	62,8±4,8	60,6±5,9
		n	3	3	4	3	3	3	3	3
		p	<0,001	<0,001	<0,001	<0,01	<0,01	<0,05	<0,001	<0,001
4th a gr.	Transplantation with reinnervation	M±m	79,2±5,5	80,6±3,9	82,8±5,2	95,8±4,2	98,6±3,1	100,4±5,3	97,9±4,6	99,2±4,8
		n	3	4	3	3	3	3	3	3
		p	<0,01	<0,01	<0,01	>0,05	>0,05	>0,05	>0,05	>0,05
4th b gr.	Transplantation with reinnervation, contralateral nephrectomy	M±m	68,9±5,0	82,8±6,2	98,2±4,6	99,0±5,0	97,8±4,2	102,3±4,5	98,8±5,1	99,5±5,0
		n	3	3	3	4	3	3	3	3
		p	<0,001	<0,01	>0,05	>0,05	>0,05	>0,05	>0,1	
5th gr.	Right side nephrectomy		100	100	100	100	100	100	100	100
		n	3	3	3	3	3	3	3	3

Table 13. Denervation in situ and autotransplantation of the kidney without and with surgical reinnervation: Correlation of their and intact kidney common excretion function (after D. Murvanidze) (%)

Kinds of operations			Terms of observations							
			2-4 days	8-10 days	1 month	2 months	4 months	6 months	1 year	2 years
1st gr.	Denervation in situ	M±m	80,4±3,5	84,5±2,7	86,3±4,9	85,1±4,7	76,5±3,5	72,4±4,4	64,5±5,2	63,3±4,0
		n	3	4	3	3	3	3	3	3
		p	<0,01	<0,01	<0,01	<0,01	<0,001	<0,001	<0,001	<0,001
2nd gr.	Denervation, reinnervation in situ	M±m	82,2±3,0	85,4±4,5	88,1±3,9	92,0±3,6	98,3±3,8	96,4±4,2	100,0±5,0	98,2±5,5
		n	3	3	4	3	3	3	3	3
		p	<0,01	<0,01	<0,01	<0,05	>0,05	>0,05	>0,05	>0,05
3rd a gr.	Transplantation without reinnervation	M±m	76,4±2,4	80,3±2,7	84,5±3,6	86,1±2,5	82,2±3,2	70,2±4,1	66,3±5,3	60,5±5,7
		n	3	4	3	3	3	3	3	3
		p	<0,001	<0,01	<0,01	<0,01	<0,01	<0,001	<0,001	<0,001
3rd b gr.	Transplantation without reinnervation, contralateral nephrectomy	M±m	80,6±3,9	83,4±4,0	86,5±4,1	92,8±3,4	94,8±3,7	90,1±3,6	83,0±2,9	75,5±3,0
		n	3	3	4	3	3	3	3	3
		p	<0,01	<0,01	<0,01	<0,05	>0,05	<0,05	<0,01	<0,001
4th a gr.	Transplantation with reinnervation	M±m	78,3±3,9	84,2±2,7	86,1±3,8	85,5±4,1	92,4±4,1	96,1±5,0	98,3±4,9	100,0±5,5
		n	3	4	3	3	3	3	3	3
		p	<0,001	<0,01	<0,01	<0,01	<0,05	>0,05	>0,05	>0,05

4th b gr.	Transplantation with reinnervation, contralateral nephrectomy	M±m n p	82,2±4,6 3 <0,01	82,1±3,2 3 <0,01	90,3±3,0 3 <0,05	96,5±4,9 4 >0,05	98,1±4,5 3 >0,05	100,0±4,5 3 >0,05	98,1±3,2 3 >0,05	98,1±5,6 3 >0,05
5th gr.	Right side nephrectomy	 n	100 3	100 3	100 3	100 3	100 3	100 3	100 3	100 3

The common excretion function of the sole autotransplanted kidney by this term was behind the function of the sole intact kidney by a marked degree (75.5±3.0%), especially by functional loading (70.7±3.4, p<0.001, Tables 13, 14).

In the fourth group ("a" subgroup), within nearly one month after the autotransplantation and surgical reinnervation of the kidney, its glomerular filtration, reabsorption and blood flow were lower as compared with the intact kidney (66.6±6.9%; 89.1±4.1% and 82.8±5.2%, respectively, p<0.01), but over time (after four months) these indices were normalized completely (Tables 10-12).

The common excretion function slightly decreased in the first four months (85.5±4.1%, 92.4±4.1%), and after six months it also became normal, including by functional loading (Tables 13, 14).

In the "b" subgroup of the fourth group a more short-term (within one month) decrease of glomerular filtration, blood flow and reabsorption of the autotransplanted sole kidney was observed (83.3±6.2%; 82.8±6.2%; 86.4±3.9%, respectively, as compared with the sole intact kidney (p<0.001). After two months they were fully normalized (Tables 10-12).

By two months the common excretion function of the autotransplanted reinnervated sole kidney also became normal, by normal conditions as well as by functional (water-milk) loading (Tables 13, 14).

3.3. Discussion of Results of Kidney Functional Investigations

The dynamics of radiorenographic data of denervated and autotransplanted kidneys in conditions of spontaneous and surgical reinnervation permits the following types of renogram to be revealed: 1) two-phase renogram with ascendant excretion segment (obturative type) (Figures 17.1-5); 2) three-phase renogram with a clear differentiation of each of them but the sharp decrease of amplitudes of vascular and secretion segments and prolongation of the excretion phase; 3) three-phase renogram with a normal level of vascular but decreased level of secretion segments and prolonged excretion phase; 4) three-phase renogram with normal indices of vascular and secretion function by amplitude and time and extension of the isopote semi-excretion period; 5) normal renogram with usual characteristics of segments after the amplitude and time.

In renoscintigrams the following types were observed: 1) rare touches with reduced dimentions of kidney functioning parenchyma; 2) the uniform rare touches with normal dimensions of kidney functioning parenchyma; 3) the normal scintigram with usual dimensions of kidney and frequent touches (Figures 17.6-8).

The first type of renogram was observed in the initial days in all groups except the "b" subgroup of the fifth group as well as in the "a" subgroup of the third group in the remote terms (one and two years) after the operation.

Table 14. Denervation in situ and autotransplantation of the kidney without and with surgical reinnervation: Correlation of their and intact kidney common excretion function (after D. Murvanidze) by the water-milk loading

Kinds of operations			Terms of observations							
			2-4 days	8-10 days	1 month	2 months	4 months	6 months	1 year	2 years
1st gr.	Denervation in situ	M±m n p	72,2±5,2 3 <0,001	76,3±4,8 4 <0,001	76,2±3,6 3 <0,001	80,4±4,2 3 <0,01	74,5±5,3 3 <0,001	70,1±4,0 3 <0,001	60,0±3,6 3 <0,001	58,5±5,5 3 <0,001
2nd gr.	Denervation, reinnervation in situ	M±m n p	76,3±3,6 3 <0,001	78,1±4,1 3 <0,001	80,0±4,0 4 <0,01	86,1±3,6 3 <0,05	96,6±3,7 3 >0,05	98,6±4,1 3 >0,05	100,0±9,0 3 >0,05	99,0±5,5 3 >0,05
3rd a gr.	Transplantation without reinnervation	M±m n p	75,5±4,7 3 <0,001	77,2±3,7 4 <0,001	78,3±3,6 3 <0,001	80,1±4,2 3 <0,01	72,2±4,6 3 <0,001	65,5±3,8 3 <0,001	60,2±4,9 3 <0,001	56,2±5,8 3 <0,001
3rd b gr.	Transplantation without reinnervation, contralateral nephrectomy	M±m n p	80,1±3,5 3 <0,01	82,3±4,8 3 <0,01	84,4±4,7 4 <0,01	90,5±3,9 3 <0,05	91,3±4,4 3 <0,05	90,4±3,5 3 <0,05	80,2±3,2 3 <0,01	70,7±3,4 3 <0,001
4th a gr.	Transplantation with reinnervation	M±m n p	74,5±3,8 3 <0,001	78,6±3,6 4 <0,001	77,3±4,1 3 <0,001	85,4±3,2 3 <0,01	93,3±3,8 3 <0,05	96,7±4,4 3 >0,05	98,8±3,9 3 >0,05	98,3±4,0 3 >0,05
4th b gr.	Transplantation with reinnervation, contralateral nephrectomy	M±m n p	82,3±3,4 3 <0,01	83,4±2,9 3 <0,01	88,3±9,2 3 <0,05	95,2±3,0 4 >0,05	98,1±3,4 3 >0,05	96,6±3,7 3 >0,05	97,5±4,0 3 >0,05	98,2±4,9 3 >0,05
5th gr.	Right side nephrectomy	 n	100 3	100 3	100 3	100 3	100 3	100 3	100 3	100 3

Table 15. Denervation in situ and autotransplantation of the kidney without and with surgical reinnervation: Correlation of their and intact kidneys' mass

Kinds of operations			Terms of observations							
			3 days	10 days	1 month	2 months	4 months	6 months	1 year	2 years
1st gr.	Denervation in situ	M±m n p	115,2±2,1 3 <0,01	113,1±1, 9 3 <0,01	114,3±2, 0 4 <0,01	106,1±1, 3 3 >0,05	92,4±1,6 3 <0,05	88,5±2,2 3 <0,01	72,0±2,1 3 <0,001	63,1±3,0 3 <0,001
2nd gr.	Denervation, reinnervation in situ	M±m n p	114,8±2,2 3 <0,01	116,0±1, 2 3 <0,01	106,1±1, 8 3 >0,05	105,4±1, 0 3 >0,05	103,3±1, 1 3 >0,05	98,0±2,0 3 >0,05	101,1±1, 9 3 >0,05	99,6±0,8 3 >0,05
3rd a gr.	Transplantatin without reinnervation	M±m n p	152,9±3,5 3 <0,001	143,4±4, 2 3 <0,001	130,3±3, 6 3 <0,001	108,4±3, 1 4 <0,05	98,1±1,1 3 >0,05	89,3±1,0 3 <0,01	71,3±1,8 3 <0,001	61,0±2,2 3 <0,001
3rd b gr.	Transplantation without reinnervation, contralateral nephrectomy	M±m n p	155,7±3,8 3 <0,001	148,0±2, 9 3 <0,001	130,4±2, 1 3 <0,001	118,3±2, 0 5 <0,001	116,0±2, 7 3 <0,01	110,1±1, 8 3 <0,01	108,0±0, 9 3 <0,05	104,4±2,0 3 >0,05
4th a gr.	Transplantation with reinnervation	M±m n p	148,8±4,2 3 <0,001	131,5±4, 0 3 <0,001	112,6±3, 1 3 <0,01	108,4±2, 1 4 <0,05	104,0±2, 0 3 >0,05	103,1±1, 1 3 >0,05	99,2±0,8 3 >0,05	101,8±0,9 3 >0,05
4th b	Transplantation	M±m	153,5±4,9	144,9±5,	125,0±3,	116,5±2,	108,8±1,	103,8±1,	104,6±1,	102,1±0,6

gr.	with reinnervation, contralateral nephrectomy	n p	3 <0,001	0 3 <0,001	9 4 <0,001	2 3 <0,01	9 3 <0,05	2 3 >0,05	0 3 >0,05	3 >0,05
5th gr.	Right side nephrectomy	 m	100 3	100 3	100 4	100 3	100 3	100 3	100 3	100 3

The first type of renal scintigram was observed in the same groups and subgroups as mentioned above. This fact testified about the common decrease of the isotope accumulation ability rather than about the local disorders in the kidney tissues. This form showed the most profound functional damage of kidneys in these groups.

The second type of renogram with a decrease of amplitudes of vascular and secretion segments and lengthening of the excretion phase testified to the considerable depression of all functions of the kidney, especially intra-renal blood circulation. But the clear differentiation of all segments in the renograms could be considered signs of the beginning of functional recovery of the kidney. This type of renogram was observed in all groups except for the fifth. In the first and third groups, after denervation and autotransplantation of the kidney without surgical reinnervation, this type of renogram had taken place in the later terms (after one and two months), and in the second and fourth groups after surgical reinnervation of the denervated and autotransplanted kidneys (ten days and one month, respectively). This type of renogram chronologically corresponded to the second type of renal scintigrams with a rare distribution of touches but normal dimensions of kidney parenchyma.

In the third type of renogram with a normal amplitude of vascular segment, the level of secretion segment and the prolonged phase of excretion decreased, providing interesting material for the interpretation of the research pathology and the dynamics of renal function recovery, as they showed an asynchronous normalization of the separate renogram segments. Since the mentioned renograms included a normal amplitude vascular segment, it can be concluded that after the operation the renal blood circulation recovered.

In the second and fourth groups, where was a surgical reinnervation of the denervated and autotransplanted kidneys, and the vascular segment of the renogram normalized within one and two months.

In the first and third groups after the denervation and autotransplantation of the kidney, the amplitude of the renogram vascular segment was firmly decreased and after four months had the worst renal blood circulation.

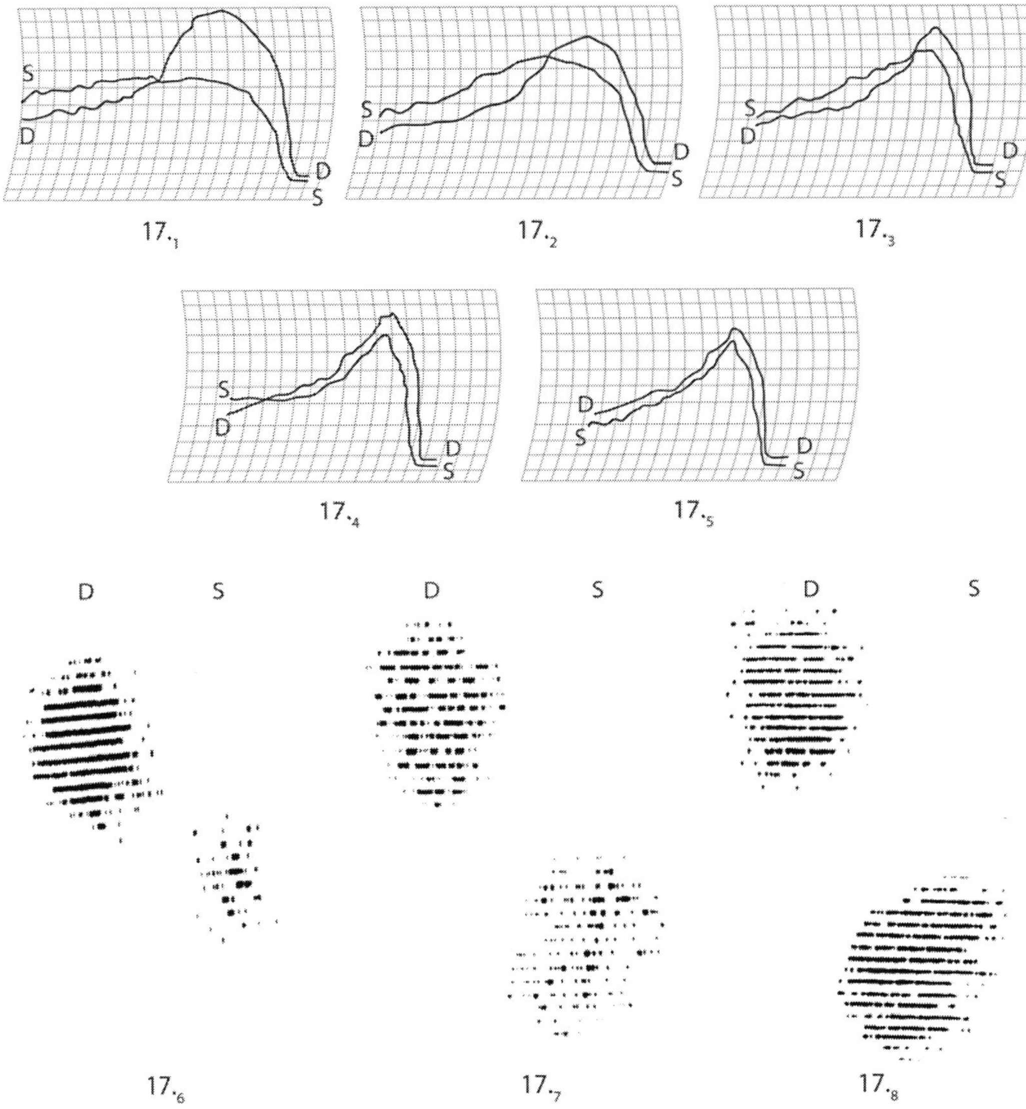

Figure 17. Types of radiorenograms and renoscintigrams after the kidney decentralization and reinnervation.
Radiorenograms: $17._1$ – 1st type; $17._2$ – 2nd type; $17._3$ – 3rd type; $17._4$ – 4th type; $17._5$ – 5th type.
Renoscintigrams: $17._6$ – 1st type; $17._7$ – 2nd type; $17._8$ – 3rd type.

The third type of renogram corresponded to the second type of scintigram with a rare distribution of touches and normal dimensions of the functioning kidney parenchyma. But it has to be mentioned that in spite of the coincidence of their common results the radiorenographic method was more sensitive than the scintigraphic.

The fourth type of renogram with normal amplitudes of vascular and secretion segments and a slightly prolonged period of semi-excretion testified to another stage of kidney functional normalization. This type of renogram had taken place in the second, and the "a" and "b" subgroups of the fourth group of experiments which were accompanied with a surgical reinnervation of the denervated and autotransplanted kidneys. Such a form of renogram was observed two, four months and one month after the operation, respectively.

The fourth type of renogram corresponded to the normal scintigrams with normal kidney dimensions and frequent disposition of touches. But as was mentioned before, the renograms gave more differentiated evaluation of kidney function than scintigrams.

Finally, the normal types of renograms and scintigrams testified to the completion of regenerative processes in the kidney and normalization of its functional state. Such radiologic data was observed in the second group, and the "a" and "b" subgroups of the fourth group of experiments four, six and two months after the operation, respectively.

In the rest (first, third) of the groups, except for the fifth (control) group of experiments, full normalization of radiologic data didn`t occur.

The functional depression of non reinnervated kidneys in these groups was confirmed by excretion urography and x-ray cinematography, which showed a more prolonged and slack excretion of the contrast medium, moderate dilatation of upper urinary ways and delay of peristaltic.

In the second and fourth groups of experiments with surgical reinnervation of the kidney within the first one to two months after the operation, we also observed the same functional disorders, but they were temporary and less expressed than in the first and third groups and were finished with full functional recovery of the kidney. Therefore these are all reasons to explain such dynamics with a beneficial influence of the surgical reinnervation.

It has to be taken into account that there is an asynchronous character of the renal functional normalization. In the first stage, the renal blood circulation and filtration ability were recovered (in the second group after one month and in "a" subgroup of the fourth group after two months), then the secretion and reabsorption functions (after two and four months, respectively) and finally, the excretion, evacuation function (after four and six months, respectively). Thanks to this dynamic a certain successiveness in the regeneration processes in the kidney can be concluded. At first the sewed nerve fibers evidently germinated along the kidney's former main nervous trunks but didn`t reach the direct functional terminals in the kidney and therefore could not exert a corresponding regulative and trophic influence on the kidney. This circumstance determined the functional depression of the kidney within the first one–two months after the operation. Later a branching of germinating nervous fibers up to the renal functional terminals occurred, which was accompanied by a recovery of renal function on the corresponding levels: initially the blood circulation and filtration were normalized, then secretion and reabsorption and finally the excretion and evacuation ability of the kidney.

The function of a sole autotransplanted reinnervated kidney was normalized in the same successiveness as by the preserved contralateral kidney, but in shorter terms. Thus, the full normalization of indices occurred within two months of the operation.

It has to be mentioned that in the "b" subgroup of the third group in which the sole autotransplanted kidney was not reinnervated, after two months its functional condition improved considerably and some indices (RI, scintigrams) approached the lower norm. Such condition went on within six months.

The comparison of the sole autotransplanted reinnervated and nonreinnervated kidneys permits one to conclude that the acceleration of the functional recovery of the reinnervated organ occurred, on the one hand, thanks to a common compensative hypertrophy of the sole kidney and, on the other hand, at the expense of an intensification of neuroregenerative processes in it. Surgical reinnervation explains the fact that in both near and remote terms, the reinnervated sole autotransplanted kidney was ahead of the sole autotransplanted nonreinnervated kidney in functional indices.

The compensative hypertrophy promoted the mobilization of reserve abilities of the sole autotransplanted nonreinnervated kidney to a certain degree, but it could not ensure a stable and full value condition of this kidney by various functional loadings; after six months exhaustion and further increase of lagging of this kidney were observed as compared with the sole autotransplanted reinnervated or the sole intact kidneys.

In this respect the investigation of the renal common excretion ability (by D. Murvanidze, 262) was very significant both under normal conditions and especially by water-milk functional loading. The distinct lagging was revealed in the period between two and six months after the operation when the other (radiologic) data of the sole autotransplanted nonreinnervated kidney were on a subnormal level.

The trials with duplication of radiorenography on the background of adrenalin injection also have to be taken into consideration. It is known [84,98,204,316,425] that denervated structures show increased sensitivity to the corresponding nervous mediators (the kidney mainly to adreanlin). Therefore, this test can be considered a significant provoking factor for the evaluation of the neuroregeneration degree in the operated kidney.

In our experiments the adrenalin injection, even in the norm, caused a decrease in basic functions of an intact kidney such as the amplitude of the vascular segment to 84%, secretion to 80%, residual radioactivity to 115%, and RI to 40.

After the operation the mentioned deviations were expressed more significantly: the amplitude of the vascular segment decreased to 40-47%, secretion to 52-65%, residual radioactivity increased to 120-135%, and RI reduced to 5–16.

Thus, the difference between the indices of the operated and intact kidneys on the basis of the adrenalin injection was 20-30%.

In the following observations the dynamics of alterations of renographic indices after the adrenalin injection in various groups was unequal.

In the first group after the kidney denervation and the "a" subgroup of the third group after autotransplantation without surgical reinnervation, the difference between the indices of the operated and intact kidneys in ranges of 20–30% was maintained over two years.

In contrast, in the second group after kidney denervation and the "a" subgroup of the fourth group after its autotransplantation and surgical reinnervation, the difference between the indices of the operated and intact kidneys in trials with adrenalin injection continued for a shorter period: the amplitudes of vascular segments of renograms became even over one to two months; of secretion segments over two to four months; and the excretion phase and RI over four to six months, respectively.

The adrenalin-test permitted us to reveal and deepen the lag of the denervated kidney, not only by the existent intact kidney when the functional asymmetry between the kidneys was distinctly expressed even without adrenalin injection, but also in the case of the sole autotransplanted nonreinnervated kidney, when during a certain period (between two and six months) the renographic indices without adrenalin injection fluctuated on subnormal levels because of compensative hypertrophy. These data testify convincingly that even in that relatively propitious period, the existent nervous apparatus of this kidney could not prevent the sensitivity to adrenalin, the organ worked on the extreme level of its reserve opportunities, which to a marked degree were exhausted after six months.

At the same time the autotransplanted and surgically reinnervated sole kidney, after two months, showed a steady normal functional level, both by ordinary radiorenography as well as with adrenalin injection, and this functional level didn`t differ from corresponding data of the sole intact kidney.

In our opinion, the mentioned results convincingly testify to the imperfection of spontaneous reinnervation of denervated and autotransplanted kidneys. In comparison, the method of surgical reinnervation used was able to ensure complex regulation of the kidney by highly differentiated functional loadings and favorable trophic influence on the kidney, which resulted, on the whole, in practically normal and stable work of the organ for a long period.

Chapter IV

Biopotentials of Nerves of Denervated and Autotransplanted Kidneys in Conditions of Spontaneous and Surgical Reinnervation

4.1. Results of Investigation of Biopotentials of the Renal Nerve

Under normal conditions the efferent impulsation of the renal nerve was represented by irregular impulses with an amplitude of 20-25 mcV, frequency of 3-5 Imp/sec and duration of each impulse of 1–2 sec (Figure 18). After intravenous injection of adrenalin in a concentration of 1:50,000 with a velocity 4 ml/sec, within 3–4 minutes a disappearance of afferent impulsation for 7–10 minutes was observed (Figure 19). After that the impulsation recovered to the initial level.

After intravenous injection of acethylcholine in the same concentration, with the velocity and duration mentioned above, the afferent impulsation became more frequent (80-90 Imp/sec) with amplitudes of 35-40 McV. Such a state was maintained for 3-4 minutes. Then the impulsation returned to the initial level (Figure 20).

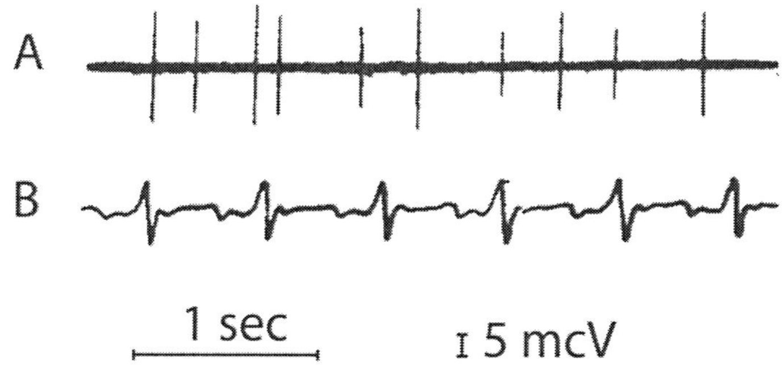

Figure 18. A-background spontaneous impulsation of the kidney nerve in the norm. B-electrocardiogram.

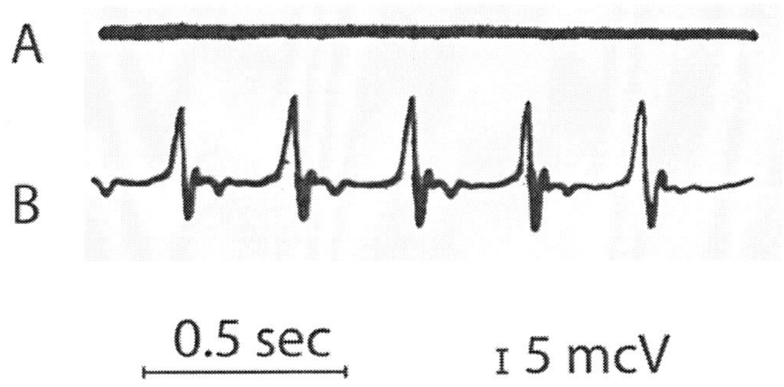

Figure 19. A-disappearance of a spontaneous impulsation of the kidney nerve after the intravenous injection of adrenalin (in the norm). B-electrocardiogram.

The increase of intrapyelon pressure by retrograde injection of water through the ureter (to 200 mm Hg pole) for 2–3 minutes also caused an increase of impulsation frequency to 90-100/sec and amplitudes of 40-42 mcV (Figure 21).

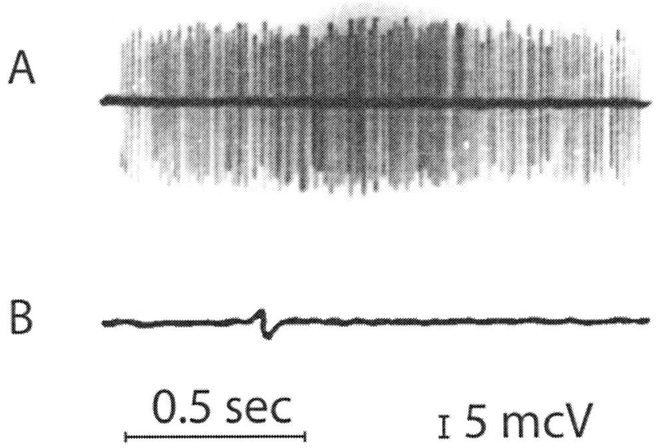

Figure 20. A-increase of the frequency of a spontaneous impulsation of the renal nerve after the intravenous injection of acetylcholine (in the norm). B-electrocardiogram.

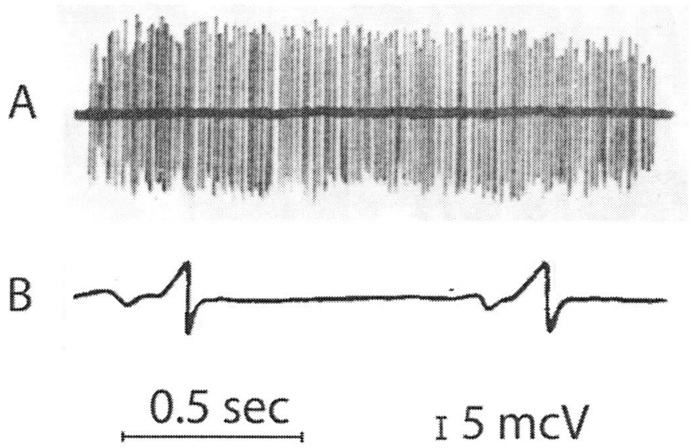

Figure 21. A-increase of the frequency of a spontaneous impulsation in answer to rising of the intrapyelon pressure (in the norm). B-electrocardiogram.

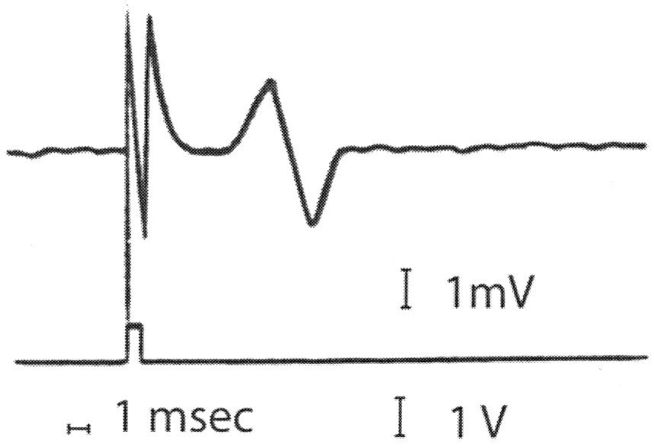

Figure 22. Threshold excitement of the renal nerve (in the norm).

By the electric irritation of the renal nerve during 0.1 m/sec the threshold of excitability fluctuated between 0.8–1.1 V, the amplitude of nerve potential was 3.2 mV (Figure 22), the time of chronaxy was 2–3 m/sec, by the increase of electric irritation the maximum nerve potential was 6.5 mV (Figure 23), and the velocity of conduction of the nerve impulse was 5 m/sec.

In the first group of experiments, three days after the kidney denervation, the impulsation from the remaining distal part of the renal nerve as in the form of a spontaneous reaction, as well as when acethylcholin injection was absent. The reactions of the renal nerve to electric irritation were also depressed. So, the threshold of excitability was 5.2 B, the amplitude of potential was 1.3 mv (Figure 25), time of chronaxy was 9.8 m/sec, maximum nerve potential was 1.5 mv and the velocity of conduction of impulse was 2.2 m/sec.

In the period from ten days to one month after the operation, neither spontaneous nor artificially stimulated impulsation was observed, it was a period of full bioelectric silence.

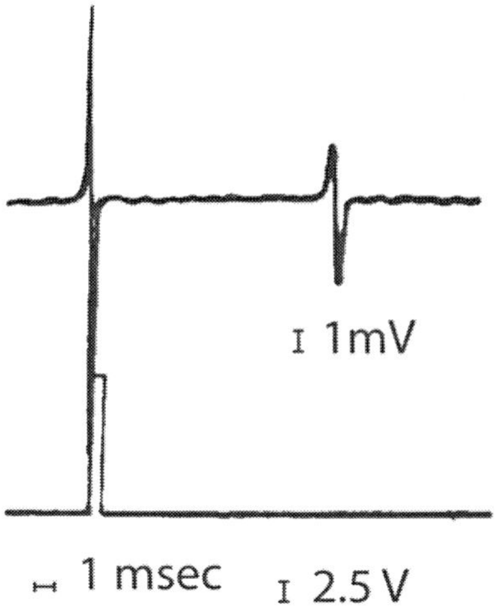

Figure 23. Increase of the renal nerve total potential amplitude by increase of its exlectric irritation (in the norm)

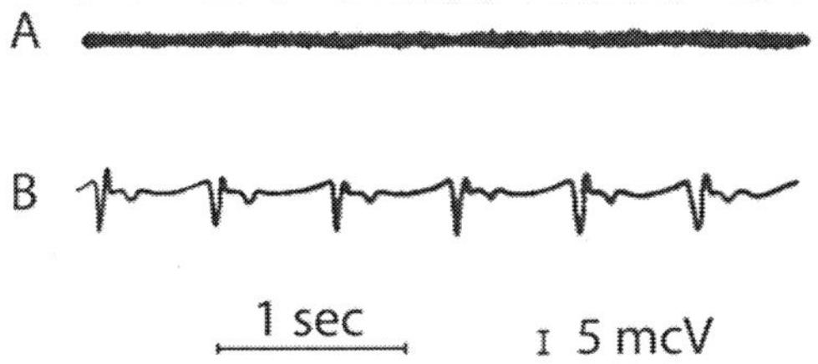

Figure 24. 3 days after the kidney denervation without surgical reinnervation.
A-spontaneous impulsation from the rest of the renal nerve is absent.
B-electrocardiogram.

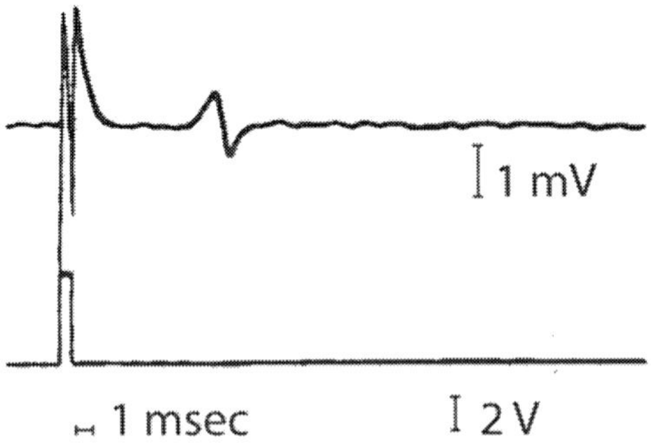

Figure 25. The same case. A threshold excitement from the rest of the renal nerve.

Two months after the operation, the impulsation of the renal nerve was not revealed as before, neither as a background nor in response to the acethylcholine injection nor to an increase of intrapyelon pressure. The irritation of the renal nerve by electrostimulator at 9.8 V caused a potential with an amplitude of 1.1 mV (Figure 26), but further increase of electric irritation didn`t lead to an increase of nerve potential. Time of chronaxy was 13.6 m/sec and the velocity of conduction of the nerve impulse was 1.8 m/sec.

Four months after the operation the state was the same on the whole. Only a slight increase of the maximum potential (1.3 mV) as compared with threshold irritation (1.0 mV) was observed.

Six months after the operation the spontaneous impulsation of the renal nerve was still not revealed. The threshold electric irritation of 7.8 V caused a potential with an amplitude of 1.2 mV, the irritation of 25 V caused a maximum potential of 1.8 mV. Time of chronaxy was slightly shortened (10.5 m/sec) and the velocity of conduction of nerve impulse increased to 2.2 m/sec.

One to two years after the operation, the spontaneous impulsation from the renal nerve was not observed, as before. The threshold electric irritation of 5.3 V caused a potential with an amplitude of 0.8 mV (Figure 27). The maximum potential of 1.3 mV could be stimulated by irritation of 21 V (Figure 28). The time of chronaxy and velocity of nerve impulse conduction did not changed compared to the previous term (10.4 m/sec and 2.4 m/sec, respectively).

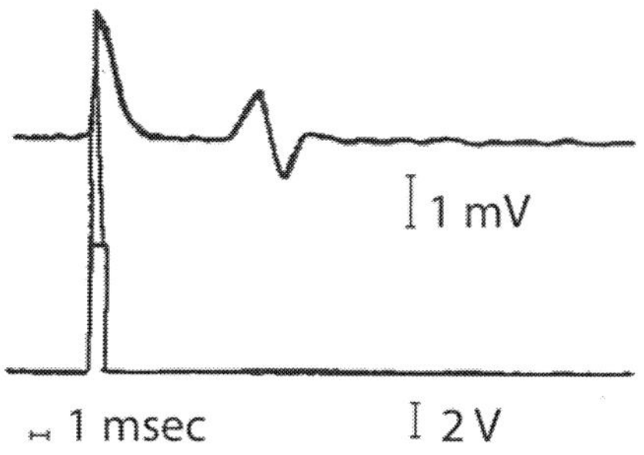

Figure 26. 2 months after the kidney denervation without surgical reinnervation. A threshold excitement from the rest of the renal nerve.

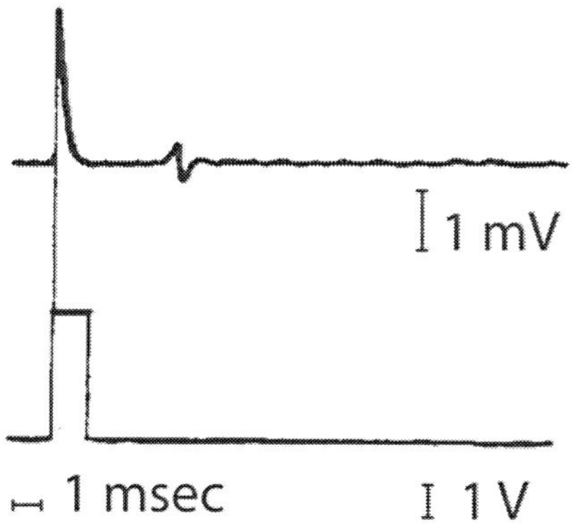

Figure 27. 2 years after the kidney denervation without surgical reinnervation.
A threshold excitement from the rest of the renal nerve.

In the second test-group, within the first month after denervation and surgical reinnervation of the kidney, the bioelectric activity of the renal nerve (distal segment) was identical with the same period of the previous group.

Two months later, spontaneous impulsation did not appear. The threshold irritation of 5.2 V caused a potential with an amplitude of 1.9 mV (Figure 29). Further increase of stimulation to 30 V led to an increase of the maximum potential to 3.2 mV. The time of chronaxy became 11.2 m/sec, and the velocity of impulse conduction increased to 3.5 m/sec.

Four months after the operation, the spontaneous impulsation from the distal part of renal nerve appeared and was represented with irregular lines with a frequency of 1.5 Hertz and an amplitude of 15 mcV (Figure 30). Intravenous adrenalin injection led to the disappearance of this spontaneous impulsation. The injection of acethylcholine, as well as the increase of intrapelvic pressure, caused an increase of the frequency of oscillation to 27.0 Hertz with an amplitude of 20 mcV (Figure 31). The threshold of excitability decreased to 3.3 V with the amplitude of potential of 2.2 mV. The maximum potential of 3.5 V was stimulated by electric irritation of 20 V. The time of chronaxy and the velocity of nerve impulse conduction became 6.5 m/sec and 3.8 m/sec, respectively.

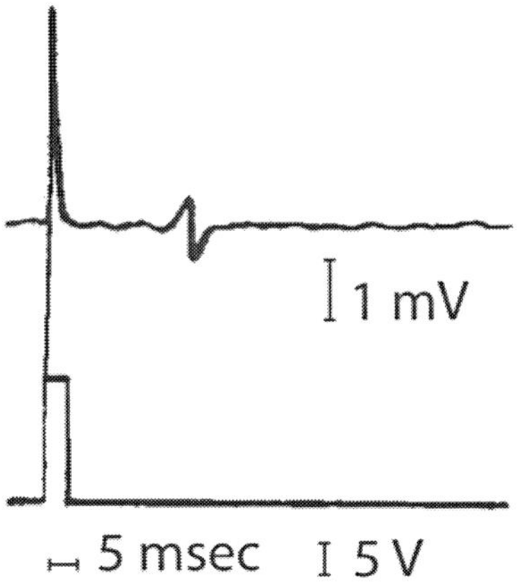

Figure 28. The same case. The increase of electric irritation causes an insignificant increase of the total potential of the renal nerve rest.

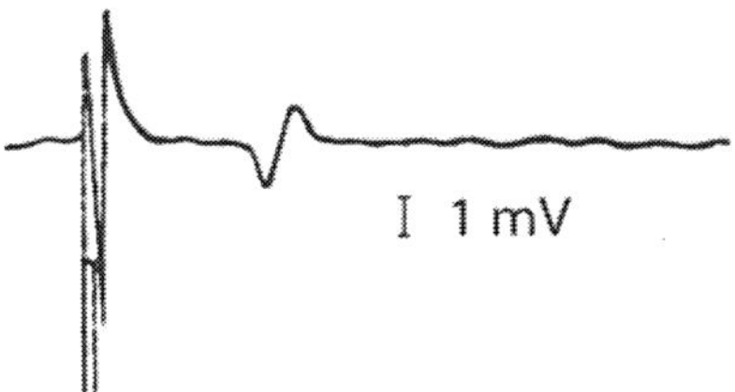

Figure 29. 2 months after the denervation and surgical reinnervation of the kidney. The threshold excitement of the renal nerve.

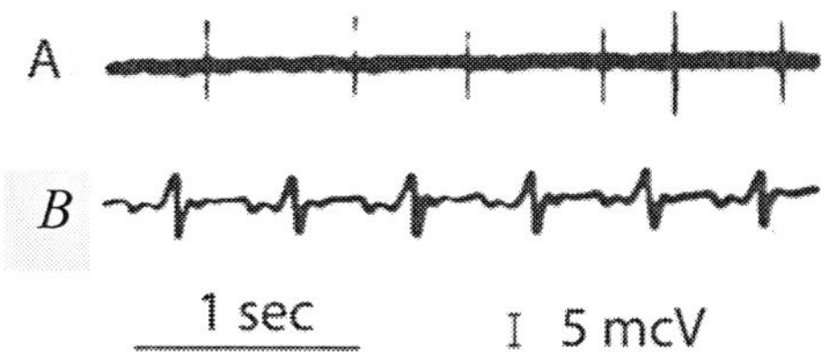

Figure 30. 4 months after the denervation and surgical reinnervation of the kidney. A-spontaneous impulsation of the renal nerve. B-electrocardiogram.

Six months after the operation, both spontaneous and evoked impulsations were observed. The background impulsation had a frequency of 3.0 Hertz and an amplitude of 17.2 mcV. The injection of adrenalin was accompanied by a disappearance of impulsation, as before. The injection of acethylcholine and an increase of intrapelvic pressure caused the more expressed increase of frequency and amplitude of impulses, as compared with the previous term (54.0 Hertz and 27.0 mcV, respectively) (Figure 32). The indices of biopotentials evoked by an electric irritation remained, as before.

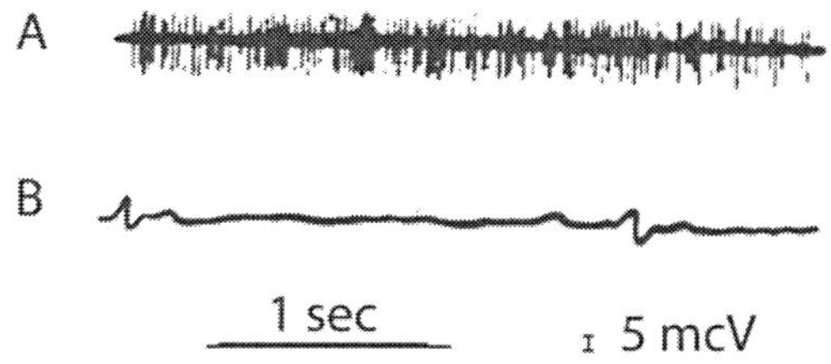

Figure 31. 4 months after the denervation and surgical reinnervation of the kidney A-increase of frequency of spontaneous impulsation from renal nerve in answer to intravenous injection of acetylcholine. B-electrocardiogram.

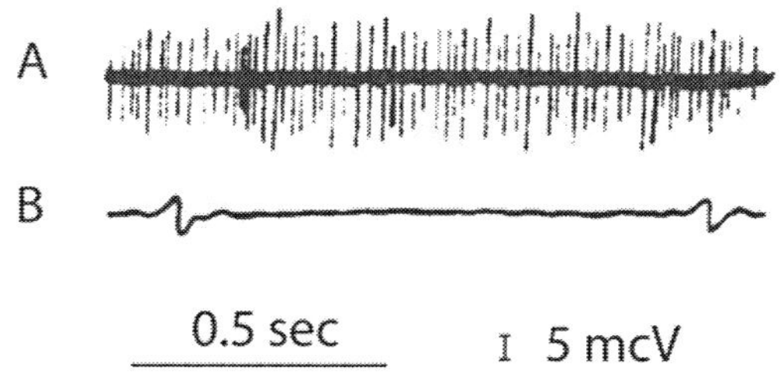

Figure 32. 6 months after the denervation and surgical reinnervation of the kidney.
A-increase of frequency of spontaneous impulsation from the renal nerve in answer to intravenous injection of acetylcholine. B-electrocardiogram.

One and two years after the operation, the characteristics of spontaneous and evoked impulsations remained, mainly without changes. In addition, a slight shortening of chronaxy time (to 5.2 m/sec) was observed.

In the third group ("a" subgroup) three days after the autotransplantation of the kidney without surgical reinnervation, the spontaneous impulsation from the rest of the renal nerve didn`t register. In response to an electric irritation of 7.4 V a potential with an amplitude of 1.2 mV was evoked, but further increase of irritation didn`t enhance the nerve potential. The time of chronaxy was 11.8 m/sec and the velocity of nerve impulse conduction was 2.5 m/sec.

The following period from ten days to one month was the period of full bioelectric silence.

Two months after the operation the spontaneous impulsation of the rest of the renal nerve didn`t appear. The electric irritation of 11.6 V was the threshold and evoked a biopotential with an amplitude of 1.2 mV; the time of chronaxy and velocity of nerve impulse conduction were 13.6 m/sec and 1.9 m/sec, respectively.

Four to six months after the operation the spontaneous impulsation of the rest of the renal nerve was absent, as before (Figure 33). By electric irritation the threshold amplitude was 1.7 mV (Figure 34) and didn`t increase more in spite of intensification of irritation up to 50 V (Figure 35). The time of chronaxy and velocity of nerve impulse conduction slightly differed from the previous term (12.5 m/sec and 2.3 m/sec, respectively).

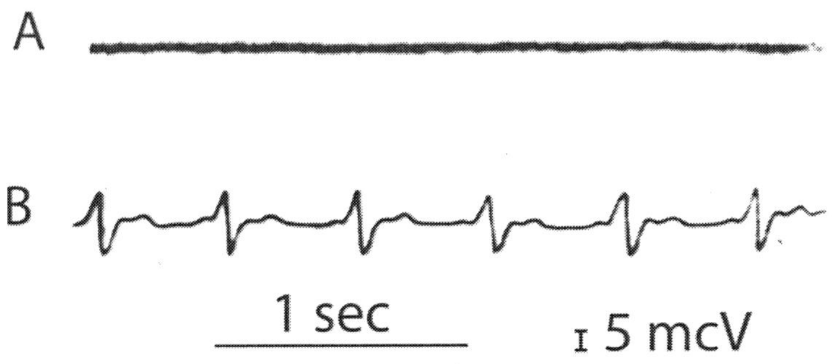

Figure 33. 6 months after the autotransplantatio of the kidney without surgical reinnervation. A-spontaneous impulsation from the rest of the renal nerve is absent.
B-electrocardiogram.

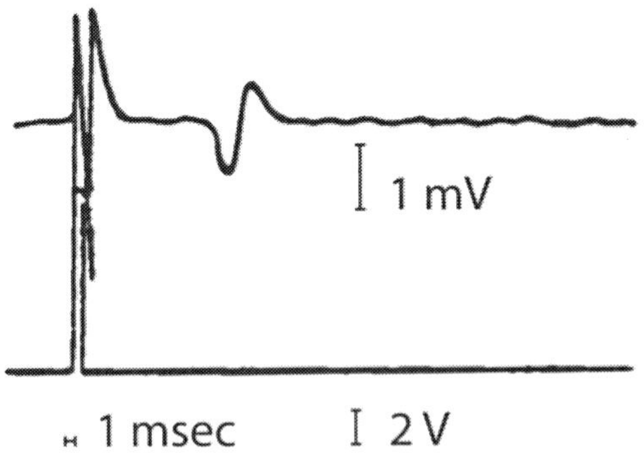

Figure 34. The same case. A threshold excitement of the renal nerve rest.

One to two years after the operation the spontaneous impulsation of the renal nerve wasn`t observed, either in the form of a background, in response to acethylcholine injection or to the increase of intrapelvic pressure. The character of reactions of the rest of the renal nerve to electric irritation remained qualitatively as previous seen, with a small quantitative difference in that the threshold decreased to 10.5 V with a maximum amplitude of biopotential of 1.6 mV; a shortening of chronaxy time (to 10.9 m/sec) and an increase of velocity of nerve impulse conduction to 2.6 m/sec were also observed.

In the "b" subgroup of the third group of experiments after autotransplantation of the sole kidney without surgical reinnervation, the same periods in the dynamics of spontaneous and evoked impulsations were observed as in the previous "a" subgroup with preservation of an intact kidney. The qualitative and quantitative characteristics of renal nerve biopotentials in both subgroups didn`t differ essentially.

In the fourth group ("a" subgroup) of experiments, three days after the autotransplantation and surgical reinnervation of the kidney, the spontaneous impulsation from the renal nerve was absent. It didn`t appear either after the acethylcholine injection or by an increase of intrapelvic pressure. The threshold irritation of 6 V caused a potential with an amplitude of 1.2 mV. The increase of electric irritation to 25 V enhanced the maximum biopotential to 1.5 mV.

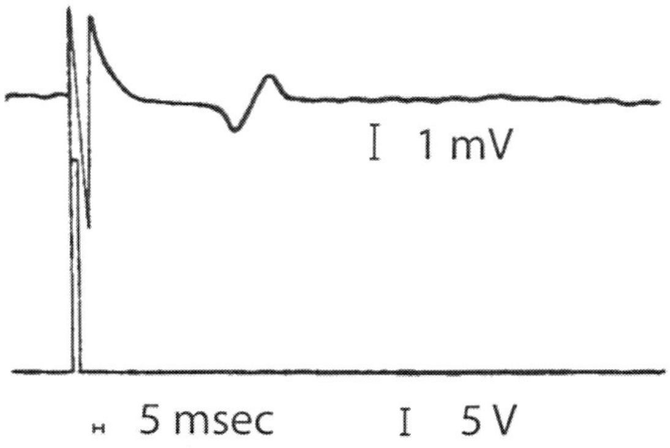

Figure 35. The same case. The increase of renal nerve rest elect5ric irritation doesn't cause an increase of its total potential amplitude.

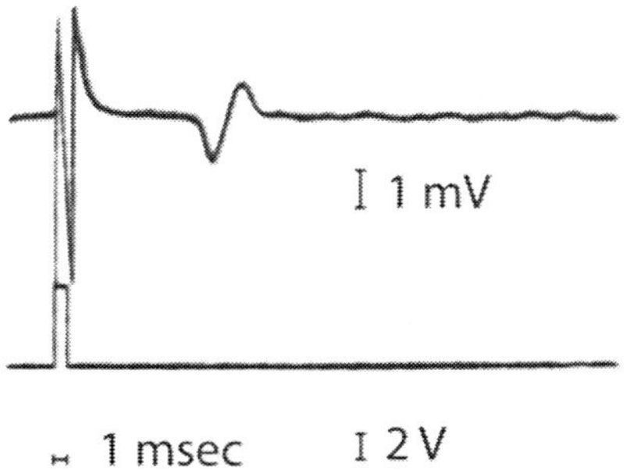

Figure 36. 2 months after the autotransplantation of the kidney with a surgical reinervation. The threshold excitement of the renal nerve.

In following observations, up to one month, a period of full bioelectric silence was observed with spontaneous as well as evoked impulsation, as before.

Two months after the operation, the spontaneous impulsation from the renal nerve didn`t appear. The electric irritation of 6.9 V caused a potential of 2.2 mV (Figure 36). The increase of electric irritation to 15 V enhanced the amplitude of biopotential to 3.2 mV (Figure 37). The time of chronaxy was 10.0 m/sec. The velocity of the nerve impulse conduction increased to 3.2 m/sec.

Four months after the operation, spontaneous impulsation began to be observed in the renal nerve on both sides, proximally as well as distally from the nerve anastomosis. This impulsation was represented by 1–2 oscillations in 1 second with an amplitude of 18.0 mcV (Figure 38). The intravenous injection of adrenalin caused a disappearance of the mentioned impulsation (Figure 39). By injection of acethylcholine, as well as by increase of intrapelvic pressure, the impulsation became more frequent (25 Hertz) with a slightly increased amplitude (22 mcV, Figure 40).

The electric irritation of the renal nerve on both sides from the nerve anastomosis was accompanied by an appearance of biopotentials. A threshold irritation of 4.2 V evoked a potential of 2.7 mV. The increase of an irritation to 20 V stimulated the maximum potential of 4.5 mV. The chronaxy time was 7.4 m/sec and the velocity of nerve impulse conduction was 3.9 m/sec.

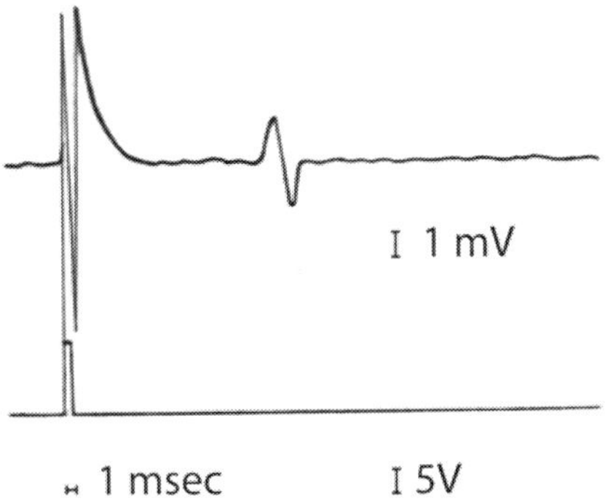

Figure 37. The same case. By increase of the electrical irritation the amplitude of the renal nerve total potential increased also.

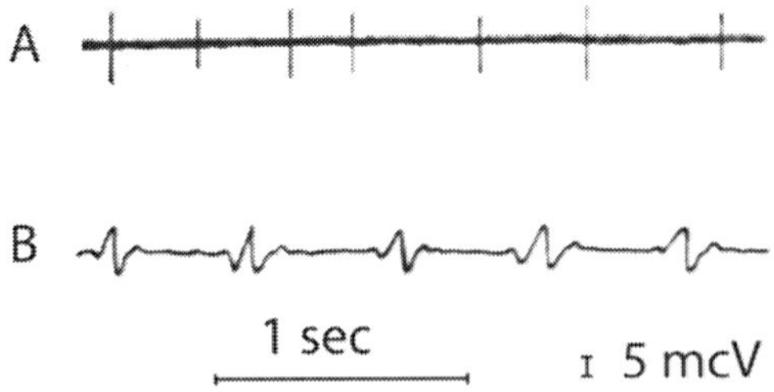

Figure 38. 4 months after autotransplantation of the kidney with a surgical reinnervation. A-spontaneous impulsation of the renal nerve, B-electrocardiogram.

Six months after the operation the qualitative characteristics of spontaneous and evoked impulsations remained the same as in the previous term. There were only quantitative differences. So, the background spontaneous impulsation was more frequent (2.5 Hertz) and high (22.0 mcV). The injection of adrenalin led to disappearance of this impulsation for 4–5 minutes and then it recovered again to the initial level. The injection of acethylcholine, as well as the increase of intrapelvic pressure, caused more significant intensification of oscillations as compared with the previous term in frequency (52.0 Hertz) as well as in amplitude (37.0 mcV, Figure 41). As for peculiarities of an evoked impulsation, the shortening of chronaxy time to 5.3 m/sec can be mentioned. The other quantitative indices remained on the level of the previous term.

One and two years after the operation the characteristics of spontaneous and stimulated impulsations remained mainly the same. The only difference was the decrease of excitability threshold to 2.1 V and of the chronaxy time to 5.0 m/sec.

In the "b" subgroup of the fourth group of experiments after the autotransplantation and surgical reinnervation of the sole kidney, nearly the same qualitative and quantitative characteristics of the spontaneous and evoked impulsations were observed, as in the previous subgroup. The only difference was the shortening of terms of recovery. So the period of full bioelectric silence continued no longer than 3 weeks, and by one month after the operation the evoked potentials were registered. Their characteristics corresponded to the data of the previous subgroup by two months after the operation.

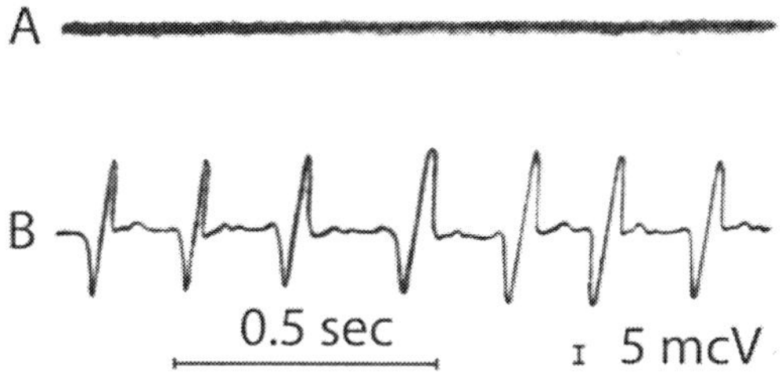

Figure 39. The same case. After the intravenous injection of adrenalin the spontaneous impulsation of the renal nerve is disappeared.

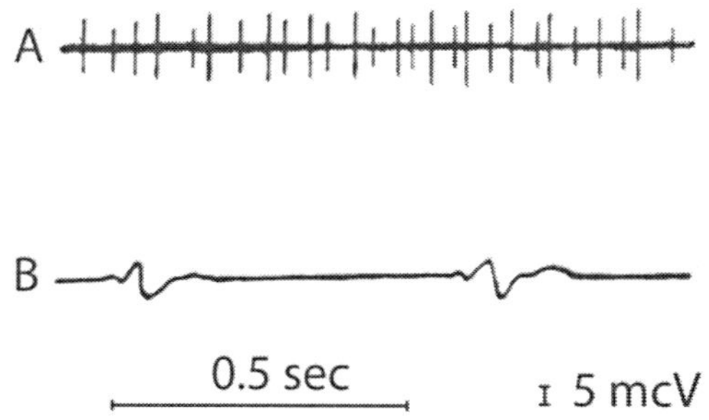

Figure 40. The same case. A-after the intravenous injection of acetylcholine the spontaneous impulsatiion of the renal nerve gets more frequent.

Two months after the operation the spontaneous impulsation appeared with specific reactions to adrenalin and acethylcholine injections.

After four months, and within all terms up to the end of experiments, the bioelectric activity of the renal nerve corresponded to qualitative and quantitative data of the previous subgroup of one and two years after the operation.

In the fifth control group of experiments, the indices of the sole kidney nerve bioelectric activity didn`t differ from the corresponding data of an intact animal with both kidneys.

4.2. Discussion of Results

The examination of the described neurophysiologic investigations in all experimental groups with decentralization of the kidney show mainly identical changes of bioelectric activity of remnants of the renal nerve in the near postoperative period (within one month). On the first stage (after three days), a disappearance of spontaneous impulsation was observed as a background as well as in response to acethylcholine injection. At the same time, the renal nerve preserved the ability to give biopotentials by electric irritation, although a distinct lag of their basic quantitative indices as compared with an intact renal nerve was observed.

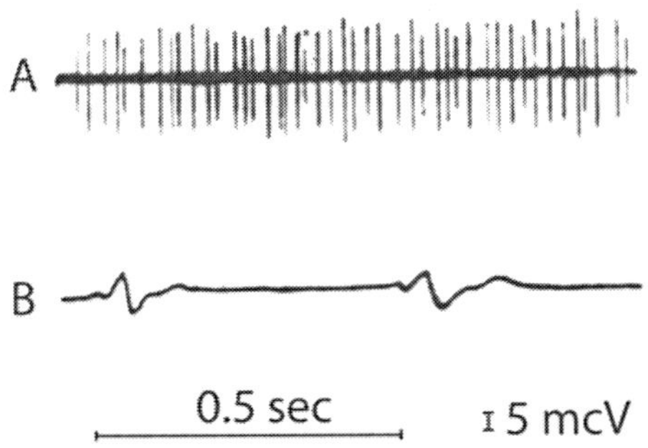

Figure 41. 6 months after the autotransplantation of the kidney with a surgical reinnervation. A-intravenous injection of acetylcholine causes the increase of a spontaneous impulsation as after the frequency as well as after the amplitude. B-electrocardiogram.

The mentioned changes have to be considered as significant disorders of bioelectric activity and evidently can be explained as a beginning of destructive alterations in amputated nerve trunks. The fact that the spontaneous impulsation disappeared while the rest of the renal nerve preserved the ability to give the biopotential in response to electric irritation and furthermore to increase the maximum amplitude by ascendant irritation, testified to an irregular course of destructive processes in cut nerve fibers.

In the next period (from three days to one month), a full bioelectric silence was observed. This phenomenon was typical for all four groups of experiments with the cutting of the renal nerve. This circumstance testified that degenerative changes in renal nerve structures during this period reached the maximum. It has to be especially emphasized that there was no difference, whether the kidney was decentralized by means of denervation in situ or in connection with autotransplantation, or whether it was surgically reinnervated or not. In all these cases a degeneration of the majority of intrarenal nerve structures inevitably occurred. Thus, within the first month after the operation in all these groups of experiments the kidney was actually deprived of nervous regulation.

The investigations performed after two months revealed a distinct difference between the groups in which the operation was either accompanied by the surgical reinnervation or not.

So, in the first group after the kidney denervation in situ and in the third group after autotransplantation without surgical reinnervation, beginning from the above-mentioned term up to two years, spontaneous impulsations were not revealed. Taking into account that the spontaneous impulsation usually characterized the state of vascular afferent receptors which are excited by extension of vascular walls and depressed by their narrowing [51,294-300], our data permit us to conclude that a decentralization of the kidney causes an upsetting of afferent impulsation from vascular receptors and their recovery didn`t occur within two years.

Two months after the operation in the first group, the electric irritation began to evoke weak biopotentials, but their amplitude didn`t increase in response to ascendant irritation. It is known that the nervous trunks usually contain a large quantity of nerve fibers of various types, each of them with its own threshold of excitement and responses to irritation according to the principle of "all or nothing". Thanks to this, by ascendant electric irritation, the excitement of various nerve fibers in accordance with their threshold occurs and as a result is accompanied by an increase of a total maximum biopotential [58].

Along with this, the increase of biopotential amplitude in answer to ascendant irritation was not registered, it can be concluded that the examined nerve trunk contained only single and evidently homogenous regenerated nerve fibers. The truth is that in the following terms (from four months to two years) an increase of biopotential amplitudes was observed, but it was possible by an electric irritation which was 4–5 times more than the threshold and the maximum potential exceeded a threshold one only by 20-30%. The lag of other neurophysiologic characteristics had also taken place: the time of chronaxy was 13.6 m/sec (by the norm 2-3 m/sec), and the velocity of nerve impulse conduction was 1,8-2,2-2,5 m/sec (by the norm 5 m/sec).

The results of experiments in the third group with autotransplantation of the kidney without surgical reinnervation mainly coincided with those of the first group. The only difference was that after two months and up to two years, the rest of the renal nerve didn`t react with any increase of biopotential as compared with threshold in spite of ascendant irritation even up to 50 V. Thus, it can be mentioned that the rest of the renal nerve of the transplanted kidney contained only single fibers which were functionally imperfect.

The difference between the results in the above-mentioned groups of experiments evidently can be explained firstly, with a more complete decentralization of the kidney by its transplantation and secondly, with less favorable conditions for its spontaneous reinnervation as compared with the kidney that underwent a simple denervation in situ. In the latter case, on the one hand, some nerve fibers located in the muscular wall of the magistral renal blood vessels were preserved untouched, and on the other hand, the renal blood vessels themselves were a peculiar directive framework which created certain conditions for a partial spontaneous reinnervation all along. In this respect the transplanted kidneys were in less favorable conditions.

Unlike the described groups, in the second and fourth groups two months after the operation, other dynamics were observed. In these groups, where the kidney denervation and autotransplantation with surgical reinnervation were performed, the spontaneous impulsation was not revealed. But the renal nerve, proximally as well as distally from the nerve anastomosis, gave a distinct reaction in response to a much lower threshold irritation (5-6 V) as compared with previous groups. It has to be noted that the renal nerve was able to increase the total maximum biopotential (by 60–70%) in response to ascendant electric irritation. It can be evidently explained by the fact that, in this term, the nerve fibers began to show activity. They were regenerated along the previous renal nervous trunks and were represented with a much higher quantity of multiform nerve fibers with various thresholds of excitement compared to the first group of experiments.

Four months after the operation, in the second and fourth test groups, spontaneous impulsation appeared. The qualitative characteristics of this impulsation were actually identical to that of the intact ones: the injection of adrenalin caused a disappearance of the background impulsation, both injections of acethylcholine and an increase of intrapyelon pressure made the impulsation more frequent. But there was a certain lag in quantitative aspects compared to the intact kidney. The amplitude of background spontaneous impulsation was 70% of the norm. The intravenous injection of acethylcholine and artificial intrapyelon hypertension made the spontaneous impulsation more frequent by only 26.2±1.5% (20-30%) as compared with an intact kidney. Furthermore, in the above-mentioned experimental groups, it didn`t increase the amplitude of biopotentials.

Six months after the operation, by injection of acethylcholine as well as by an increase of intrapyelon pressure, the increase of the frequency of spontaneous impulsation reached 51.5±2.2% (49-63%) and the amplitude of biopotentials to 69.3±4.2% (60-75%) of the norm ($p<0.01$).

In the following period (one and two years after the operation) a decrease of excitability threshold to 1 V and a shortening of the chronaxy time to 5 m/sec (by the norm 2–3 m/sec) were observed. Thus, it can be concluded that after the surgical reinnervation of the denervated and autotransplantaed kidneys, the regeneration of most of the various efficient nerve fibers along the intraorganic nervous trunks was complete by six months, on the whole. Then only a further growth of quantitative indices of their activity had taken place.

It has to be especially noted, there were essential differences in neuroregeneration processes in the "b" subgroups of the third and fourth groups of experiments with a removal of an intact kidney. As in the third group, after the kidney autotransplantation without reinnervation, the regeneration of only single and functionally insufficient nerve fibers occurred. In the fourth group with surgical reinnervation of the autotransplanted sole kidney, not only quite healthy nerve fibers regenerated but also an intensification and acceleration of neuroregeneration precesses were observed.

The latter circumstance, on the one hand, could be explained by common reasons of rebuilding of a sole kidney in connection with a compensative hypertrophy, but actually it was determined mainly by favorable anatomic conditions which were made thanks to sewing of perivascular fascial shreds of anastomosed blood vessels in combination with the ordinary sewing of renal large nerve trunks.

The described neurophysiologic investigations permit us to express an opinion in some cardinal questions which determined the principal direction of our work: Does the sewing of fascial shreds of anastomosed blood vessels constitute real grounds for efficient artificial reinnervation of the kidney transplant? In what terms does the germination of nerve fibers into the kidney occur? What are the dynamics of regeneration of adrenergic and cholinergic, afferent and efferent nerve fibers? How adequate is the resulting surgical reinnervation for the normal work of the kidney transplant in qualitative and quantitative respects?

The above described data and their analysis permit us to conclude that after the surgical reinnervation of denervated, as well as autotransplanted kidney simultaneously with a degeneration of intraorganic nervous apparatus, the germination of sewed nerve fibers had taken place. They could be registered after their bioelectric activity. Taking into account that the impulsation evoked with electric irritation was recovered in two months, and spontaneous impulsation within four months, the level of nerve fiber germination into the kidney in various terms after the intervention can be concluded.

The character of bioelectric signals and described successiveness of their appearance testifies to that within the first two months the sewed nerve fibers germinated into the kidney along the previous intrarenal nerve channels and by four to six months they reached up to the level of renal functioning terminals.

Thus, the method of kidney surgical reinnervation used ensured the recovery of the intraorganic nervous apparatus approximately equaled the volume and level of reflex arc of ordinary neuroplastic operations [7,182,290].

The performed investigations permitted a differentiated evaluation of adrenergic and cholinergic nervous structures in the course of regeneration. Beginning from the fourth month after the surgical reinnervation of the autotransplanted kidney, the spontaneous bioelectric impulses could be registered from the renal nerve, both from the proximal and distal segments from the place of nerve anastomosis. Furthermore, the intravenous injection of adrenalin caused a disappearance of this impulsation and injection of acethylcholine, on the contrary, caused its intensification of frequency and amplitude. It is known that the spontaneous impulsation of the renal nerve characterizes the state the bioelectric activity of renal vascular afferent terminals and this activity is reduced by contraction of renal blood vessels and increased by their widening [91,92,184]. It is also known that adrenalin is a specific mediator for the conduction of nervous impulses through contacts of adrenergic nerve fibers, and acethylcholine is the specific cholinergic mediator [184]. The fact that by four to six months the renal blood vessels reacted quite adequately on specific nervous mediators and it was further expressed in specific changes of renal nerve bioelectric activity, which testifies about the normal relations between the adrenergic and cholinergic nerve structures in the transplanted kidney up to the level of the vascular terminals.

The fact that these relations can not be explained only by humoral reactions and were determined mainly by the successful regeneration of adrenergic and cholinergic nerve fibers that occurred are convincingly seen by comparison of these data with results of the first and third groups of experiments performed without surgical reinnervation of the kidney. In the latter groups, firstly a background spontaneous impulsation was not observed and secondly the injection of acethylcholine didn`t cause its appearance and moreover its intensification. Thus, it can be supposed that without a direct surgical reinnervation of the kidney neither anatomic recovery of afferent vascular terminals nor the achievement of normal relations between the adrenergic and cholinergic nervous elements would occur.

Furthermore, we obtained the direct and clear data concerning the dynamics of regeneration of afferent and efferent nerve fibers. The condition of an afferent innervation was evaluated after a background spontaneous impulsation, impulsation by adrenalin, acethylcholine injections, increase of intrapyelon pressure and after electrically evoked biopotentials.

In the first and third groups of experiments performed without surgical reinnervation of the kidney, the spontaneous impulsation of the renal nerve specific to the afferent innervation was absent during the whole period of observation. Two months after the operation only single biopotentials evoked by electric irritation could be revealed, but they were weak, imperfect and incapable of conducting a normal afferent impulsation.

In comparison with that in the test-groups, with the surgical reinnervation of the kidney two months after the operation, an artificially evoked impulsation appeared, then (after four months) a spontaneous impulsation and two years of observations of their qualitative characteristics didn`t differ from the standard. There was only a certain lag in quantitative respects.

Thus, in our opinion, the above-mentioned results testify convincingly about a successful recovery of the majority of afferent nervous strictures which reacted specifically enough on various medicaments and mechanical irritation.

As for a comparative rate of regeneration of afferent and efferent nerve structures, there is evidence that their recovery proceeded parallel with the same speed. This phenomenon can be explained by the fact that efferent and efferent nerve fibers are usually located in the common nerve trunks and in equal conditions for regeneration [182].

Finally, the data permit us to answer the main question—how perfect is the resulting surgical reinnervation in qualitative and quantitative respects for the normal work of a transplanted kidney? There are reasons for a positive answer, because in the second and fourth groups with the kidney surgical reinnervation, the nerve fibers germinated up to the level of terminals and by this term the regeneration of adrenergic and cholinergic, afferent and efferent nerve structures were completed with effective specific bioelectric activity. It has to be mentioned that if the qualitative bioelectric characteristics of regenerated renal nerves actually didn`t differ from the standard by electric, medicinal or mechanic irritations, the quantitative characteristics were slightly behind the norm. The amplitude of background spontaneous impulsation was 15-18 mcV, the norm was 22-25 mcV, the increase of its frequency by acethylcholine injection was 42 and 53 Hertz, the norm was 80 and 90 Hertz, respectively, the ratio of a total biopotential to threshold was 150–160% , the norm was 210%, the chronaxy time was 5.2 m/sec of the norm of 3 m/sec, the velocity of nerve impulse conduction was 3.8-4.1 m/sec of the norm of 5 m/sec.

To some degree this small lag of quantitative neurophysiologic data could influence the perfectness of the regenerated nervous apparatus on the kidney condition and would be concluded definitively by comparison of these data with parallel functional and morphologic results. In the given chapter we can compare them only with results of similar neurophysiologic investigations made on the model of neuroplastic operations. So, the results [182] show that even by direct sewing of large nerves "end to end", full regeneration of all nerve fibers didn`t occur and the indices of their bioelectric activity five months after the operation were 52.5-70.8-84.9% of the background level.

According to results [237], after the epineural anastomosis, only 70% of nerve fibers germinated from the central to distal part of the nerve.

As an important peculiarity of reinnervated organs, particularly in intestinal autotransplant, it has to be mentioned that even by relatively insufficient capacity of germinated nervous wisp, if only a part of the regenerated axons reached the terminal level, each of them came into axodendric contact with several neurons according to the rule of "multiplication phenomenon". Thanks to this, they were able to ensure a satisfactory innervation of the whole transplant [205,311].

It can be supposed that the mentioned "multiplication phenomenon" is widespread in the kidney, too. Moreover, the conduction of nervous impulses to functional units of even the normal kidney is carried out not only through direct contact with nervous terminals but also by means of nervous mediator diffusion [374].

Thus, the obtained qualitative and quantitative results of neurophysiologic investigations and their comparison with the known literature information testify that, after the surgical reinnervation of the denervated as well as autotransplanted kidneys by I.D. Kirpatovsky [189], the ends of the vegetative nervous plexus were in the same relation as in the case of direct sewing of nervous trunks "end to end". Furthermore, the character and volume of regeneration of the intraorganic nervous apparatus created favorable conditions for its normal adaptive and trophic influence on the kidney [356].

Chapter V

The Morphologic State of Denervated and Autotransplanted Kidneys by Spontaneous and Surgical Reinnervation

The examination of the microscopic structure of the kidney parenchyma and its nervous apparatus was performed for the control and research of the morphologic background of the obtained functional results. On the one hand, it permitted us to answer the main practical question, is the surgical reinnervation of transplanted organs needed or not and on the other hand, would it enrich to a certain degree the existent knowledge about the intricate pathologic-anatomic nature of the nervous and trophic regulation of the kidney tissue.

The importance and complexity of this aim dictated the use of special modern neurohistologic research methods related to the field of "functional morphology," in addition to traditional methods. Therefore, the kidney common morphologic state, structure of its nervous apparatus, differentiated evaluation of adrenergic and cholinergic elements, transport function of afferent nerve fibers and renal ultrastructure were examined.

5.1. The Structure of Dogs Intrarenal Nervous Apparatus in the Norm

The complex description of intact dogs' intrarenal neurohistology was determined by necessity to have a normal background for comparison with denervated cases and a lack of such data in available literature. Various nerve plexus take part in the kidney innervation: pl.pl renalis, solaris, intermesentericus, aorticus abdominalis, hypogastricus, pelvicus, lienalis (or hepaticus), and pancreaticus [369-371,375]. They contain mainly unmyelinized adrenergic and cholinergic elements. In the field of renal gate, the magistral nerve trunks and fibers are located on the front and back surface of the renal artery, furthermore, they are distributed through the fat tissue and penetrate the kidney in the composition of the connective tissue skeleton which is the couch for blood, lymphatic vessels and are the initial section of urinary pathways [66,88,89,140,160,170,331,332,369,409,419]. Inside the kidney the nerve fibers are also spread along the blood vessels, urinary pathway walls and also across the renal capsule, through peculiar hatches, in the places of connection of capsular blood vessels with those of the renal cortical substance [26,34,68,85,140,141,306,321,381,397].

After the division of the main renal artery the branches of the renal nervous plexus anastomose between themselves and abundantly cover the front and back branches of the renal artery. Also, a big quantity of nervous terminals are observed in the kidney connective tissue skeleton along the blood vessels. After the penetration of nerve fibers in the kidney depth, on the level of interlobular arteries a part of the nerve fibers come out in perivascular tissue, and cross to renal channels and reach glomerulas here and there. The intrarenal venous channel is innervated very scantily, compared with the arterial channel, and contain mainly unmyelinized nerve fibers and afferent terminals. Their typical peculiarity is the presence of polyvalent receptors [338,339,347,369,370].

As for innervation of the main morphofunctional unit of the kidney-nephron, there is quite contradictory literature. Some authors [3,181,269,271,367-370] found nerve elements penetrated into the renal channels and glomerulas. At the same time other authors denied their existence [88,89,263,427]. The main explanation of this discrepancy can be considered by the methodical imperfection of the neurohistologic techniques used, particularly of thin histologic cuts. Sufficiently thick cuts (100-180 mcm) and preliminary fixation of morphologic material in the substance AFA permitted a very fine and abundant innervation of nephron various segments to be revealed [369,370].

The nerve fibers reach the glomerulas by various ways. The afferent fibers accompany the interlobular arteries, then the arterioles of the glomerulas give the terminals in the direction of adjoining proximal channels and small blood vessels. Near the glomerulas the afferent nerve fibers give branches to the glomerular capsule, juxtaglomerular complex and neighbouring channel walls.

In the kidney medullar layer, the nervous apparatus is represented more scantily than in the cortical layer. The Henle loops are innervated at the expense of dispersed afferent terminals which are also in contact with many channels.

The innervation of the nephron distal segment is made by nerve fibers going from its initial segments. Furthermore, the distal segments become the nerve branches from the neighboring pyelon walls.

The collective tubules are supplied by afferent nerve terminals as well as by the finest fibers. At the same time the typical parallel disposal of collective tubules determines the corresponding orientation of their nerve fibers.

In the perinipple zone and on the walls of collective tubules there are also circular and button form nerve terminals which represent the polyvalence receptors and play an important role in the coordinated urine production and evacuation [181,183,367].

For the receptory nervous apparatus of the pyelon is typically a successive offshoot of afferent terminals from one common myelinized nerve fiber to various layers of the pyelon walls such as the mucosal, muscular and adventitial membranes.

The authors [367,378] explain this phenomenon with the display of a polyvalent reception which is necessary for perception of the whole pyelon as one functional unit and is very important for the pyelon coordinated contractions.

It has to be mentioned that just as receptors in the pyelon have a linear orientation, those in the juxtapyelon segment of the ureter have a circular disposition. In one author's [367] opinion, this peculiarity corresponds to the stretch lines of connective tissue and smooth muscle elements in this segment of the upper urinary tract.

One of disputable theoretical questions of kidney neurohistology is the existence and character of intraorganic ganglions. This argument has more than one century of history and reflects mainly on the contradiction between two conceptions. On the one hand, [85,307,340,385] is an advanced hypothesis about the automatic activity of the upper urinary tract. On the other hand are those who didn`t find nerve elements in the upper part of the ureter suggesting a myogenous hypothesis of ureter contraction. According to this the contraction waves arise directly in the smooth muscle of the ureter without participation of ganglions [152,167,308,422].

As for adrenergic and cholinergic innervation of the kidney in modern neurohistologic methods, there is little information [134-139,384,387-390]. It was determined with an absence, for much time, of objective and sufficiently sensitive methods for differentiated and specific evaluation. This flaw was corrrected in the last years thanks to new specific neurohistologic methods [9,22,70,71, 100-102,180].

The most sensitive method for examination of catecholamines, the formaldehyde method [100-101] is considered. It permits the presence of 5-10-7 ng noradrenaline to be revealed in a single sympathetic nerve [116].

A detailed description of adrenergic and cholinergic nerve structures in a dog's normal kidney was made by several authors [134-139,358,359,377-379,384,387-390].

The adrenergic and cholinergic nerve fibers penetrate the kidney in composition of plexus renalis mainly along the renal artery. They create in the kidney external periarterial nervous nets which accompany a.a. interlobulares, arcuatae. Their lateral branches represent their own adrenergic and cholinergic innervation apparatus in various structures of the organ.

Along the whole preglomerular arterial channel its external side is surrounded with a dense adventitial nerve plexus. It gives the adrenergic nerve fibers in the direction of efferent arterioles and proximal channels. These fibers enter then into the cortico-medullar nervous net. Distinguished in this area are firstly, periarteriolar nerve fibers along the vasa recta vera et spuria and secondly, nerve fibers in the direction of the marginal zone of the kidney juxtamedullar layer. The cholinergic nerve elements are represented here more scantily than the adrenergic elements. At the same time it has to be mentioned that channel adrenergic nerve fibers didn`t form, as a rule, the nervous nets, they mainly make synaptic contacts with channel walls and sometimes with blood vessel walls.

The system of adrenergic nerve fibers in the pyelon wall is represented mainly with branches going from interlobar periarterial nervous net. The distribution of cholinergic nerve fibers is the same.

Based on modern scientific data the conception of chemical transfer of a nervous irritation and homeostatic function of peripheric neurons can be considered in the following way. The intimate topographic-anatomic relations of terminal nerve fibers with blood vessel smooth muscle is regarded, by a majority of authors, as morphological evidence of vasomotor function. In this way the renal nervous apparatus exerts its regulation of kidney functions, which directly or indirectly, are connected with macro- or microblood-circulation. They are the distribution of blood in the kidney, its inflow in glomerulas, glomerular filtration, effective filtration pressure, and definitive formation of urine [113,138,224,387,388,390].

Furthermore, this nervous regulation is, on the one side, by a vasomotor mechanism controlling the renin-angiotensin system, general blood pressure in the organism and final composition of the urine, and on the other hand, the nervous mediators noradrenalin and acethylcholine directly influence the ion transport through the cellular membranes of kidney structures which are in the diffusion zone of these mediators [135,387-390].

The presence of a large quantity of nerve fibers in the pyelon and on the border between the calices and papillas are connected by authors with their active participation in the intricate and coordinated function of urodynamics. There is an opinion that these nervous structures are the main components of a so-called rhythm-initiator which regulates the complex peristaltic motions of the pyelon and ureter [110,369,370].

The authors connect the purpose of nerves accompanying the glomerular arterioles with their regulative influence on the kidney juxtaglomerular apparatus. They particularly regulate the secretion of a monoamine, arterial blood pressure changes and so on [27-29,99,133,222, 258, 268,273,302,306,424,436].

5.2. The Ultrastructure of the Dog Intact Kidney

The description of the normal kidney submicroscopic structure of the dog is still insufficient and scanty and a need to have a control for experimental groups dictated the exposition of our own corresponding material.

The kidney glomerula (Figure 42) contains a capillary ball covered with a capsule which has parietal and visceral sheets. The first is external, but the second is internal and covers the capillary loops. There is a Bowman cavity (BC) between these sheets. The walls of the ball capillary contain four components: endothelium (En), basal membrane (BM), visceral epithelium (VE) and mesangial cells (MC). The endothelial cell covers the capillary (C) from the inside and has cytoplasma and a nucleus (N). The cytoplasma contains a wide part (around the nucleus) and a flat part, the cytoplasmatic plate (CP). The latter has a thickness of 200-300 A°, is pierced with pores and covers the internal surface of the basal membrane (BM). The basal membrane itself has three layers, a middle one which is electronic dense and 300-500 A° wide, and two external ones which are light. The basal membrane limits the capillary space (C) from the Bowman cavity (BC). In the Bowman cavity there are the cells of the visceral epithelium called podocytes (Pc) located on the basal membrane. Their cytoplasma creates shoots called trabeculas (T), which give the thin stickshape formations, the pediculas (Pd). They are divided with pores and directly contact the basal membrane. In the space between the capillaries there are the mesangial cells (MC) which also give single shoots in the direction of a capillary.

The nephron tubular apparatus contains a proximal segment with winding and straight parts, thin segments, distal segments with straight and winding parts and collective (straight) tubules.

Epithelial cells from one side are limited with a basal membrane which is a sequel of the basal membrane of the Bowman capsule parietal sheet and from the other (apical) side are directed to the tubular channel.

The typical peculiarity of proximal segment epithelial cells (Figure 43) is the presence of a brush border (BB), which is the system of micropiles covered with a membrane. In the same place the cell cytoplasma also contains pinocytose vesicles (PcV). In the opposite (basal) space of the cytoplasma are where the oblong mitochondrias (M) with a clear system of cristas (Cr) are located. The cytoplasma contains ribosomes (R), Goldgi complex (GC), lysosomes (L), and single cisterns of the endoplasmatic net (ENC). The cell nucleus (N) has an oval form and contains a uniformly distributed chromatin.

The nephron thin segment (Figure 44) is represented with relatively little epithelial cells. Their cytoplasma is organelle poor, containing single mitochondrias (M), ribosomes (R) and cisterns of an endoplasmatic net (ENC). The cellular apical surface is uneven because of stickform branches protruding in the direction of tubular channels.

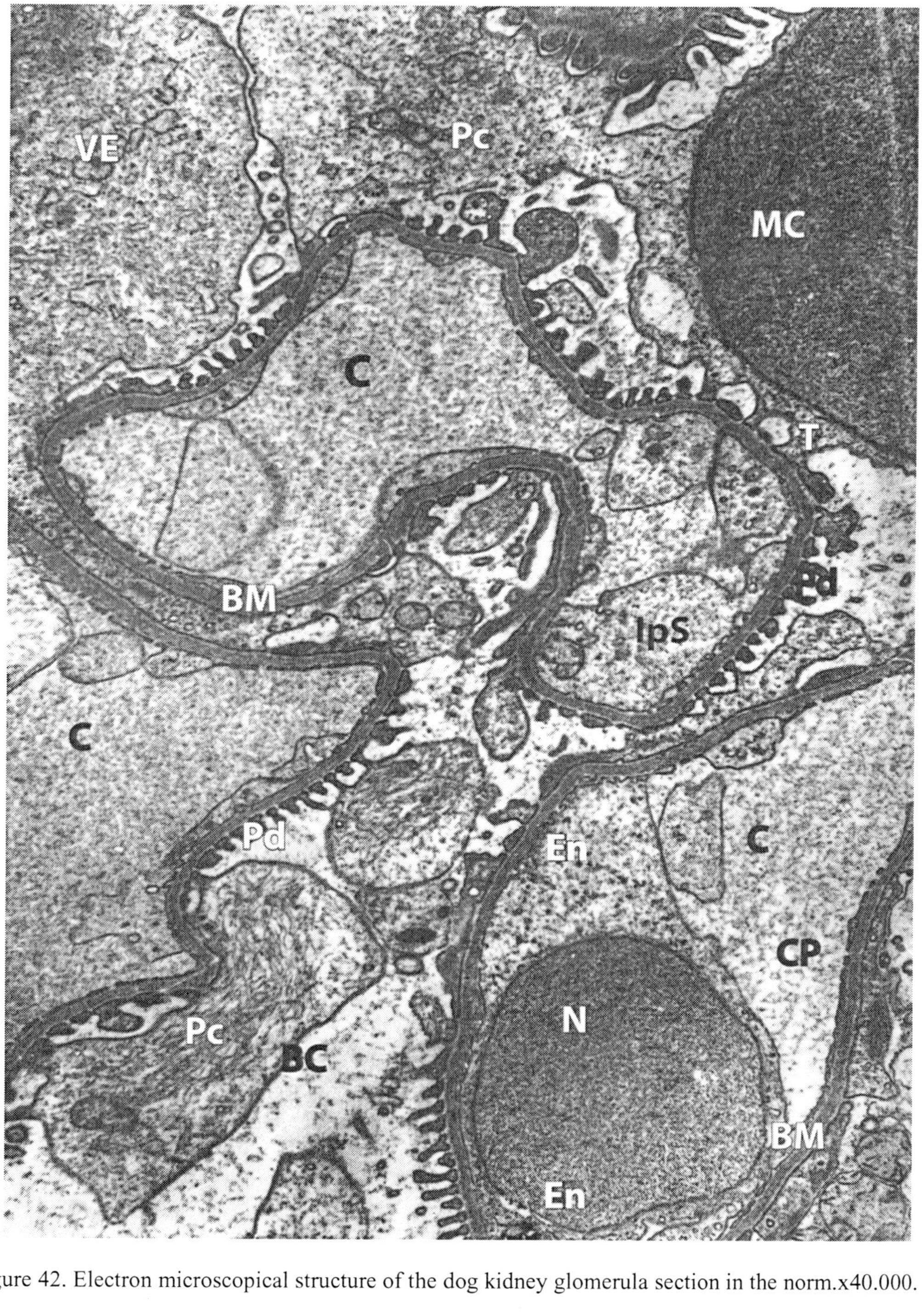

Figure 42. Electron microscopical structure of the dog kidney glomerula section in the norm.x40.000.

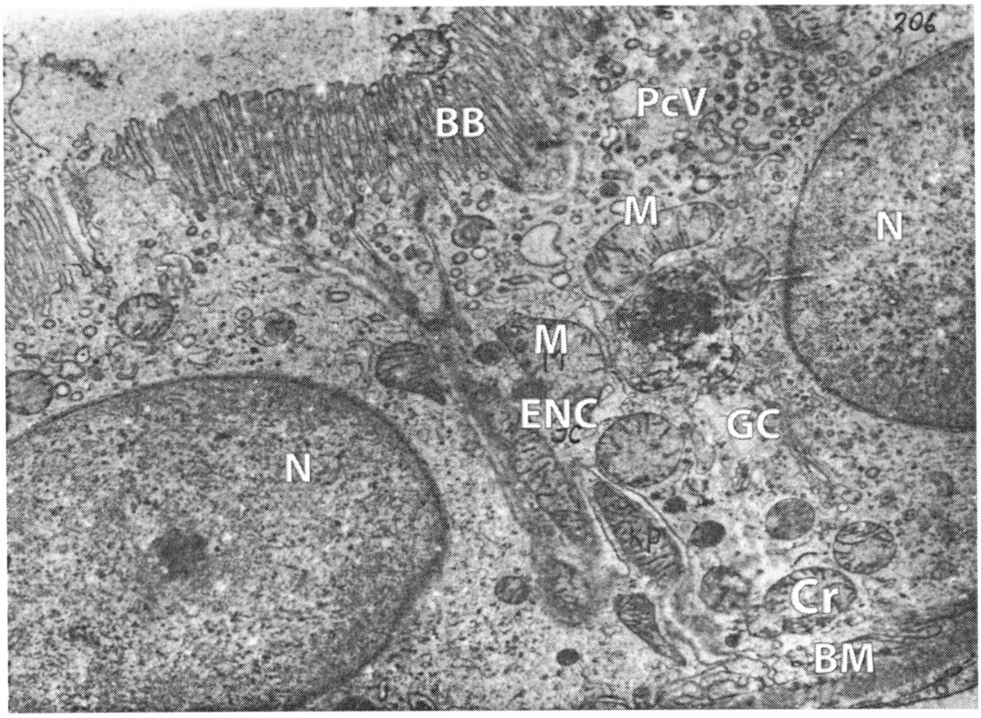

Figure 43. Ultrastructure of the dog kidney nephrom proximal segment epithelial cell section in the norm.x18.000.

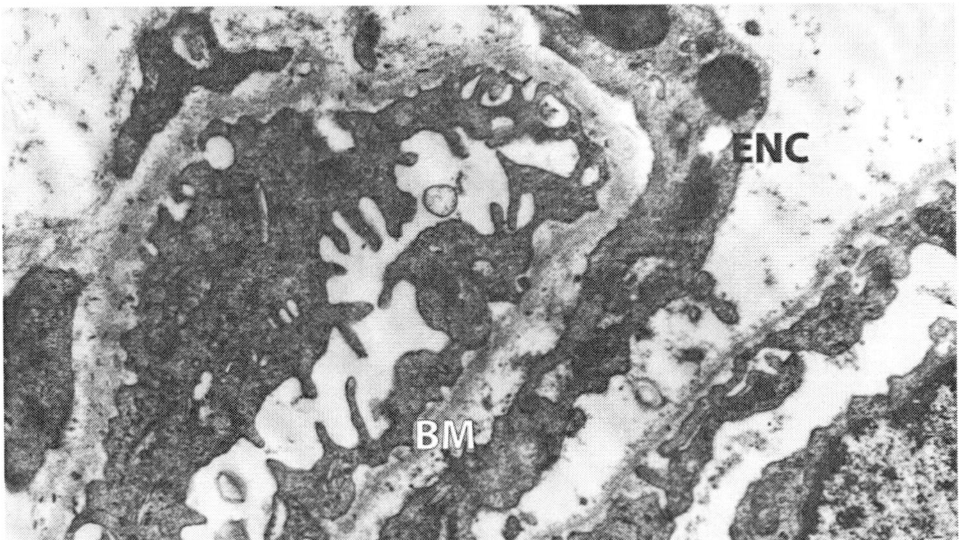

Figure 44. Ultrastructure of the dog kidney nephron thin segment epithelial cell section in the noerm.x10.000.

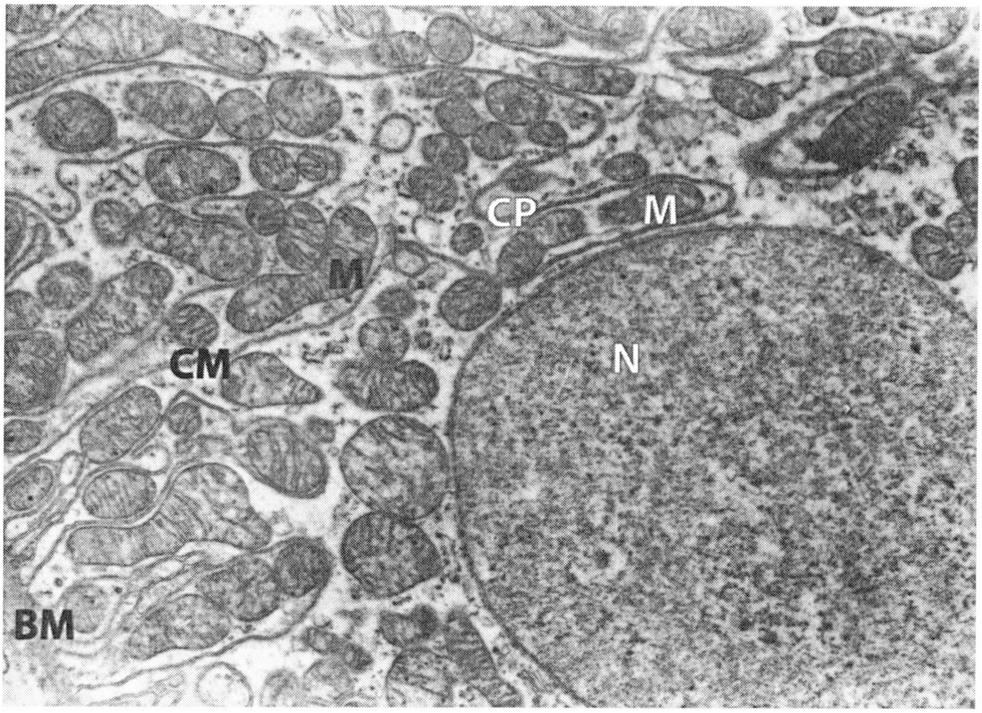

Figure 45. Ultrastructure of the dog kidney nephron distal segment epithelial cell section in the noerm.x18.000.

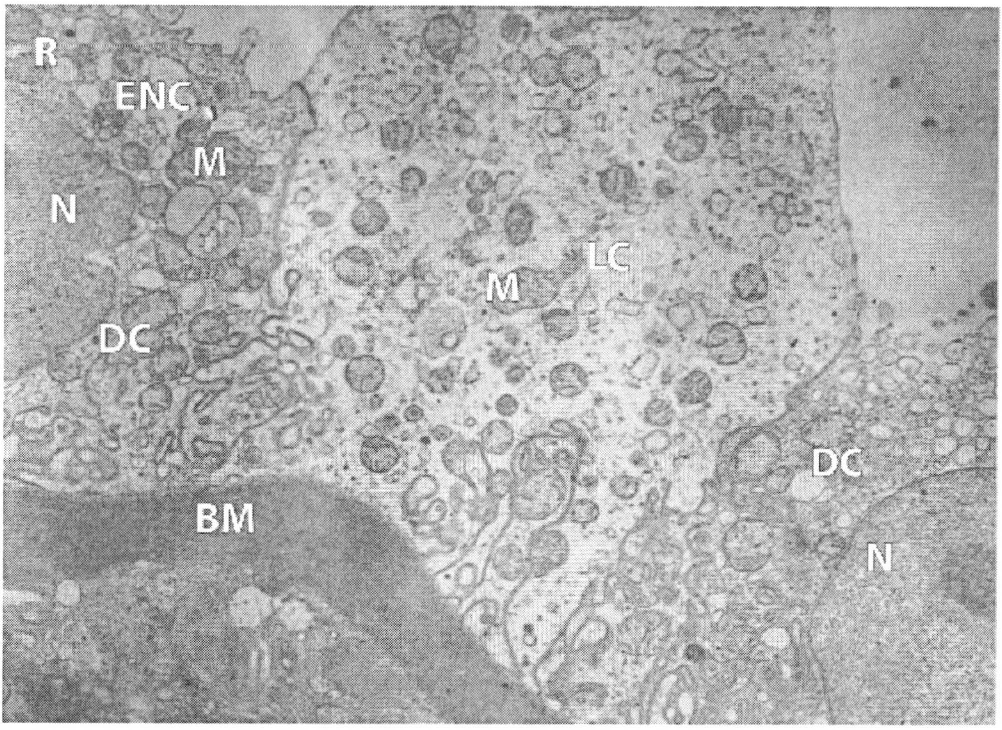

Figure 46. Ultrastructure of the dog kidney collective tubules cell section in the norm.x22.000.

The structure of the nephron distal segment (Figure 45) resembles the proximal one but in contrast, the latter contains a greater quantity of oblong mitochondrias (M) located between the folds of the cytoplasmatic membrane (CM) and occupied the largest part of the cell, sometimes from its basal to apical field. Furthermore, the brush border (BB) is absent in the distal segment.

The collective tubules (Figure 46) are distinguished with the presence of light (LC) and dark (DC) cells. The light cells have a cubic form, with a smooth apical surface, contain a small quantity of mitochondrias (M) without distinct orientation, cisterns of the endoplasmatic net (ENC) and ribosomes (R). The dark cells are more planar and contain the same organelles located more compactly.

Thus, the ultrastructure of a dog's intact kidney doesn`t differ essentially from known literary data [225,303,322,348,400,443] and can be considered as an initial background state for comparison with experimental groups.

5.3. The State of the Kidney after Denervation In Situ

In the first group three days after the kidney denervation, it was united with surrounding tissue; its mass was 115.2+/-2.1% of that of the intact kidney ($p<0.01$, Table 15). Microscopically, a moderate hyperemia was revealed in the cortical as well as in the medullar substances of the kidney. The big, middle and small arteries were overcrowded with blood. Intertubular capillaries were also widened and contained deformed erytrocytes. Here and there the appearance of a diapedesis was observed.

In the perivascular kidney cortical substance, around the glomerulas and along tubules, a lymphoid infiltration was revealed. The glomerulas themselves were slightly full-blooded, the Bowman cavity was widened, the proximal and distal segments of the nephron were subjected to dystrophic changes, and sometimes contained hyaline cylinders.

In the juxtamedullar zone and medullar substance of the kidney the lymphoid infiltration was expressed less than in the cortical substance. The nephron thin segment and straight tubules were slightly widened, their epithelial cells were dystrophic, and sometimes their channels contained hyaline cylinders. The calices and pyelon walls were swelled. Here and there accumulations of lymphoid cells were observed.

Along the big blood vessels in longitudinal and cross-sections, the nerve bunches were seen. Their composition was not homogeneous. Side by side with relatively intact unmyelinized nerve fibers, swelled myelinized fibers with signs of degeneration were found. Also, the spherical growths in the field of preterminals attracted attention.

The specific fluorescence of catecholamines in the kidney parenchyma wasn't observed. The cholinergic nerve fibers were represented by single fibers along the big blood vessels. A decrease in color intensity as compared with the norm should be mentioned.

By electron microscope, within epithelial cells of the nephron proximal and distal segments, a swelling of mitochondrias and vacuolization of cytoplasma and osmiophyle granule inclusions (OGI) were observed (Figure 47). The other segments of the nephron were relatively intact.

Ten days after the kidney denervation its mass exceeded the contrary kidney. Their ratio was 113.1±1.9%, $p<0.01$, (Table 15). Histologic examination revealed a stagnation of the blood which in the medullar substance of the kidney was expressed more than in the cortical (Figure 48). At the same time the lymphoid infiltration in the latter was expressed more. One part of glomerula was full-blooded, with some shrinkaged, but the majority of them were quite intact. The nephron proximal and distal segments were dystrophic, single hyalinic cylinders were seen in their channels. The thin segment and straight tubules didn`t suffer any essential changes. The calices and pyelon walls were the sites of inflammation.

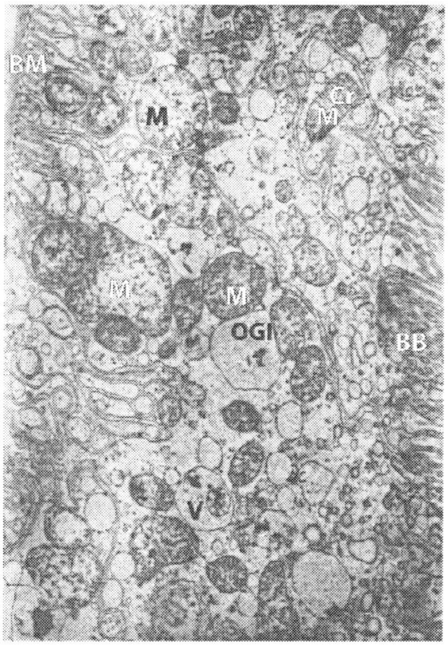

Figure 47. Ultrastructure of the nephron proximal segment epithelial cell section 3 days after the kidney denervation without surgical reinnervation. A swelling of some mitochondrias (M) and a cytoplasma vacuolization (V) are observed.x22.000.

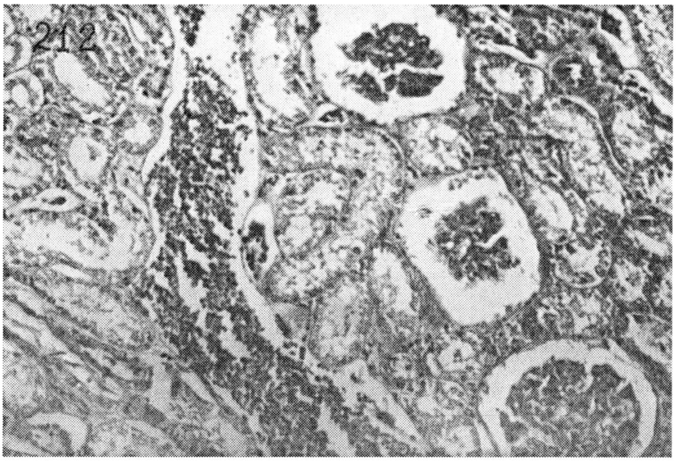

Figure 48. Microphotogram of the kidney 10 days after its denervation without surgical reinnervation. A blood stagnation in the parenchyma is observed. Painted with hematoxilin a.eosin.x200.

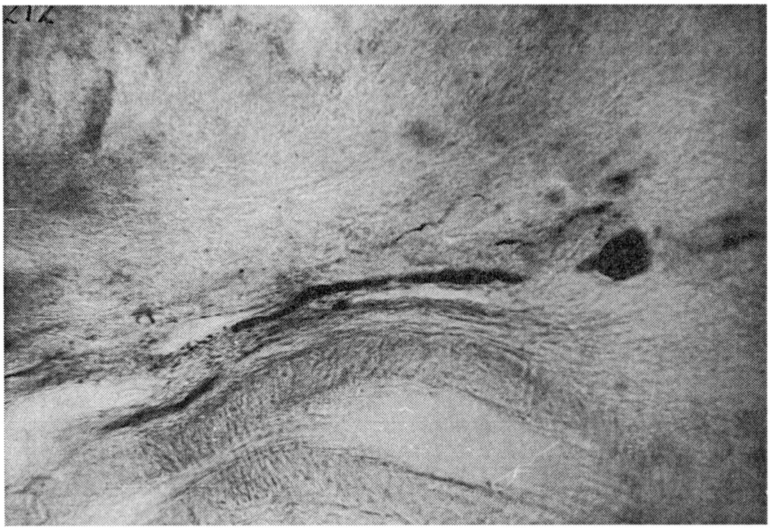

Figure 49. Microphotogram of the kidney 10 days after its denervation without surgical reinnervation. A degeneration of nerve fibers in the field of kidney blood vessels and pyelon is observed. Painted after Bilshovsky-Gross-Lavrentiev.x200.

The main part of intrarenal nerves was degenerated. This process was expressed irregularely. Some of them were quite intact, but their quantity was less than in the previous term (Figure 49).

48 hours after the intrarenal injection of the horse radish peroxidase, its presence in the ganglion cells of the spinal brain and border symphathetic trunk on the ThIX-LIII level was not observed (Figure 50). The adrenergic nerve fibers had not been revealed, as before (Figure 51). Single cholinergic nerve fibers were seen only along the big blood vessels. The ultrastructure of the kidney on the whole corresponded to that observed in the previous term.

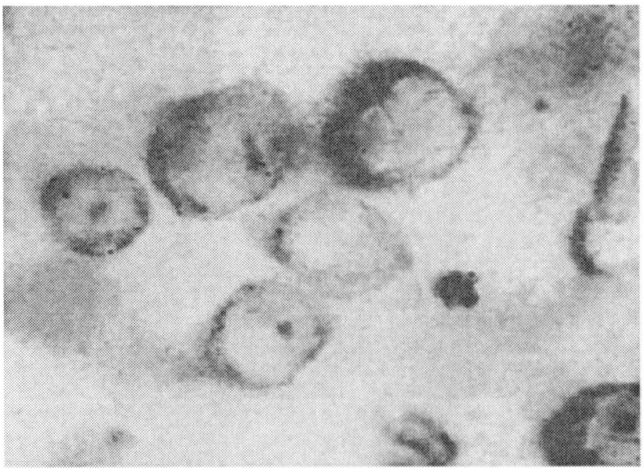

Figure 50. A section of the sympathetic trunk on the level of L1 10 days after the kidney denervation without surgical reinnervation. Ganglion cells do not contain the horse radish peroxidase granules. Painted after Mesulam.x900.

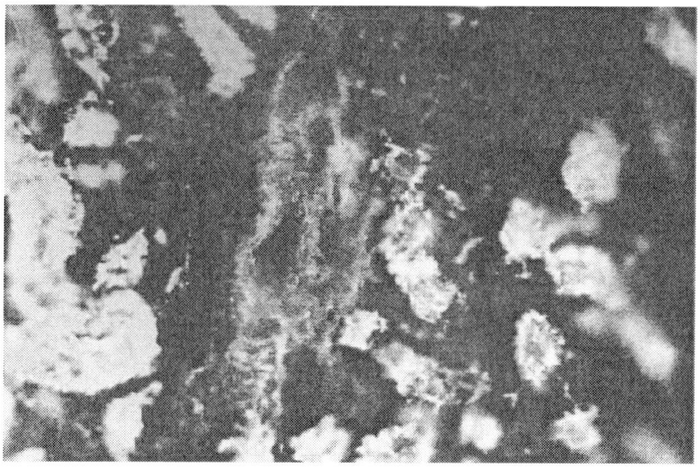

Figure 51. Microphotogram of the kidney 10 days after its denervation without surgical reinnervation. The catecholamines specific luminescence along the blood vessels and tubules is absent. Luminescent microscopy after Falck a. Owman. LUMAM I-1.x200.

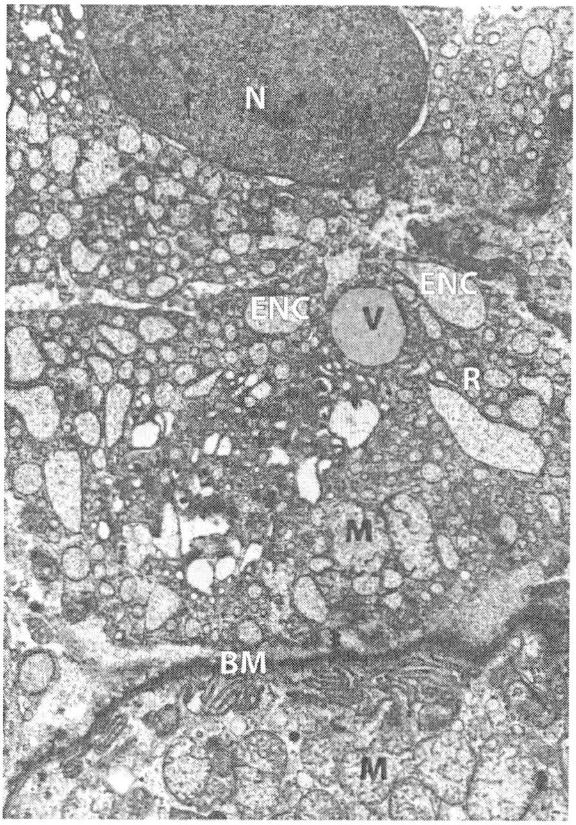

Figure 52. Electronogram of the nephron proximal segment epithelial cell section 1 month after the kidney denervation without surgical reinnervation. A swelling of some mitrochondrias (M), widening of endoplasmatic net cisterns (ENC) and accumulation of ribosom (R) on their external membranes are seen x20.000.

One month after the kidney denervation its mass ratio to the opposite kidney, as before, was 114.3±2.0%, p<0.01, Table 15). In the whole kidney parenchyma an expressed blood stagnation was seen. The development of young connective tissue around the blood vessels and lymphoid infiltration in the juxtamedullar zone were observed. A part of the glomerulas was shrunken but the rest was relatively intact. The nephron proximal and distal segments were subjected to hyalinic dystrophy. Its thin segment was without essential deviations. The straight tubules were surrounded with young connective tissue and contained single hyaline cylinders in their channel.

Almost all nerve elements in the kidney were degenerated. Neither fluorescent adrenergic nor cholinergic nerve fibers were observed.

Epithelial cells of the nephron's proximal and distal segments with swelled mitochondrias and widened cisterns of the endoplasmatic net with ribosomes accumulated on the external membrane were observed (Figure 52). The glomerulas, epithelial cells of the thin segment and the collective tubules were not changed much.

Two months after the denervation the kidney mass didn`t differ reliably from the intact side (106.1±1.3%, p>0.05, Table 15). The magistral blood vessels at the site of anastomosis were passable, their intima wall was smooth. In the kidney cortical and medullar substances the stagnation of blood, diapedesis, and lymphoid infiltration were revealed.

The walls of big, middle and small blood vessels were thickened. The connective tissue around them was matured (Figure 53).

In the kidney cortical and juxtamedullar zones the centres of sclerosis were observed. A part of the glomerula was hyperemized. The epithelial cells of the nephron tubule was in a state of albuminous dystrophy. Thickened layers of connective tissue were often found in the intertubular space.

Along the big blood vessels, side by side with empty nerve membranes, the single regenerating nerve fibers with growth heads were seen, but the fluorescent adrenergic nerves were absent (Figure 54). At the same time, single cholinergic nerve fibers were observed in the field of big blood vessels, the juxramedullar zone and in the pyelon wall. The ultrastructure of the kidney didn`t differ essentially from that of the previous term.

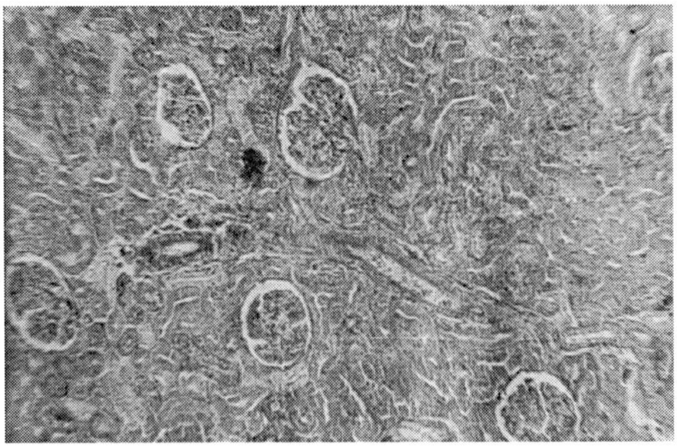

Figure 53. Microphotogram of the kidney 2 months after its denervation without surgical reinnervation. A blood stagnation is still remained in the parenchyma. Perivascularly and periglomerularly layers of a connective tissues are revealed. Painted after Mallory.x120.

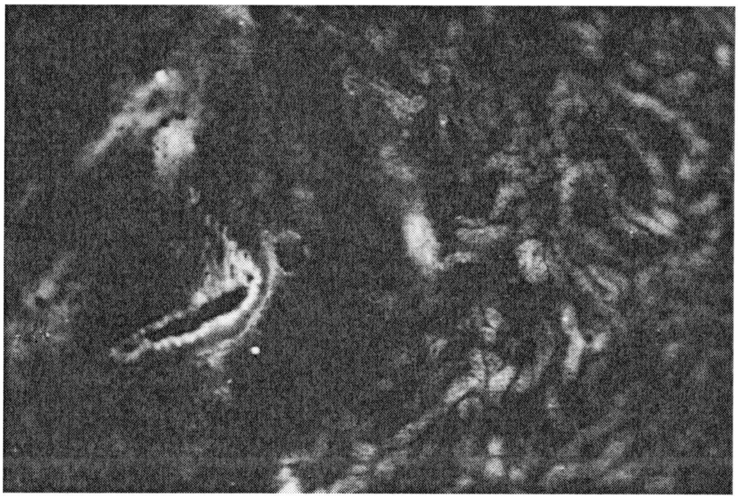

Figure 54. The same case. A specific luminescence of catecholamines along the blood vessel is absent. Luminescent microscopy after Fulck a. Owman. LUMAM I-1.x120.

Four months after the denervation the kidney had a slack consistency and its mass slightly lagged from the intact side (92,4±1,6, p<0,05, Table 15). In the juxtamedullar and medullar substances the blood was stagnated and the blood vessels walls were thickened. A diffusive development of rough connective tissue in the cortical substance and especially around the blood vessels and glomerulas was observed. The cortical substance on the whole was atrophic. The nephron proximal and distal segments and straight tubules suffered albuminous dystrophy, and the tubular channels became friable.

On the border between the cortical and medullar substances and along the arc arteries the germination of single unmyelinized nerve fibers was observed, but they were finished in the perivascular connective tissue. A specific luminescence of catecholamines in the kidney parenchyma and pyelon was not revealed. Around the blood vessels single cholinergic nerve fibers were seen.

By electron microscope a vacuolization in glomerular mezangial (Figure 55) and endothelial cells (Figure 56) attracted attention. The nephron epithelial cells of proximal and distal segments were characterized by a sharp widening of endoplasmatic net cisterns with circumferential accumulation of ribosomes on the external membrane. Furthermore, autophagic vacuoles (APV) were found there (Figure 57). The thin segment and collective tubules had a low electronic density and were subjected to the cell cytoplasma vacuolization.

Six months after the denervation, the kidney parenchyma was distinguished by low density as before, its mass was less than that of the opposite kidney (88.5±2.2%, p<0.01, Table 15). The diffusive, perivascular sclerosis and signs of atrophy in the glomerulars, nephron proximal segments and distal segments was observed.

The structure of the kidney nervous apparatus didn`t differ essentially from the previous term (Figure 58, 59). The transfer of horse radish peroxidase from the kidney parenchyma to ganglion cells of the spinal brain didn`t occur. Electron microscopic pictures on the whole were the same as in the previous term (Figure 60, 61). The kidney ultrastructure was relatively intact.

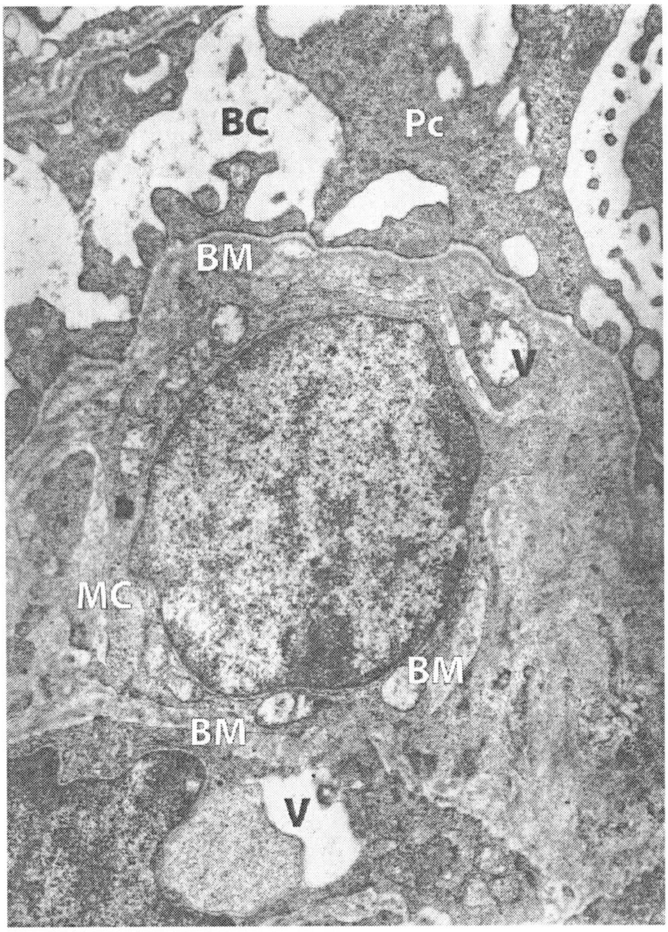

Figure 55. Electronogram of the kidney glomerular section 4 months after its denervation without surgical reinnervation. The vacuolization (v) of a mesangial cell (MC) is observed.x30.000.

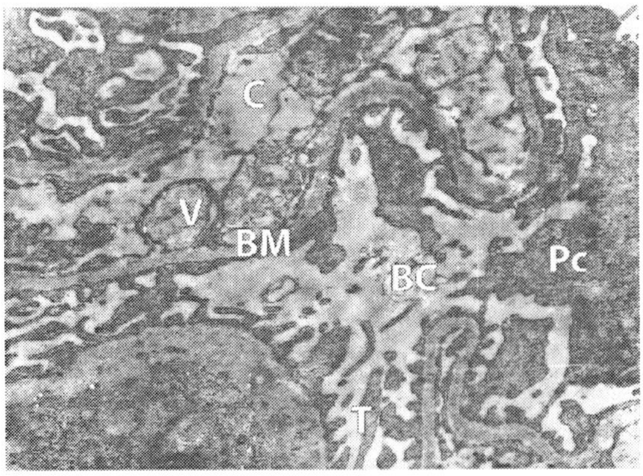

Figure 56. Electronogram of the kidney glomerula section 4 months after its denervation without surgical neinnervation. In some places the cytoplasmatic membrane of the capillary (C) endothelial cell is exfoliated from the basal membrane (BM) and creates finger-like growings with vacuoles (V) inside.x8000.

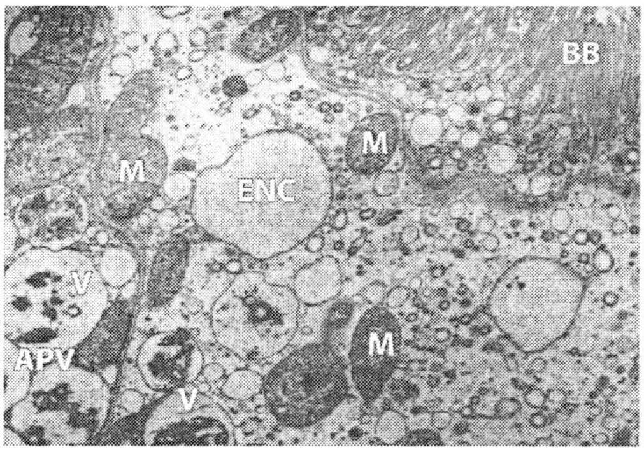

Figure 57. The same case. in the epithelial cell of the nephron proximal segment a widening of endoplamsatic net cisterns (ENC), swelling of mitochondrias (M) and appearance of autophagic vacuoles (APV) are observed.x12.000.

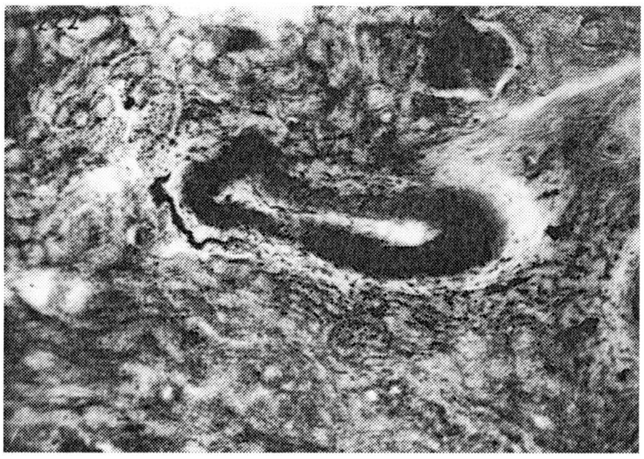

Figure 58. Microphotogram of the kidney 6 kidney 6 months after its denervation without surgical reinnervation. In the field of the pyelong blood vessel single nerve fibers are revealed. Panted after Bilshovsky-Gross-Lavrentjev.x200.

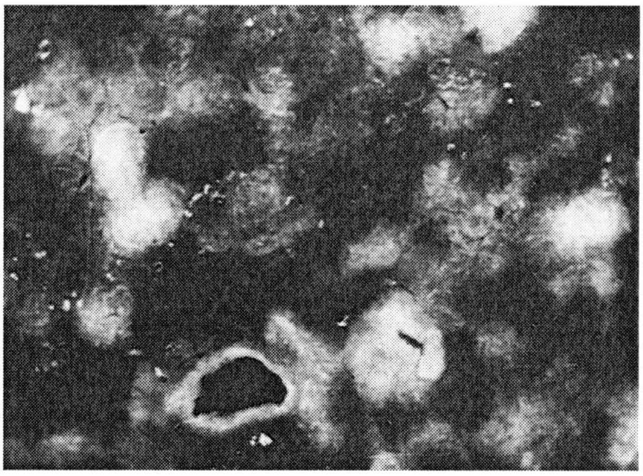

Figure 59. The same case. The catecholamines specific luminescence along the blood vessel is absent. Luminescent microscopy after Falck-Owman. LUMAM I-1.x200.

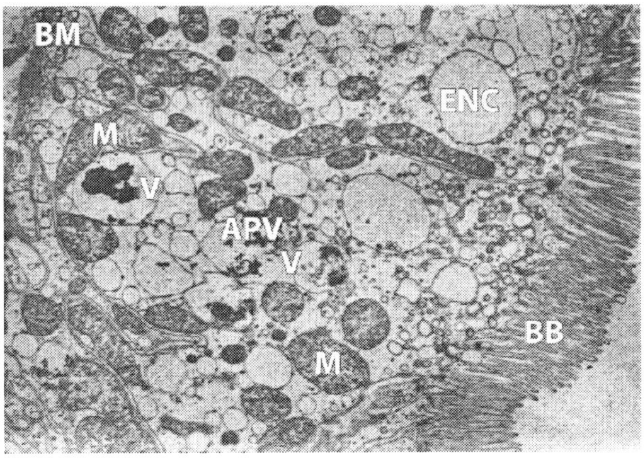

Figure 60. Electronogram of an epithelial cell section of the nephron proximal segment 6 months afater the kidney denervation without surgical reinnervation. A vacuolization (V) of cytoplasma at the expense of widening of endoplasmatic net cisterns (ENC), swelling of mitochondrias (M), in some cases their destruction with autophagocytosis (APV) are observed.x12.000.

One year after the operation the kidney, seen macroscopically, was atrophied, had a soft and slack consistency, and was behind the opposite kidney in size and mass (72.2±2.7%, $p<0.001$, Table 15). Histologic examination revealed the blood stagnation, diapidesis and advanced diffusive sclerosis in the kidney cortical substance. A part of the glomerulas was hyperemized, atrophied, surrounded with thickened, with a sclerosed capsule. The epithelium of the nephron proximal and distal segments suffered various degrees of dystrophy from parenchymatous to hyalinous.

On the border between the cortical and medullar substances the scared tissue was expressed much more. The channels of straight tubules were widened and their epithelial cells atrophied. The walls of calices and pyelon were also partially sclerosed and atrophied.

Along the big blood vessels there were the nervous fibers with single branches which were lost in the connective tissue.

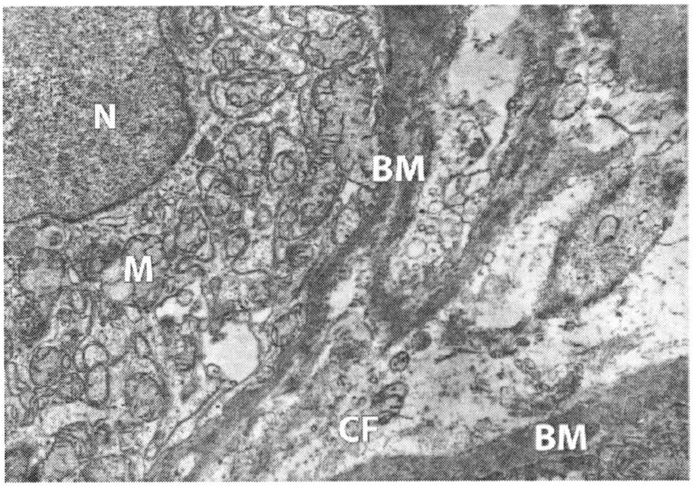

Figure 61. The same case. Intertubular splits contain a large quantity of collagen fibers (CF).x11.000.

In the cortical and medullar substances of the kidney, as well as in the field of the glomerulas and tubules, regenerated nervous elements were not found out.

The luminescent adrenergic nerves were also not detected. A cholinergic innervation was represented very scantily, and was only along the pyelon blood vessels. The ultrastructure of the kidney was not changed as compared with the previous term.

Two years after the denervation the kidney showed shrinkage and was atrophied with a slack consistency. Its mass was 63.1±3.0% of the opposite kidney mass ($p<0,001$, Table 15, Figure 62). In the kidney parenchyma there was blood stagnation, and local and diffusive sclerosis. The rough scared tissue was mainly expressed in the blood vessels walls, around them and on the glomerulas. Many glomerulas were atrophied, others were full-blooded or hyalinized. But half of the glomerulas were relatively preserved. Proximal and distal segments of the nephron were dystrophic.

The nerve elements of the kidney were represented mainly with empty Shwann membranes and single regenerated nerve fibers along the blood vessels and in the connective tissue skeleton of the kidney. In the field of the glomerulas and tubules the nerve elements including the fluorescent adrenergic elements were not detected. Cholinergic nerves were seen only along the big blood vessels in the kidney pyelon. 48 hours after the horse radish peroxidase intrarenal injection, penetration to the ganglion cells of the spinal brain and sympathetic trunk was not found (Figure 63). By electron microscope, dystrophic and sclerotic changes were observed in the kidney, as in the previous term.

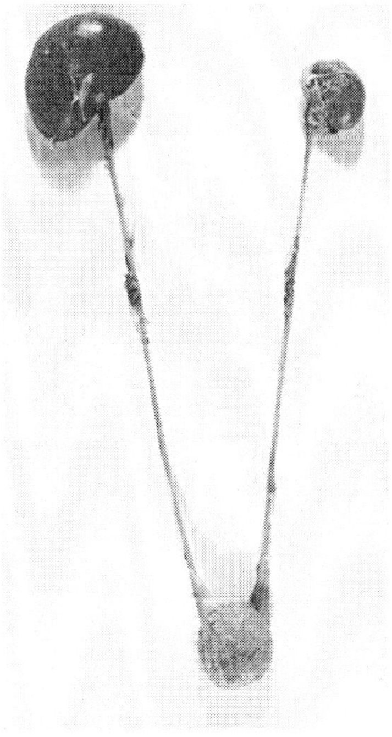

Figure 62. A macromorphologic preparation of kidneys 2 years after denervation of the left kidney without its surgical reinnervation. A considerable atrophy of an operated (left) kidney and a vicarious hypertrophy of an intact (right) kidney are observed.

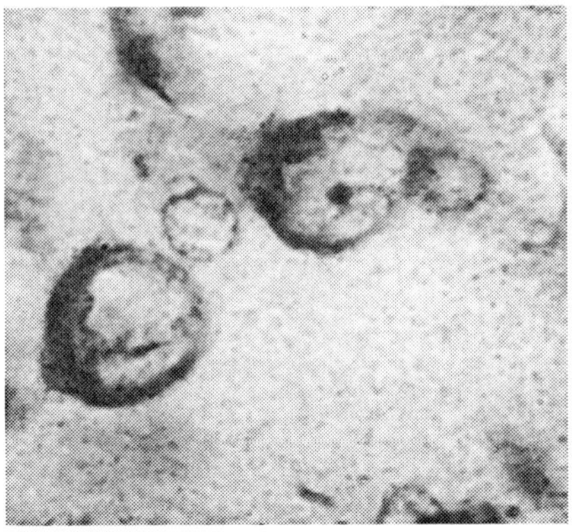

Figure 63. Section of a lateral horn of the spinal brain on the level of L1 2 years after the kidney denervation without surgical reinnervation. The granules of a horse radish peroxidase are not revealed in the ganglion cells. Painted after Mesulam.x900.

5.4. The State of the Kidney after Denervation in Situ and Surgical Reinnervation

In the second group of experiments, within the first ten days after the denervation and surgical reinnervation of the kidney, its mass was slightly increased compared to the opposite side (114.8±2.2, $p<0.01$, Table 15). In the cortical substance a somewhat expressed hyperemia and local lymphoid infiltration were observed. Capillaries of some glomerulas were full-blooded, but the majority of them had a normal structure. The epithelial cell of the nephron proximal segment were not changed much, at the same time in the distal tubules, signs of hyalinous dystrophy were observed. The nephron thin segment was relatively intact but in collective tubules the epithelial cells were swelled and their channels were narrowed. The walls of the kidney calices and pyelon were hyperemiezed and lymphoid infiltration was seen in the submucosal layer.

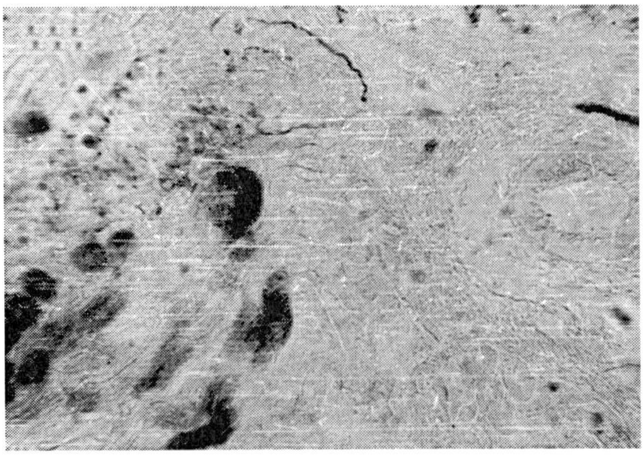

Figure 64. Microphotogram of the kidney 10 days after its denervatioN and surgical reinnervation. Degenerating nerve fibers are seen along the blood vessels. Painted after Bilshovsky-Gross-Lavrentjev.x200.

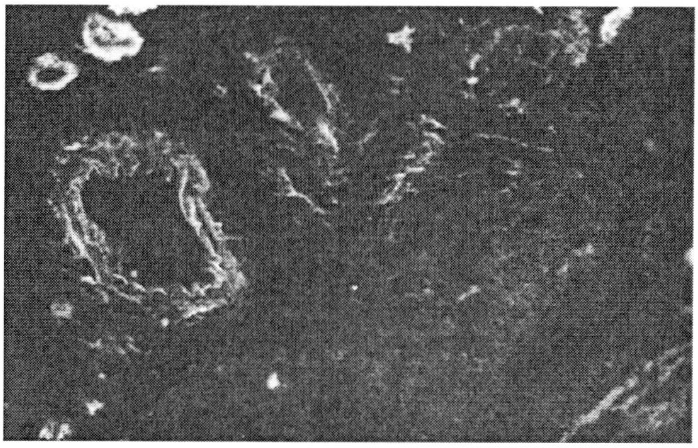

Figure 65. The same case. A specific luminescence of catecholamines along the blood vessels is absent. Luminescent microscopy after Falck a. Owman. LUMAM I-1.x200.

The nervous trunks were found along the big blood vessels, a considerable part of them was degenerated (Figure 64), while others were intact but the specific luminescence of catecholamines were not detected (Figure 65). In the pyelon walls and along the big blood vessels single cholinergic nerve fibers were observed. The trial with the transport of horse radish peroxidase was negative.

By electron microscope, some kidney glomerulas were hyperemized. In the epithelial cells of the nephron proximal and distal segments a vacuolization of cytoplasma and swelling of mitochondrias were observed (Figure 66). In the thin segment and collective tubules such changes were uncommon.

One month after the operation the kidney didn`t differ from the opposite one in size or mass (Table 15).

Microscopically, in the kidney cortical substance a moderate hyperemia, blood stagnation, and rare places of lymphoid infiltration near the glomerulas were observed. Parts of the glomerulas were full-blooded, but the majority of them were intact.

In various parts of the proximal nephron, thin and distal segments, hyalinous dystrophy was revealed, but their channels were preserved. In the kidney calices and pyelon, mainly in the submucosal layer, the signs of blood stagnation and lymphoid infiltration were sometimes observed.

Neurohistologic examination revealed the beginning of nerve fiber regeneration along the big blood vessels and in the pyelon wall, but the specific luminescence of catecholamines was not detected. The cholinergic nerve fibers formed nets in the walls of the calices, pyelon and around the big blood vessels.

The ultrastructure of the kidney was essentially not changed compared to the previous term.

Two months after the operation the operated and intact kidneys didn`t differ in size, consistency or mass (Table 15). Microscopically, only a small part of the glomerulas were full-blooded, while the others were quite intact. The nephron proximal, thin and distal segments were subjected to hyalinous dystrophy. In the juxtamedullar and medullar substances a small hyperemia was still preserved, but lymphoid infiltration was not observed there. The straight tubules were without visible pathologic changes. The calices and pyelon walls were slightly hyperemized.

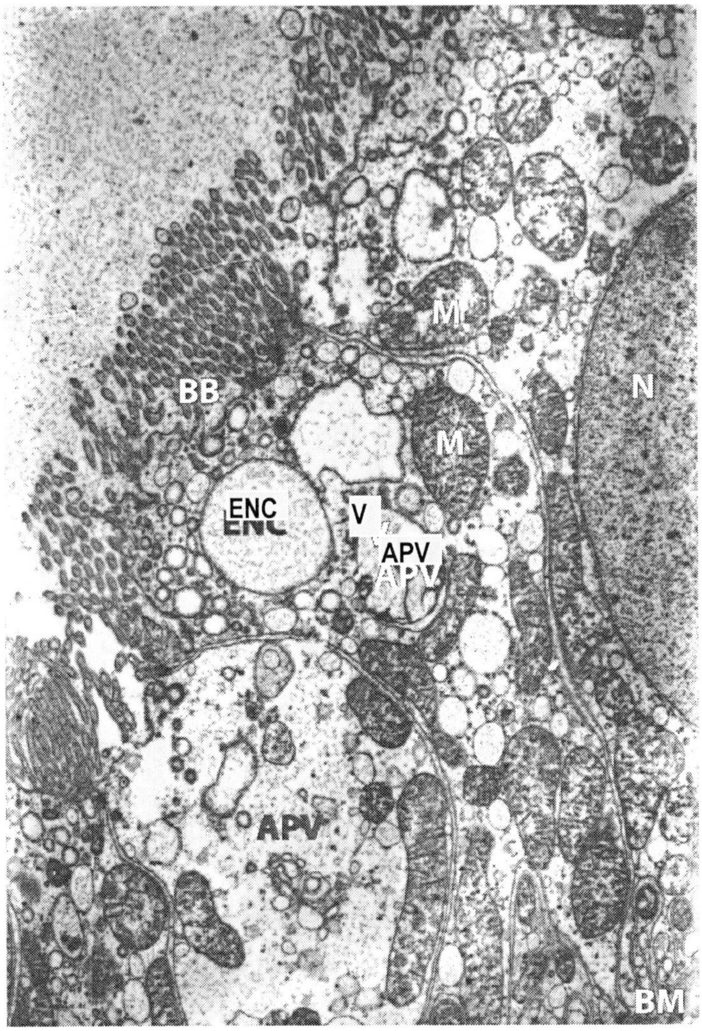

Figure 66. Electronogram of an epithelial cell section of the nephron proximal segment 10 days after the denervation and surgical reinnervation of the kidney. A vacuolization (V) of cytoplasma and swelling of some mitochondrias (M) are observed.x15.000.

Along the arc arteries the large nerve trunks were detected, they made thin branches oriented with the glomerulas and pyelon. Some of them had "growth heads". In the field around the arc arteries a weak specific luminescence of catecholamines was detected (Figures 67,68). The localization and structure of the cholinergic nerve fibers didn`t differ from the previous term.

Four months after the operation the operated kidney had the same size, consistency and mass as the opposite intact kidney (Table 15). Histologically most of the glomerulas didn`t show any pathologic changes. The interstitial tissue was free from sclerotic processes. The juxtamedullar zone, medullar substance, and the walls of the calices and pyelon were without any pathologic deviations.

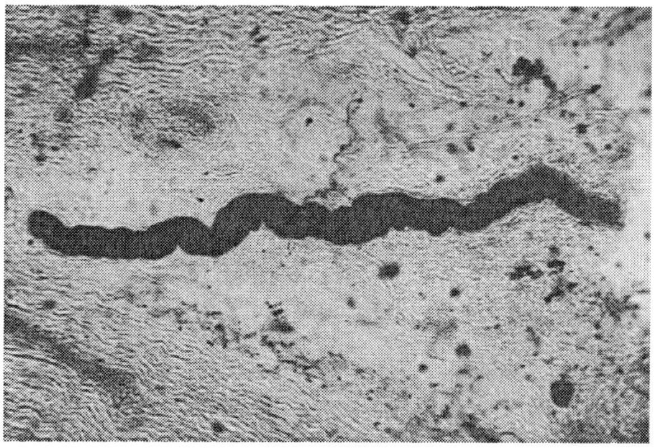

Figure 67. Microphotogram of the kidney 2 months after its denervation and surgical reinnervation. In the field of the pyelon the germination of a thin nerve fibers from the large nerve trunk is observed. Painted after Bilshovsky-Gros-Lavrentjev.x200.

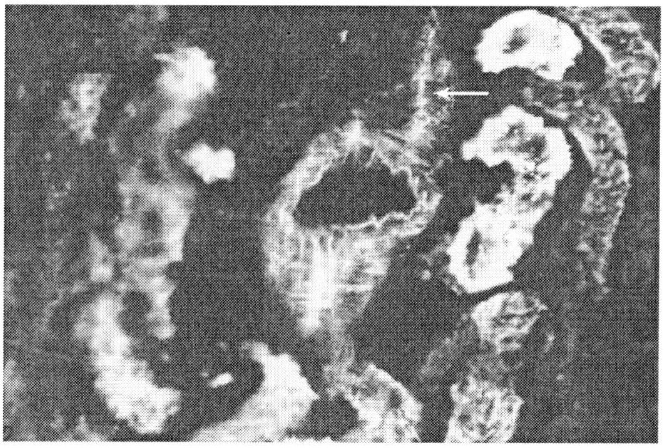

Figure 68. The same case. A weak luminescence in the vascular adventitial layer is traced (indicated with an arrow). Luminescent microscopy after Falck a. Owman. LUMAM I-1.x200.

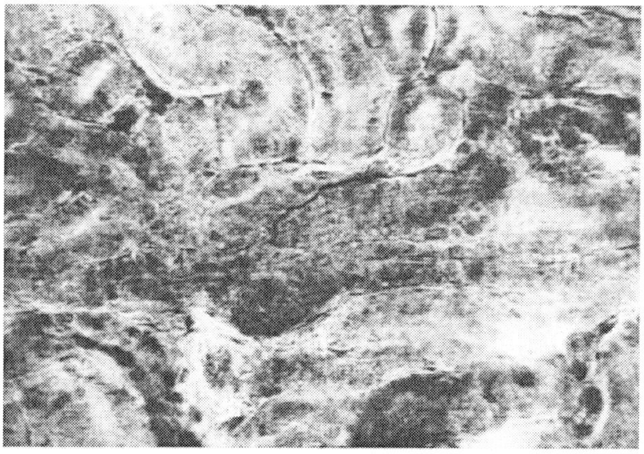

Figure 69. Microphotogram of a kidney 4 months after its denervation and surgical reinnervation. Germinating nerve fibers arrive at tubules. Painted after Bilshevsky-Gros-Lavrentjev.x200.

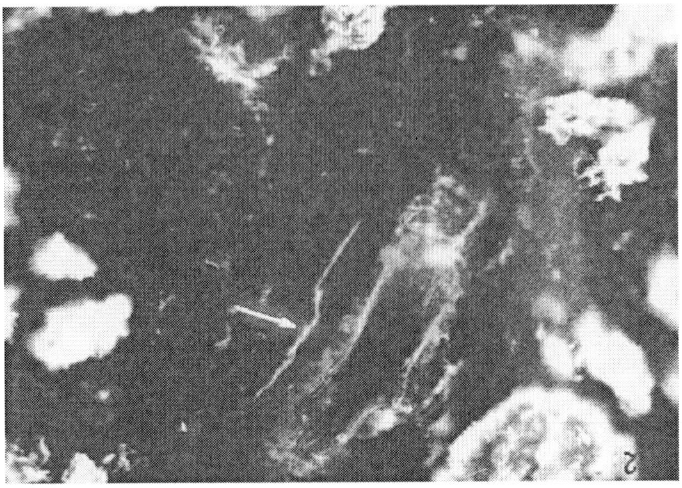

Figure 70. The same case. A luminous adrenergic nerve fiber is seen along the blood vessel (indicated with an arrow). Luminescent microscopy after Falck a. Owman. LUMAM I-1.x200.

Along the big arteries and arterioles, in longitudinal and cross-sections, regenerated nervous trunks were often found, they made branches which reached the glomerulas, tubules and pyelon walls with their terminals (Figure 69). On the border between the cortical and medullar substances a weak specific luminescence was observed (Figure 70). The structure of cholinergic nerve fibers was, as before.

The kidney ultrastructure corresponded to the standard (Figure 71).

Six months after the operation the general morphologic and neurohistologic structure of the kidney didn`t differ essentially from the previous term (Figure 72). Two days after the intrarenal injection of horse radish peroxidase its granules were detected in ganglion cells of the lateral horns of the spinal brain and sympathetic trunk on the level of ThXII-LII (Figure 73).

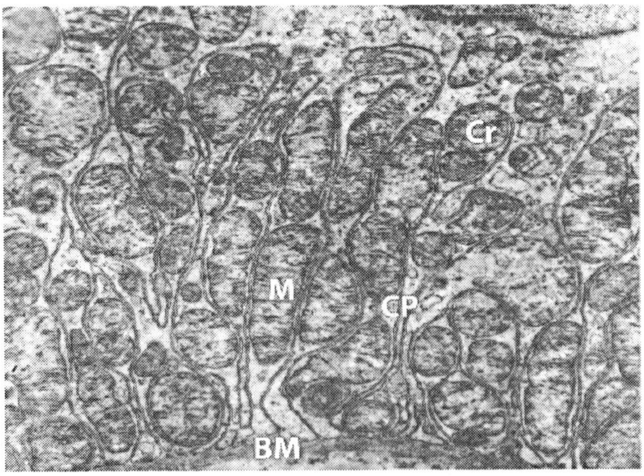

Figure 71. Electronogram of an epithelial cell of the nephron distal segment 4 months after the denervation and surgical reinervation of the kidney. Any essential pathology is not revealed.x15.000.

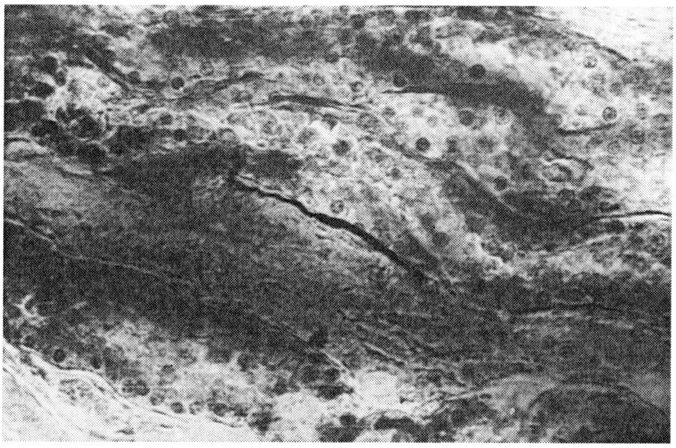

Figure 72. Microphotogram of a kidney 6 months after its denervation and surgical reinnervation. In the field of nephron tubules a germinated nerve fiber is seen. Painted after Rasskasova.x200.

One to two years after the operation, macroscopically, the kidney didn`t differ from the opposite one in size, consistency or mass (Table 15). The blood vessels had an histologically elastic structure. The interstitial tissue did not experience sclerosis. The glomerulas were surrounded with an elastic membrane. The epithelial cells of the nephron proximal, thin and distal segments didn`t show any visible pathology. The walls of the kidney calices and pyelon had a normal structure.

Along the blood vessels the nerve trunks were observed with branches germinated up to the glomerulas, tubules and pyelon.

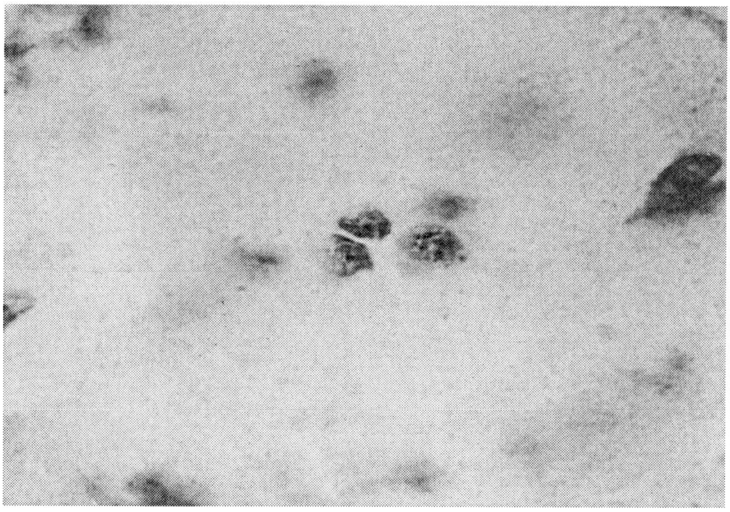

Figure 73. Section of a lateral horn of the spinal brain on the level of L1 6 months after the kidney denervation and surgical reinnervation. Small granules of the horse radish peroxidase are revealed in the ganglion cells. Painted after Mesulam.x600.

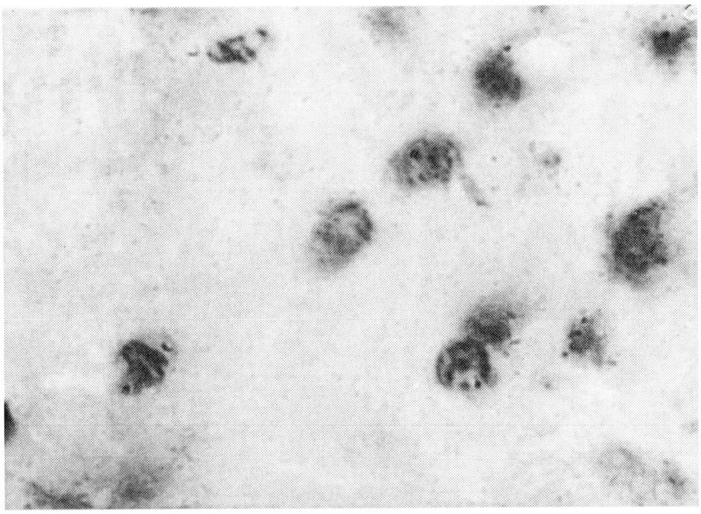

Figure 74. Section of a lateral horn of the spinal brain on the level of L1 2 years after the denervation and surgical reinnervation of the kidney. Granules of the horse radish peroxidase are seen in the ganglion cells. Painted after Mesulam.x600.

Adrenergic nerve fibers were represented with intensive luminescent adventitial nets around the kidney arc arteries. Some thin branches reached the glomerulas and tubules. In the pyelon walls and along the big and middle arteries the cholinergic nerve fibers were seen, their structure didn`t differ from the standard.

Two days after the injection of the horse radish peroxidase into the living kidney, from the two year test-group, the small granules (0.1-0.5 mcm size - the product of the reaction of peroxidase with diaminobenzidyne) were found in ganglion cells of the lateral horns of the spinal brain and homolateral sympathetic trunk on the level of ThXII-LII (Figure 74).

The ultrastructure of the kidney was quite normal.

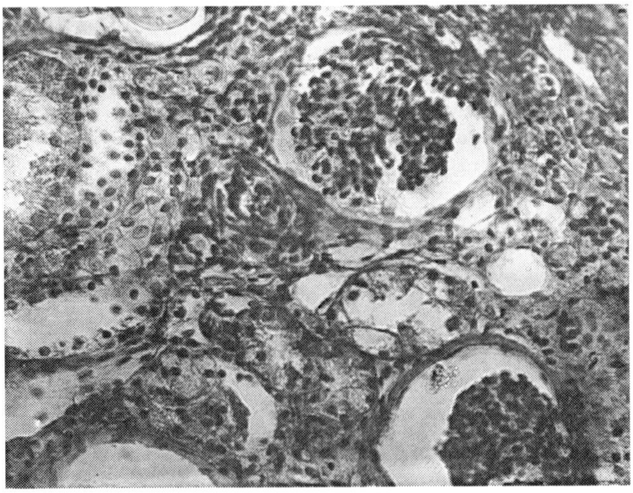

Figure 75. Microphotogram of a kidney 10 days after its autotransplantation without surgical reinnervation. A local lymphoid infiltration and dystrophy of a tubular epithelium are revealed in the cortical substance. Painted with hermatoxilin a. eosin.x250.

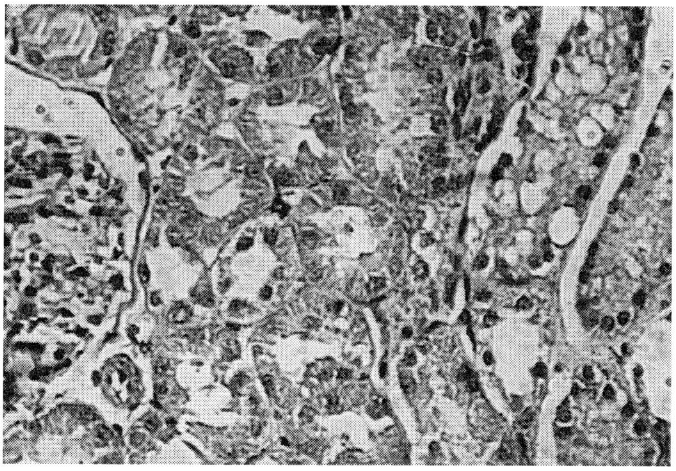

Figure 76. The same case. A dystrophy and vacuolization of the tubular epithelium are seen in the kidney cortical substance. Painted with hematoxilin a. eosin.x400.

5.5. The State of Autotransplanted Kidney

In the third group of experiments after kidney autotransplantation without surgical reinnervation in the first ten days the kidney increased in size and mass compared to the intact kidney (152.9±3.5, $p<0.001$, Table 15). Histologically, stagnation of blood with erythrocyte diapedesis in the transplant juxtamedullar amd medullar substances was observed. At the same time, lymphoid-cell infiltration and dystrophy in the kidney cortical substance were more expressed (Figure 75, 76). The nephron thin segment and collective tubules were relatively intact. Small lymphoid infiltrates in the calices and pyelon walls were observed.

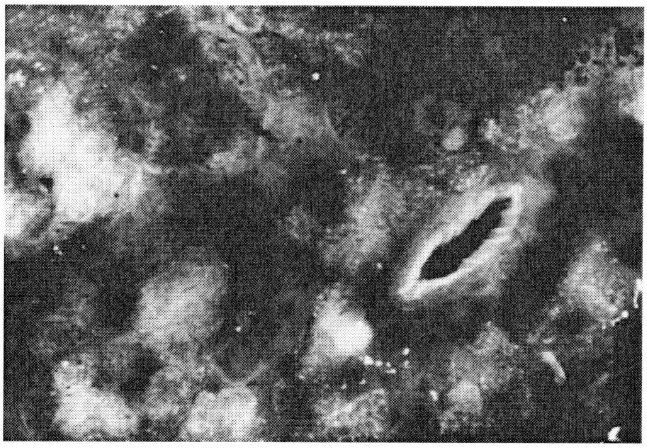

Figure 77. Microphotogram of a kidney 10 days after its autotransplantation without surgical reinnervation. A specific catecholamine luminescence in the periadventitial tissue is absent. Luminescent microscopy after Falck a. Owman. LUMAM I-1.

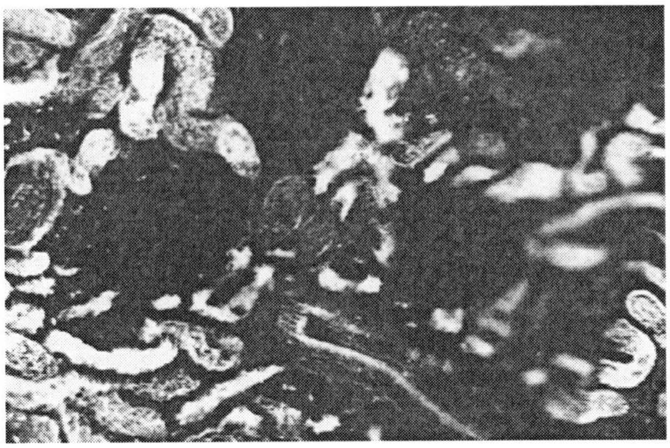

Figure 78. The same case. A specific catecholamineluminescence in the field of tubules, glomerulas, juxtamedullar apparatus is also absent. Luminescent microscopy after Falck a. Owman. LUMAM I-1.x200.

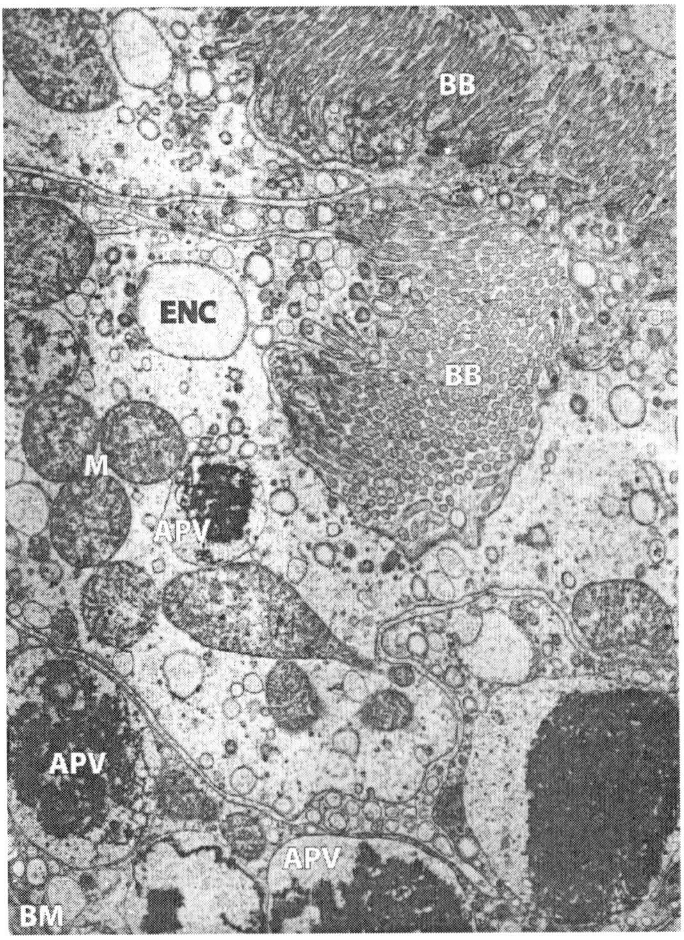

Figure 79. Electronogram of the nephron proximal segment epithelial cell 10 days after the autotransplantation of the kidney without its surgical reinnervation. A swelling of mitochondrias (M) and appearance of autophagic vacuoles (APV) are revealed.x20.000.

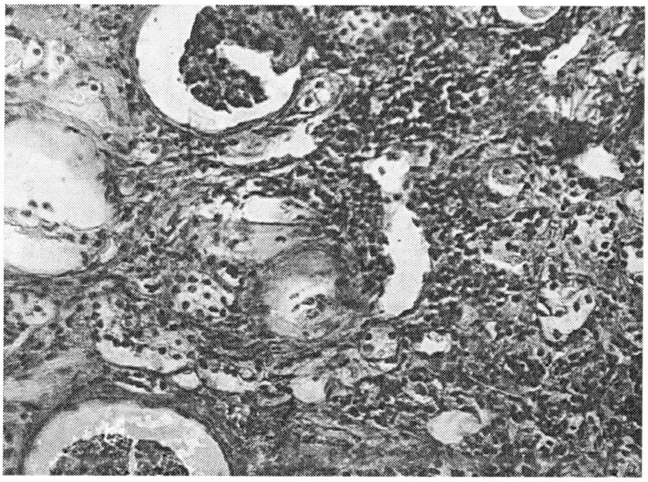

Figure 80. Microphotogram of a kidney 2 months after its autotransplantation without surgical reinnervation. A local lymphoid infiltration and perivascular sclerosis are observed in the cortical substance. Painted with hematoxilin a. eosin.x200.

The majority of the kidney nerve fibers underwent degeneration, but only one of them were preserved. Adrenergic nerves had lost their ability for luminescence (Figure 77,78).

Some cholinergic nerve fibers along the big arteries were safe.

The test with the horse radish peroxidase was negative.

By electron microscope, epithelial cells of the nephron proximal and distal segments showed slightly swelled mitochondrias and autophagic vacuoles (Figure 79). The thin segment and collective tubules didn`t suffer any essential changes.

One to two months later the operated kidney surpassed the intact one in mass (130.3±3.6%, $p<0.001$, Table 15).

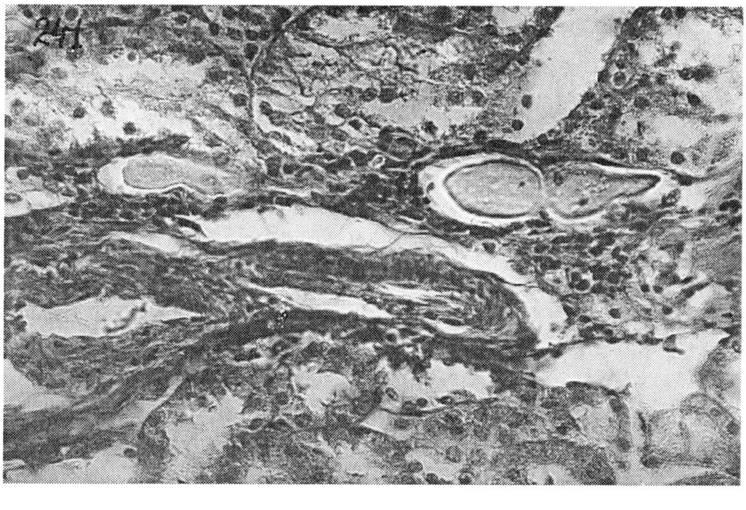

Figure 81. The same case. A connective tissues is traced around the blood vessel. Painted after Van-Gison.x200.

Microscopically, in the kidney cortical and medullar substances, blood stagnation and local infiltration were observed. The walls of big, middle and small arteries and veins were thickened. Partially in the cortical and medullar substances, and essentially in the juxtanedullar zone, a local sclerosis was detected (Figures 80, 81). Parts of the glomerulas were hyperemized, while others were atrophied or oblitered, but nearly half of them remained safe. Epithelial cells of various segments of the nephron suffered albuminous dystrophy.

If after one month the nerve elements of the kidney were degenerated, two months later the single regenerating nerve fibers with growth heads appeared. They germinated through the empty nerve membranes along the big blood vessels.

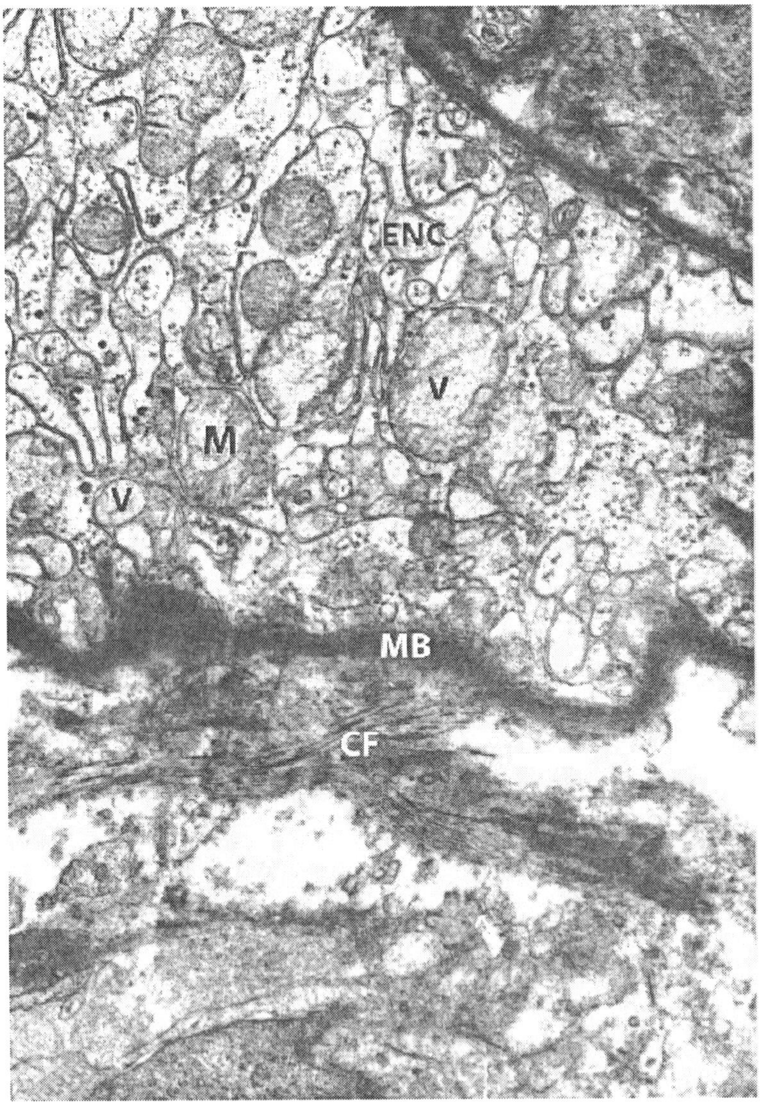

Figure 82. Electronogram of the nephron distal segment epithelial cell 4 months after the autotransplantation of the kidney without its surgical reinnervation. A swelling of mitochondrias (M), vacuolization (V) of cytoplasma, formation of collagen fibers 9CF) in the intertubular space are observed.x20.000.

The adrenergic nerves with a specific luminescence were not detected, as before. At the same time single unmyelinized cholinergic nerve fibers were seen in the juxtamedullar zone, pyelon and along the big arteries of the kidney.

The ultrastructure of the kidney was mainly the same as the previous term.

Four months later the operated kidney became equal to the intact kidney in mass (98.1±1.1%, p>0.05, Table 15). In comparison to the previous terms, the initial signs of diffusive sclerosis have to be mentioned, especially around the blood vessels in the kidney cortical substance.

Along the big blood vessels in the juxtamedullar zone there were slightly more germinated unmyelinized nerve fibers as compared with the previous term, but they stopped in the connective tissue and didn`t reach the nephrons. The luminescent adrenergic nerve fibers were not detected in the kidney parenchyma and pyelon. Now and then single cholinergic nerve fibers were seen around the big arteries and in the pyelon wall.

By electron microscope, in the epithelial cells of the proximal and distal segments of the nephron, swelling of the mitochondrias, cytoplasma vacuolization, and the appearance of connective tissue in the intertubular space were observed (Figure 82).

Six months after the operation the kidney had a slack consistency. Its mass was lower than the intact kidney (89.0±1.0, p<0.01, Table 15).

Histologically, parts of the blood vessels had sclerosed. Furthermore, diffusive sclerosis was observed in the entire kidney parenchyma. In the cortical substance of the kidney local upsettings were mentioned. Parallel with normal and even hypertrophied glomerulas, there were also atrophied and empty structures with small local necroses. It seems that an embolization of nourishing blood vessels occurred with subsequent necroses in the cortical substance. The proximal and distal segments of the nephron were subjected to dystrophy and contained hyalinous cylinders in their channels. In the juxtamedullar and medullar substances of the kidney a blood stagnation was seen and blood vessel sclerosis. The channels of straight tubules were widened and gaped.

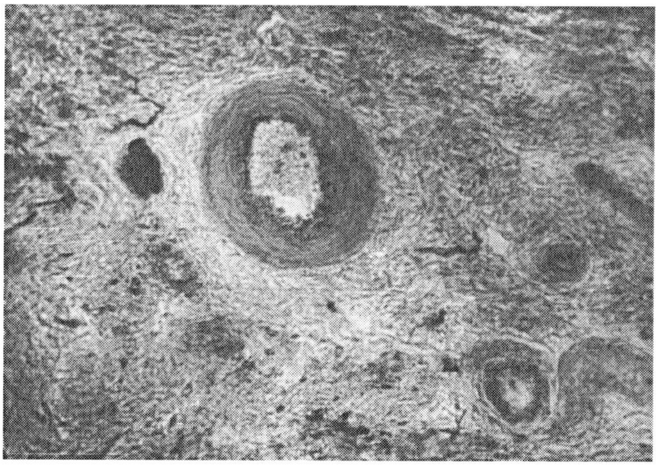

Figure 83. Microphotogram of the kidney 6 months after its autotransplantation without surgical reinnervation. Single thin nerve fibers are traced in the perivascular connective tissue. Painted after Bilshovsky-Gros-Lavrentjev.x200.

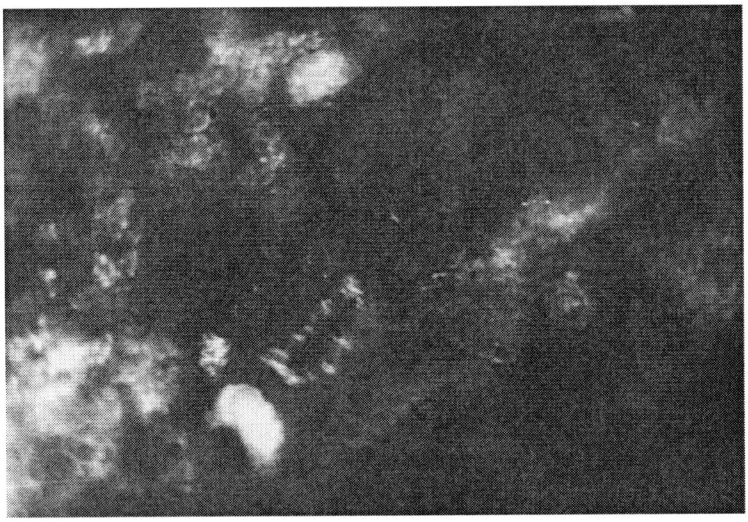

Figure 84. The same case. The catecholamine specific luminescence in he perivascular field is absent. Luminescent microscopy after Falck a. Owman. LUMAM I-1.x150.

In the calices and pyelon walls, scared tissue was seen. The single unmyelinized nerve fibers, germinated along the blood vessels, reached the pyelon walls but they didn`t run through the kidney connective tissue skeleton to its parenchyma (Figure 83). The luminescence reaction for catecholamines was negative, as before (Figure 84). Poor development of cholinergic nerve fibers along the big renal arteries and the pyelon walls was seen. The horse radish peroxidase test didn`t detect any transport ability of the renal afferent nerve elements (Figure 85).

Election microscope pictures, on the whole, corresponded to the previous findings (Figure 86).

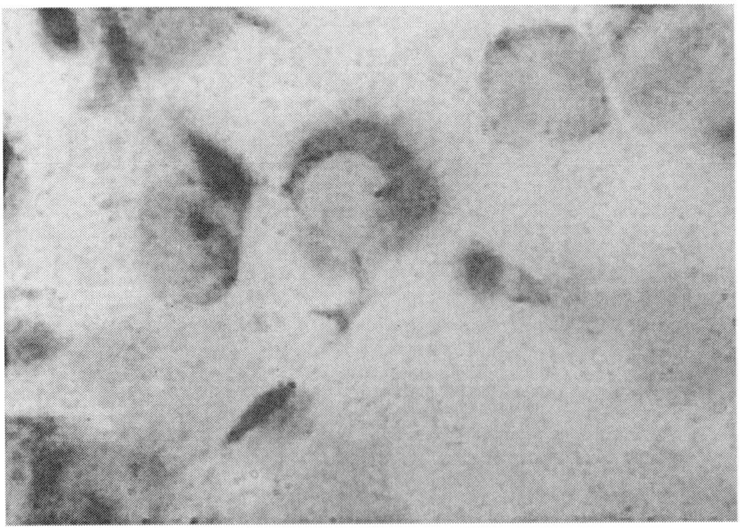

Figure 85. The section of the spinal brain lateral horne on the level of L1 6 months after the kidney autotransplantation without surgical reinnervation. Granules of horse radish peroxidase in the ganglion cells are not found. Painted after Mesulam.x900.

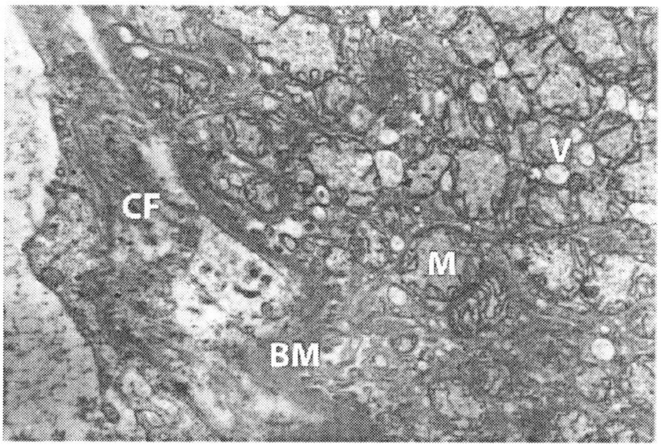

Figure 86. Electronogram of the nephron proximal segment epithelial cell 6 months after the kidney transplantation without surgical reinnervation. A swelling of mitochondrias (M), vacuolization 9V) of cytoplasma, formation collagen fibers 9CF) in the intertubular space are mentioned.x15.000.

One year after the transplantation the kidney had a slack consistency, was atrophied, and its mass was 71.3+/-1.8% of the opposite intact kidney (p<0.001, Table 15).

Microscopically, in the kidney cortical and medullar substances and on the border between them, blood stagnation and diapedesis were maintained. In the entire parenchyma and especially in its cortical substance, diffusive sclerosis was expressed more than before (Figures 87, 88). The walls of the calices and pyelon were also sclerosed and atrophied.

Partially regenerated nerve fibers along the magistral renal blood vessels were observed. They gave single unmyelinized nerve branches ending in the connective tissue, which didn`t reach the glomerulas and tubules. The specific luminescence of catecholamines was absent, as before. Single cholinergic nerve fibers were found now and then around the blood vessels and in the field of the pyelon.

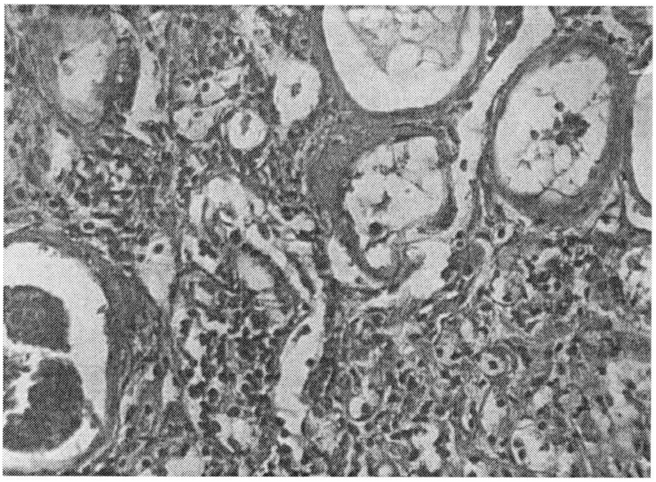

Figure 87. Microphotogram of the kidney 1 year after its autotransplantation without surgical reinnervation. A periglomerular sclerosis and atrophy of the tubular epithelium are observed. Painted after Mallory.x300.

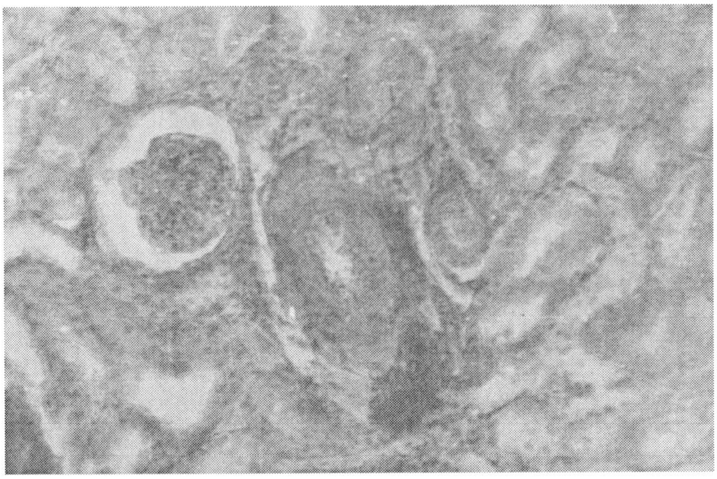

Figure 88. The same case. An expressed perivascular sclerosis is seen. Painted after Van-Gison.x250.

Two years after the operation the kidney was shrunken much more and atrophied, its mass was 61.0±2.2% of the opposite kidney ($p<0,001$, Table 15). Moderate blood stagnation, local and diffusive sclerosis, and atrophy of parts of the glomerulas and epithelial cells were seen on the background of others hyperthrophy (Figures 89, 90).

A nervous apparatus was represented scantily, with empty nerve membranes and a small quantity of regenerated unmyelinized nerve fibers. They sometimes reached the pyelon walls. Single thin cholinergic nerve fibers were only found along the magistral renal blood vessels. The testings with catecholamins luminescence and horse radish peroxidase were negative, as before.

By electron microscope, the changes mentioned above were maintained. The sclerosis process advanced much more in the intertubular space (Figure 91). At the same time there were cells with relatively intact ultrastructure.

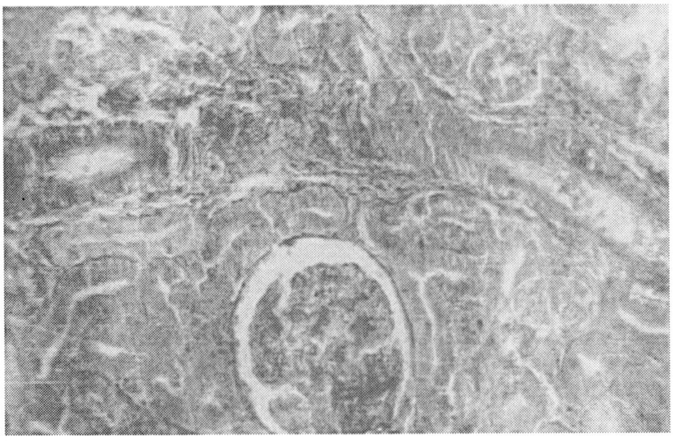

Figure 89. Microphotogram of the kidney 2 years after the kidney autotransplantation without surgical rinnervation. A blood stagnation in the cortical substance is observed. Painted after Mallory.x300.

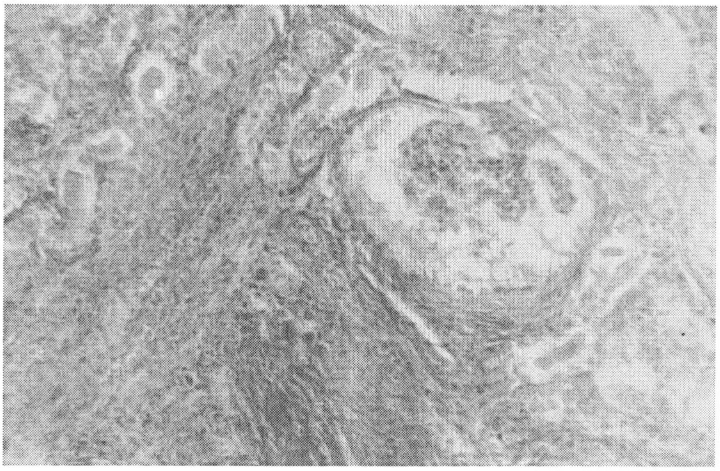

Figure 90. The same case. A growing periglomerular, local and diffusive sclerosis, atrophy of some glomerulas and epithelial cells are observed. painted after Van-Gison,x300.

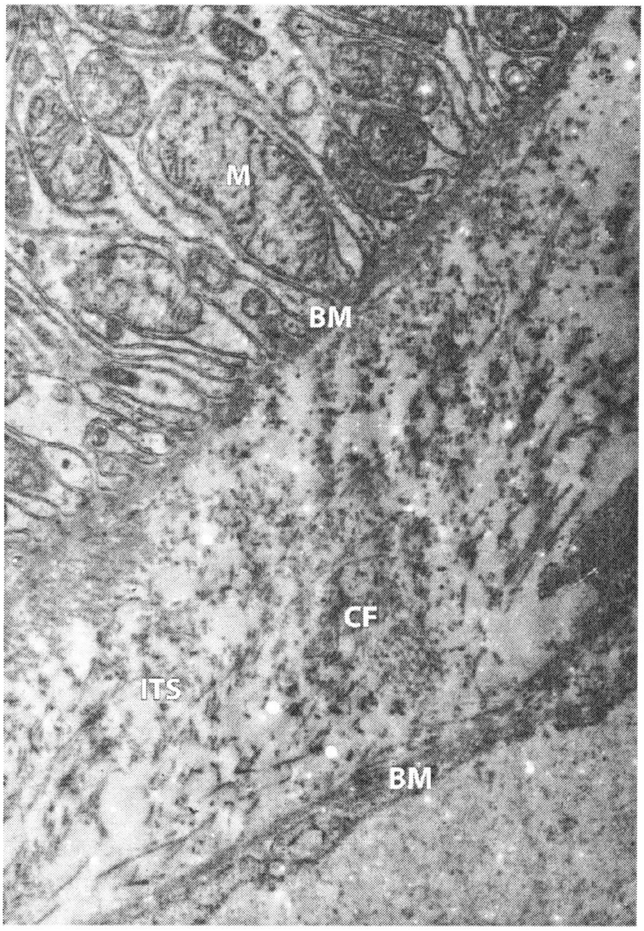

Figure 91. Electronogram of the nephron distal segment epithelial cell 2 years after the kidney autotransplantation without surgical reinnervation. An intertubular space (ITS) contains a large quantity of collagen fibers (CF).x20.000.

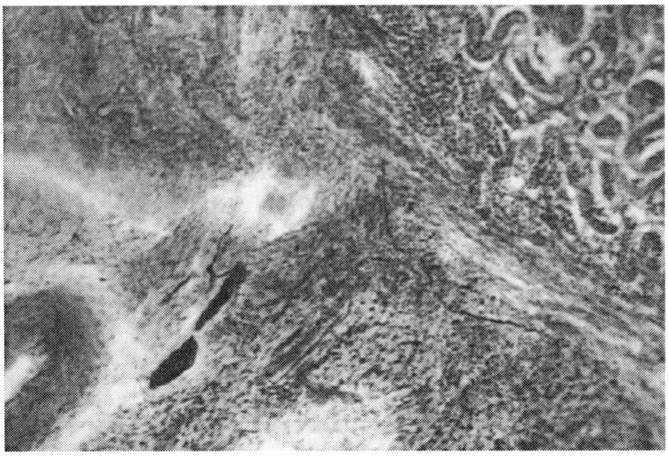

Figure 92. Microphotogram of the kidney 10 days after its autotransplantation and surgical reinnervation. Partially preserved nervefibers are seen in the f8ield of pyelon and tubules. Painted after Rasskasove.x150.

In cases when, together with the kidney autotransplantation, the opposite kidney was removed, the dynamics of morphologic changes were mainly the same as in the previous subgroup of experiments The difference was that in the sole autotransplanted kidney the various segments of the nephron that were not experiencing atrophy and sclerosis, were hypertrophied more, while kidney size and mass didn`t differ from that of the sole intact kidney (Table 15).

5.6. The State of the Kidney after Autotransplantation and Surgical Reinnervation

In the fourth group of experiments the autotransplanted and surgically reinnervated kidney, in the first ten days, was somewhat increased in size and mass compared to the intact opposite kidney (148,8±4,2, p<0,001, Table 15). In the cortical and medullar substances, and on the border between them, a moderate hyperemia and local lymphoid infiltration were observed.

Along the big blood vessels, nerve trunks with degenerating fibers were detected (Figure 92). The luminescent adrenergic nerve elemenets were not revealed (Figure 93). Only single cholinergic nerve fibers were seen along the big arteries and in the pyelon.

By electron microscope, in epithelial cells of the proximal and distal segments of the nephron, a vacuolization, mitochondrial swelling, and an increase of cisterns of the endophasmatic net were observed, as in the previous groups (Figure 94).

One month later the operated kidney continued to have slightly more mass than the opposite intact kidney (112,6±3,1%, p<0,01, Table 15). In the cortical, juxtamedullar and medullar substances, and the calico-pyelon system, a slight blood stagnation, local lymphoid infiltration, hyperemia of a part of the glomerulas and a dystrophy in the proximal and distal tubules were maintained.

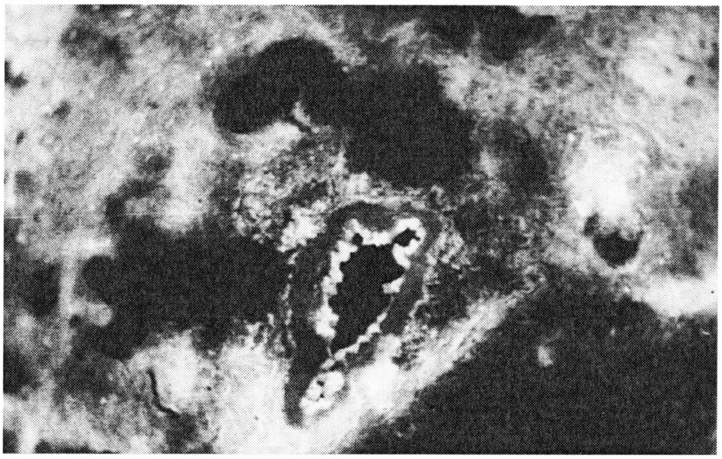

Figure 93. The same case. The catecholamine specific luminescence in the periadventitial layer is not detected. Luminescent microscopy after Falck a. Owman. LUMAM I-1.x200.

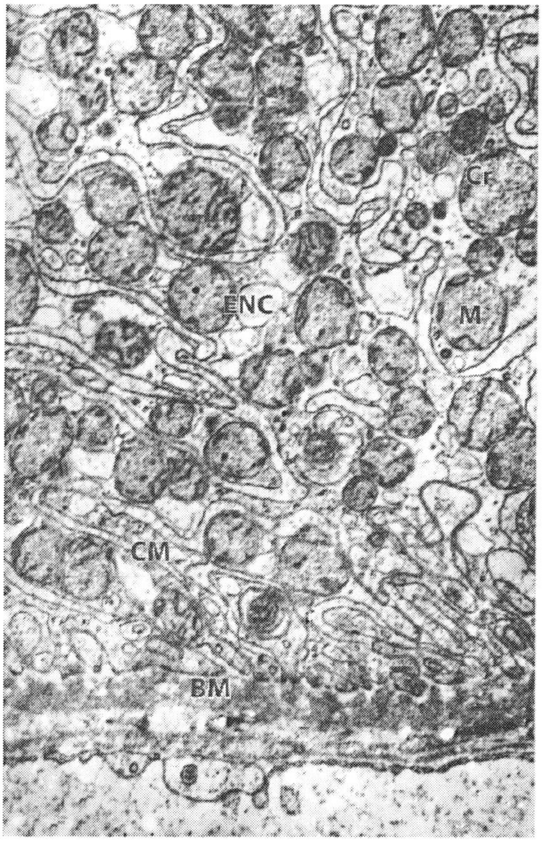

Figure 94. Electronogram of the nephron distal segment epithelial cell 10 days after the autotransplantation and surgical reinnervation of the kidney. A moderate swelling of some mitochondrias 9M) with peripheric disposition of cristas in them, widening of endoplasmatic net cisterns (ENC) are observed.x20.000.

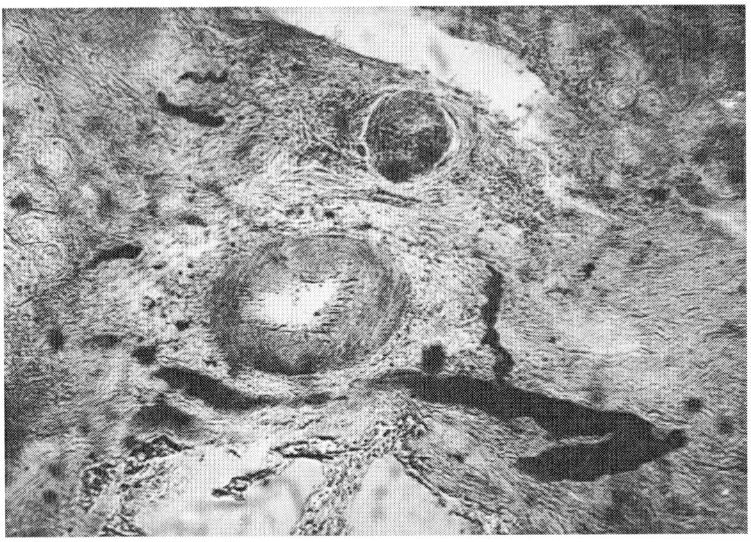

Figure 95. Microphotogram of the kidney 2 months after its autotransplantation and surgical reinnervation. In the perivascular field regenerating nerve fibers are grown out from the large nerve trunk. Painted after Bilshovsky-Gros-Lavrentjev.x150.

The majority of the intrarenal nerve fibers were degenerated. In other respects the common morphologic and electron microscopic structure of the kidney didn`t differ from the previous term data.

Two months later the mass of the operated kidney slightly exceeded the mass of the intact kidney (108.4±2.1, $p<0.05$, Table 15). Histologically, regenerating nerve fibers with branches to the pyelon were revealed (Figure 95). It has to be especially distinguished that at this time a faint specific luminescence of catecholamins around the big arteries in the juxtamedullar zone could be detected (Figure 96). Cholinergic nerve fibers mainly in the field of the pyelon blood vessels were observed.

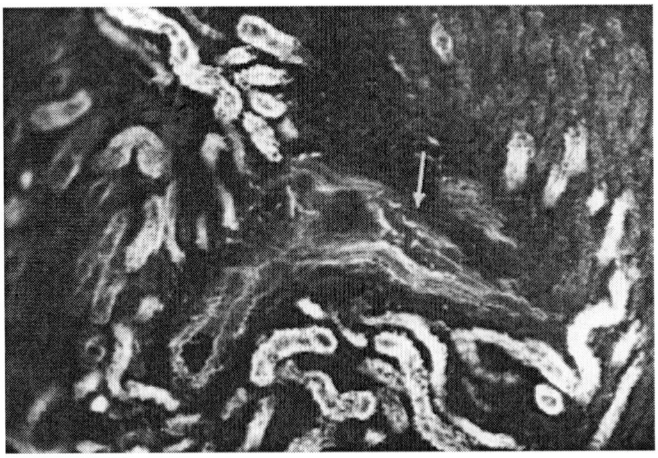

Figure 96. The same case. In the periadventitial layer of the blood vessel a weak specific luminescence is traced (indicated with an arrow). Luminescent microscopy after Falck a.Bowman. LUMAM I-1.x120.

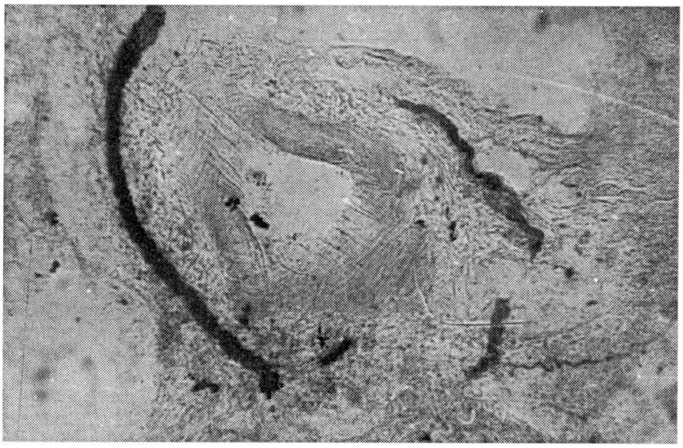

Figure 97. Microphotogram of the kidney 4 months after its autotransplantation and surgical reinnervation. around the artery there is a big quantity of large myelinized nerve fibers with regenerating shoots in direction of the pyelon. Painted after Bilshovsky-Gros-Lavrentjev.x200.

Evidenced by electron microscope, the kidney glomerulas were safe. In the epithelial cells of the proximal and distal segments of the nephron, a swelling of parts of the mitochondrias and widening of cisterns of the endoplasmatic net were observed. Epithelial cells of the thin segment and straight tubules were, on the whole, intact.

Four to six months after the operation the kidney didn`t differ from the intact one in size and mass (Table 15). The main part of the kidney parenchyma and its interstitial tissue was free of the sclerotic processes. Along the renal big arteries and arterioles, a great number of regenerating unmyelinized nerve fibers were observed. Their terminals germinated up to the level of the glomerulas and tubules, penetrating the pyelon wall (Figures 97-100). Along the big arteries, mainly in the juxtamedullar zone, the adrenergic nerve fiber nets with specific luminescence were detected (Figures 101-105). The cholinergic nerve fibers were also observed in the pyelon wall (Figure 106).

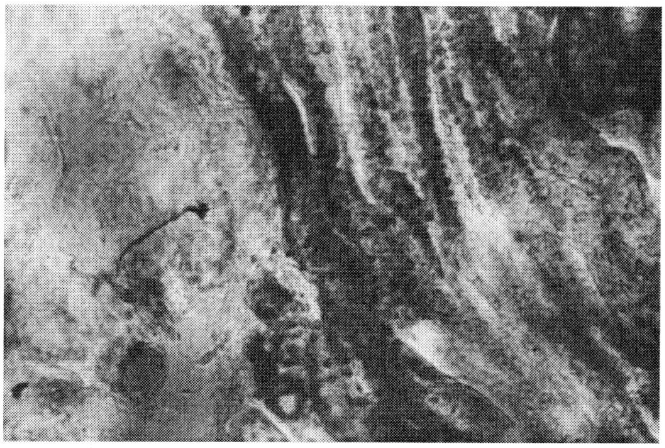

Figure 98. The same case. Nerve fibers germinating in direction of tubules are seen. Painted after Rasskasova.x200.

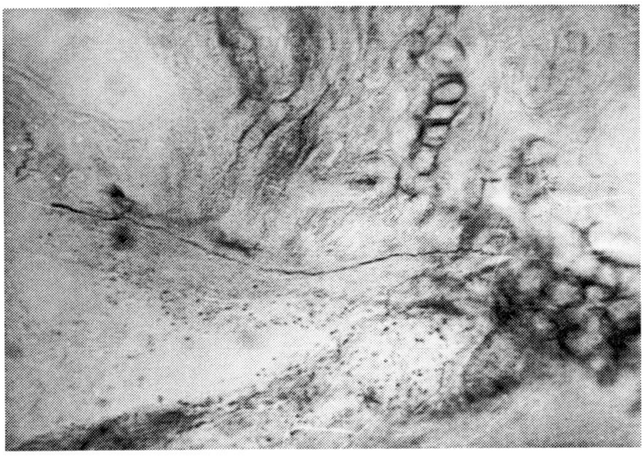

Figure 99. Microphotogram of the kidney 4 months after the autotransplantation and surgical reinnervation of the kidney. Regenerating nerve fibers arrive at pyelon walls and tubules. painted after Bilshovsky-Gros-Lavrentjev.x150.

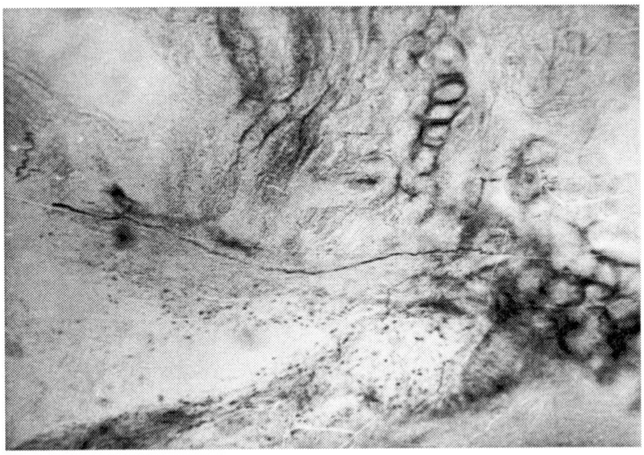

Figure 100. The same case.x300.

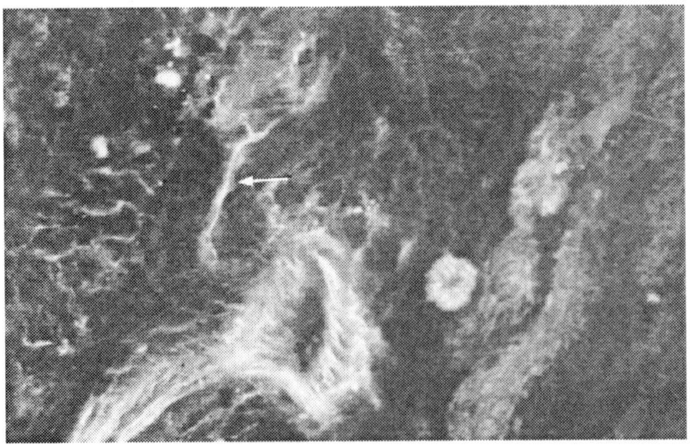

Figure 101. microphotogram of the kidney 4 months after its autotransplantation and surgical reinnervation. in the field of tubules along the artery a weak specific luminescence is seen (indicated with an arrow). Luminescent microscopy after Falck a. Owman. LUMAM I-1.x200.

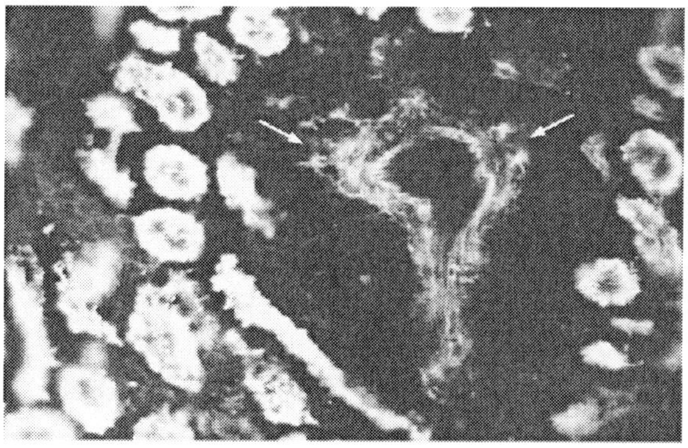

Figure 102. Microphotogram of the kidney 6 months after its autotransplantation and surgical reinnervation. In the periadventitial tissue the sections of a luminescent adrenergic nerve plexus are seen (indicated with arrows). Luminescent microscopy after Falck a. Owman. LUMAM I-1.x200.

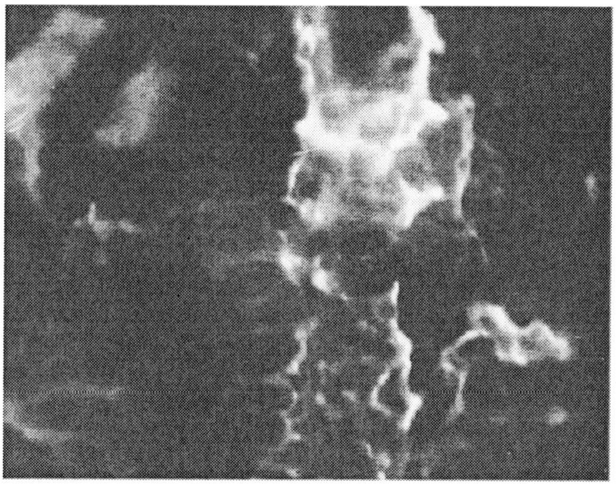

Figure 103. Microphotogram of the kidney 6 months after its autotransplantation and surgical reinnervation. Luminescent adrenergic nerve fibers are seen in the field of arc arteries and tubules. Luminescent microscopy after Falck a. Owman. LUMAM I-1.x400.

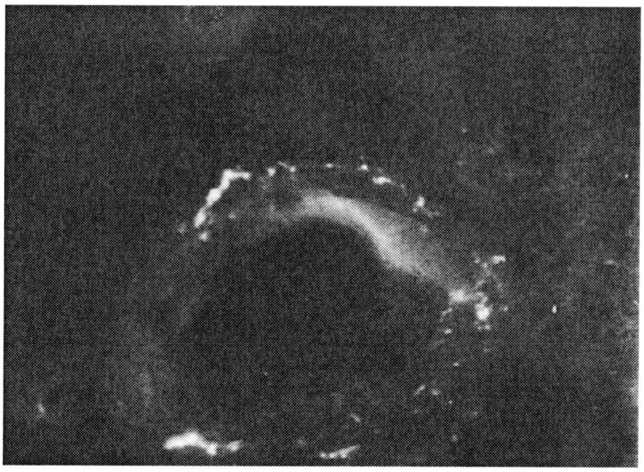

Figure 104. The same case. A luminescent adrenergic nervous plexus is observed around the artery. Luminescent microscopy after Shvalev a. Juchkova. LUMAM I-1.x400.

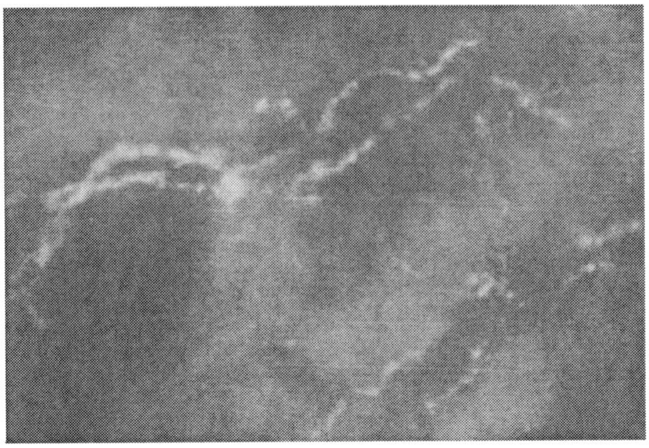

Figure 105. The same case. A luminescent adrenergic nervous plexus is traced int he field of tubules. Luminescent microscopy after Shvalev a.Juchkova. LUMAM I-1.x400.

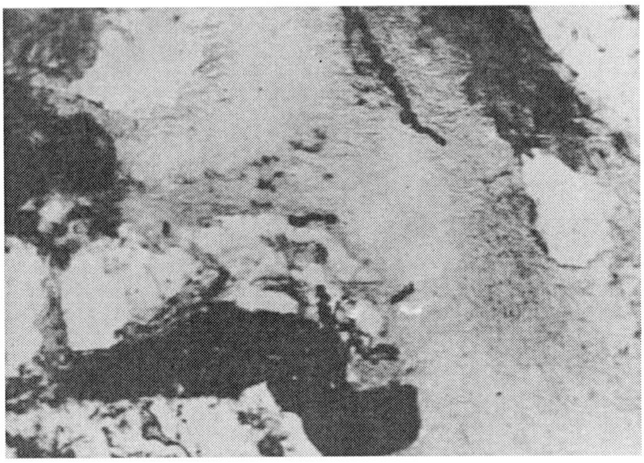

Figure 106. The same case. In the field of kidney pyelon single cholinergic nerve fibers are observed. painted after Karnovsky a. Roots.x200.

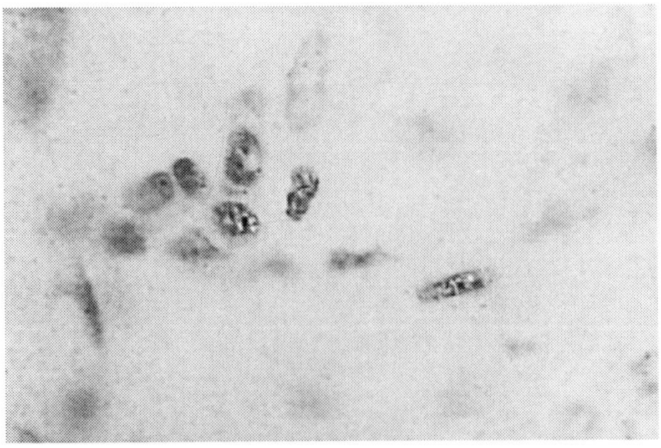

Figure 107. Section of a sympathetic trunk on the level of L1 6 months after the transplantation and surgical reinnervation of the kidney. The ganglion cells contain the granules of a horse radish peroxides. painted after Mesulam.x600.

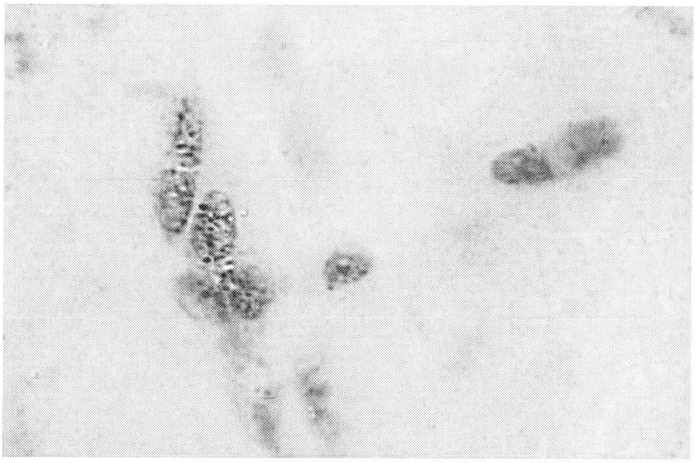

Figure 108. the section of the spinal brain lateral horn on the level of L1 6 months after the transplantation and surgical reinnervation of the kidney. The ganglion cells contain the specific granules of horse radish peroxidase. Painted after Mesulam.x600.

Two days after the supravital injection of horse radish peroxidase into the kidney parenchyma, the product of its reaction with diaminobenzidyne, in the form of small granules in the ganglion cells of the lateral horns of the spinal brain and the border sympathetic trunk on the level of ThXII-LII, was detected (Figures 107, 108). There were not any upsettings in the kidney ultrastructure (Figures 109, 110).

One to two years after the operation the macro-, micro- and ultrastructure of the kidney, on the whole, didn`t differ from the opposite intact kidney (Figure 111).

Along the intrarenal blood vessels, the nerve fibers were observed with branches in the direction of the pyelon, glomerulas and nephron tubules (Figures 112, 113).

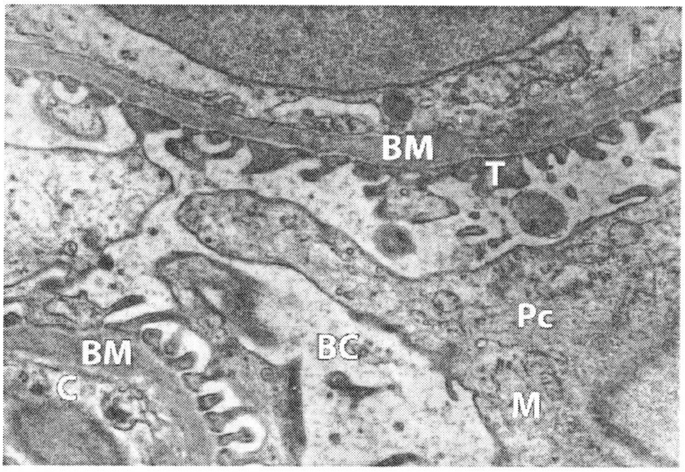

Figure 109. Electronogram of glomerula section 6 months after the autotransplantation and surgical reinnervation of the kidney. Any essential pathology is absent.x15.000.

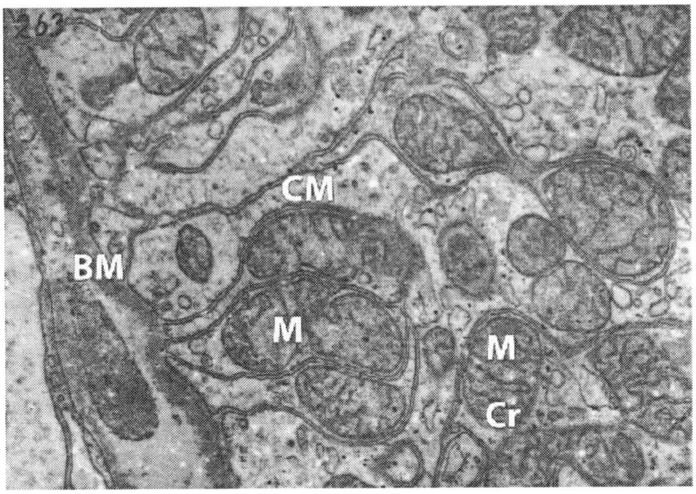

Figure 110. Electronogram of the nephron distal segment epithelial cell 6 months after the kidney autotransplantation and surgical reinnervation. There are not the signs of an intertubular sclerosis. mitochondrias (M) have a dense matrix and regular system of cristas (Cr). x15.000.

In the nerve fiber nets around the renal arc arteries, a specific luminescence of cathecholamines was seen. Their thin branches were located close to the glomerulas and tubules (Figures 114, 115). Localization and cholinaesterase activity in the kidney corresponded to the standard.

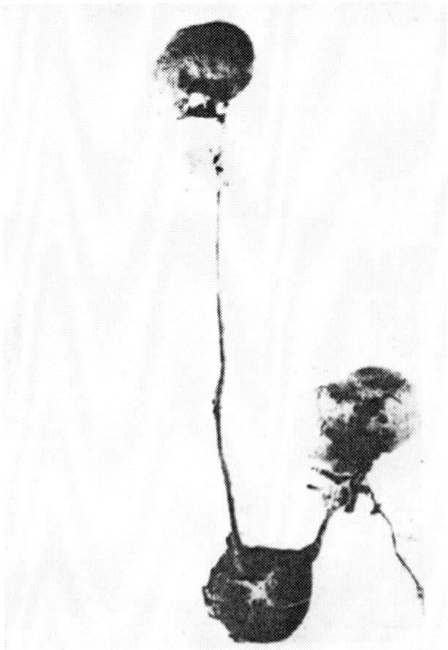

Figure 111. Macromorphologic preparation of an urinary ftract 2 years after the autotransplantation and surgical reinnervation of the left kidney. A preserved section of the nerve anastomoses is seen. Any atrophy of the transplanted (left) kidney is not observed.

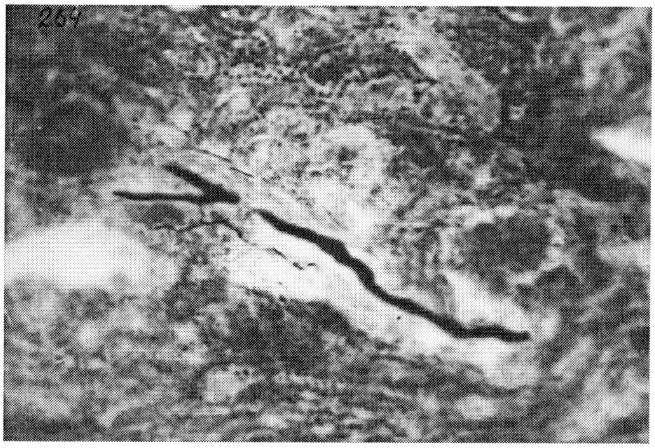

Figure 112. Microphotogram of the kidney 1 year afater its autotransplantation and surgical reinnervation. In the field of tubules and glomerulas regenrating myelinized nerve fibers are observed. Painted after Rasskasova.x200.

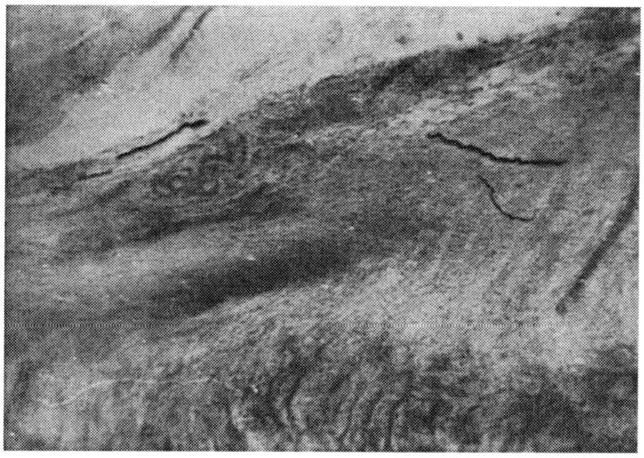

Figure 113. The same case. In the kidney pyelon wall and near the tubules myelinized and unmyelinized nerve fibers are seen. Painted after Bilshovsky-Gros-Lavrentjev.x150.

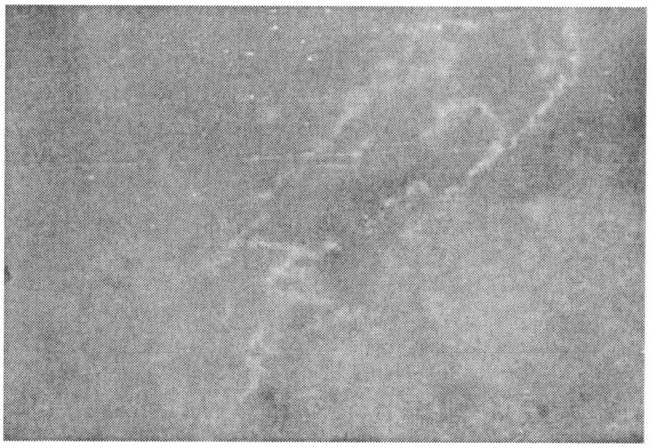

Figure 114. Microphotogram of the kidney 1 year after its autotransplantation and surgical reinnervation. Among the two glomerulas a luminescent adrenergic nervous plexus is observed. Luminescent microscopy after Shvalev a. Juchkova. LUMAM I-1.x400.

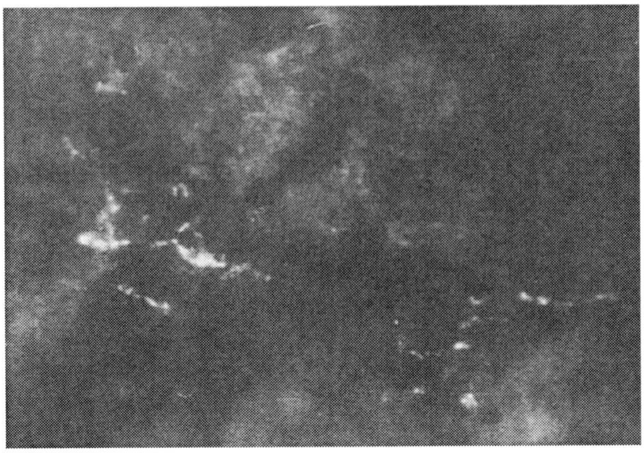

Figure 115. The same case. A luminescent adrenergic nervous plexus in the field of glomerulas and tubules is observed. Lumionescent microscopy after Shvalev a. Juchkova. LUMAM I-1.x400.

As in the previous term, normal transport of horse radish peroxidase from the nerve terminals located in the kidney parenchyma up to the ganglion cells on the level of ThXII-LII was observed (Figure 116).

In experiments with reinnervation of an autotransplanted kidney and contralateral nephrectomy, the same dynamics were observed, as in the cases without removal of an intact kidney. But the common reactive changes, such as blood stagnation and lymphoid infiltration, in the sole kidney were expressed slightly more within the first month after the operation.

On the other hand, the active regeneration of nerve fibers, including luminescenting adrenergic fibers, were detected earlier, two months after the operation. Four months later the structure of the autotransplanted and reinnervated sole kidney didn`t actually differ from the intact sole kidney (Figure 117).

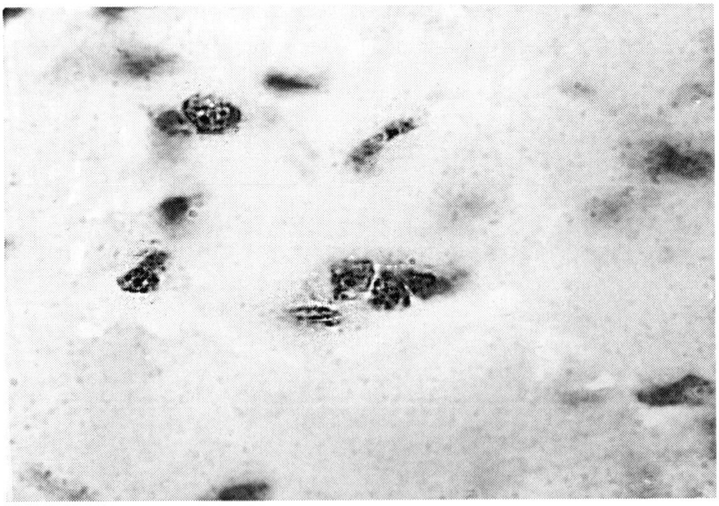

Figure 116. Section of the sympathetic trunk on the level of L1 2 years after the autotransplantation and surgical reinnervation of the kidney. Granules of the horse radish peroxidase are seen in the ganglion cells. Painted after Mesulam.x600.

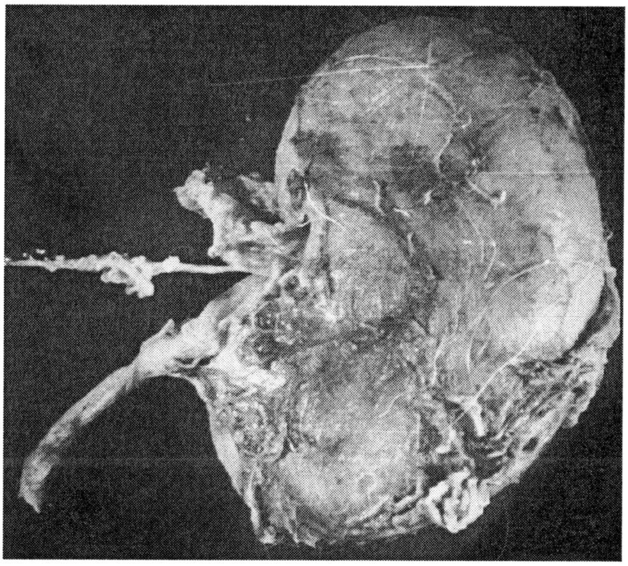

Figure 117. Macromorphologic preparation of the kidney 2 years after its autotransplantation with surgical reinnervation and contralateral nephrectomy. A renal nerve with anastomosis section is seen. The kidney is hypertrophied.

5.7. The State of a Sole Intact Kidney

In the fifth group of experiments with one side experiencing nephrectomy, four to six months later, the signs of compensative hypertrophy in the sole intact kidney are an increase of glomerular and tubule diameter and an expressed impregnation of nerve fibers were mentioned. Retrograde transport of horse radish peroxidase from the kidney to the ganglion cells of the lateral horns of the spinal brain and sympathetic trunk on the level of ThXII-LII was observed (Figure 118).

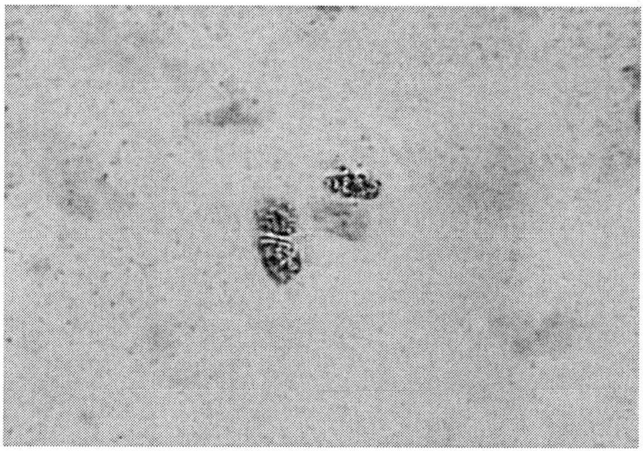

Figure 118. Section of the sympathetic trunk on the level of L1 on the side of the sole intat kidney. in the ganglion cells granulas of the horse radish peroxidase are detected. Painted after Mesulam.x600.

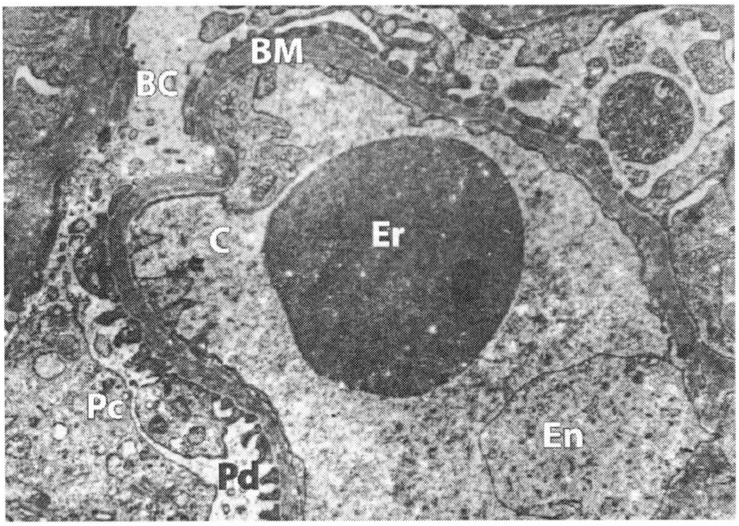

Figure 119. Electronogram of an intact kidney glomerula 4 months after the contralateral nephroctomy. There is not any essential pathology.x15.000.

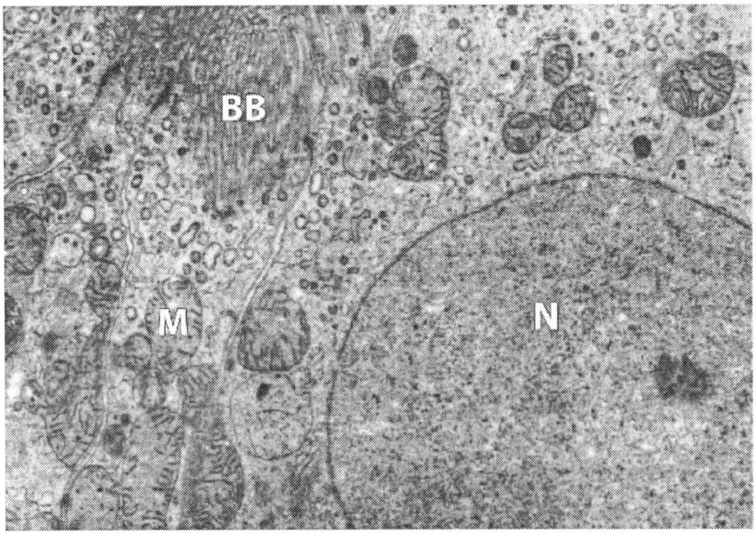

Figure 120. Electronogram of the nephron proximal segment epithelial cell 4 months after the contralateral nephrectomy. There is not any pathology.x15.000.

The ultrastructure of this kidney didn`t differ from the standard (Figures 119, 120).

5.8. Discussion of Morphologic Results

The described morphologic investigations permitted to the discovery of natural laws in the dynamics of changes in the kidney parenchyma and its nervous apparatus, and to notice an evident dependence between them. So, in all four groups of experiments after the denervation or autotransplantation of the kidney, with or without its surgical reinnervation during the first month, blood stagnation, lymphoid infiltration and various degrees of the kidney dystrophy were observed. But after two months a distinct difference was observed between the groups. In the first and third groups of experiments, made without surgical reinnervation, the signs of blood stagnation and lymphoid infiltration maintained, while the dystrophy advanced gradually and was finished with an atrophy and sclerose of a considerable part of the kidney including the glomerulas, nephron segments and blood vessels.

In the second and fourth groups after the same operations, but accompanied by surgical reinnervation, the slightly expressed signs of hemostasis and dystrophy were maintained within two months, but four to six months later the structure of the kidney on the macro-, micro- and ultrastructural levels didn`t actually differ from the intact kidney.

Parallel neurohistologic investigations in all four mentioned groups showed a gradual degeneration of most of the intraorganic nervous apparatus within the first month, but after two months a clear dissociation was revealed in their dynamics.

In the first and third groups was observed a germination of single unmyelinized nerve fibers along the big blood vessels which stopped in the connective tissue and didn`t reach the nephrons. In the second and fourth groups, intensive regeneration of nerve fibers occurred, which by four to six months germinated up to the glomerulas, tubules and pyelon walls of the kidney.

The very interesting and important results of the kidney nervous apparatus examination with horseradish peroxidase must be emphasized. 48 hours after intrarenal injection, its granules were detected in the ganglion cells of the spinal brain and sympathetic trunk on the level of ThXII-LII. This fact has to be considered firstly as direct evidence of recovery of anatomic wholeness of the postganglion nervous apparatus of the kidney up to its cortical substance; secondly it testified to the normal transport function of regenerated nerve fibers; thirdly these data showed that the kidney parenchyma was sufficiently saturated with nerve terminals able to absorb the neurotropic substances.

In the first and third groups of experiments performed without surgical reinnervation the same examination was negative for two years.

Hence it follows that the surgical reinnervation created favorable conditions for directed germination of a great quantity of nerve fibers along the natural phylogenetic pathway from the kidney gate up to the basic functional and structural units of the kidney.

Some natural questions come up: what are the morphologic evidences of the regenerated nerve fibers perfection? Is it justified to connect the observed dynamics and character of neuroreggenerative processes with the character of common structural changes in the kidney?

These questions are closely connected with one of the interesting sections of neurophysiology and neurohistology, the doctrine on the adaptive and trophic influence of the nervous system on the organs. In accordance with this theory, founded by L.A. Orbeli [283], the nervous system, except of motor, blood vessel contractive, secretory and sensitive functions, exerts an adaptive and trophic influence on the organs, tissues and cells. The first means the ability to ensure an accommodation of various organs to permanently changing functional demands, while the trophic influence signifies an intimate regulation of physical and chemical condition, metabolism and nourishment of tissues and cells of organs. What`s more, both these factors play an independent role. It means that for ensuring normal conditions of organs and their tissues not only functional loading, but also the trophic influence of the nervous system is necessary [18,302,429-431].

This influence is realized through the system of adrenergic (sympathetic) and cholinergic (parasympathetic) nerves which are in intimate and intricate relations, and after a majority of their manifestations act in contrary directions. The adrenergic and cholinergic nerves realize their specific function through production of the corresponding nervous mediators, catecholamines and acethylcholine.

Catecholamines are represented with noradrenalin, adrenalin and intermediate products of metabolism such as dophamin, S-hydroxitriptamin dehydroadrenalin, dehydronoradrenalin, adrenochrom, noradrenochrom, adrenolutine and noradrenolutine [21,98,102,143,144,188, 230,284,319,320,406-408,411]. There is vast literature about the increase or decrease of nervous mediator action. But the final results of such influence were not described for more than 100 years, and there are few works about the intimate physical and chemical processes which are the basis of the metabolism and nourishment of tissues. It was established that cathecholamines regulate the content of energetic resources in tissues (glycogen, creatinphosphate, adenosinethreephosphate acid), the activity of phosphorilase, lipase, and cuccinatdehydrogenase [4,30,31,95,96,115,143,144,309,378].

An increase of catecholamine concentration or stimulation of adrenergic nerves causes an intensification of the utilization of these substances, a decrease of their level in tissues, and activation of phosphorilase, lipase, and succinat-dehydrogenase [4,69,144,229,309,313-315].

On the contrary, the desympathization of organs or the introduction of ganglioblockers (reserpine) causes a weakening of the utilization of glycogen, creatinphosphate, ATP and an increase of their content in tissues. What`s more, these biochemical changes are reflected morphologically in various degrees of dystrophy, connective tissue (lipoid) degeneration, swelling, and atrophy of tissue structures. Dystrophic alterations and the loss of contractive ability of blood vessel walls in connection with desympathization are accompanied with sharp full-bloodness [47,143,144,301].

It has to be noted that although cathecholamines, except adrenergic nerve terminals, are produced in the supraren cortical substance and chromaphin cells of the organism and can reach desympathized organs and tissues through humoral pathways, their concentration is so scanty that they can not compensate for the trophic influence of adrenergic nerves. Therefore even through safe humoral delivery of cathecholamines to a desympathized organ, the typical dystrophic changes appear [144]. The authors explain this fact in that the concentration of cathecholamines in the field of adrenergic nervous terminals exceeds their concentration in the blood by 1000-10000 times and reaches 3-30 mg for each gram of nervous tissue [98,100,102,144].

As for cholinergic nerves, there are less comprehensive and more contradictory data. It was stated that the stimulation of a wandering nerve or introduction of acethylcholine causes an increase in glycogen, creatinphosphate, ATP concentration, activity of succinatdehydrogenase, cytochromoxidase and a decrease of oxygen utilization in tissues [79]. What`s more, the action of acethylcholine is changeable considerably depending on the introduced mediator dose. Moderate doses of acethylcholine cause an increase of glycogen content in the dog heart [325]. Large doses of acethylcholine, on the contrary, decrease the glycogen level. The authors explain this phenomenon as a disturbance of physiologic coordination between the glycogen and breathing [313,315].

There is not a solid common opinion as to the switching of cholinergic nerves of the kidney. One group of authors observed the dystrophic changes in the kidneys after the vagotomy [5,12]. Other authors [369,370] consider that the kidney has mainly adrenergic innervation, and the cholinergic nerves are represented very scantily, therefore their upsetting doesn`t cause essential morphologic changes in the kidney.

There is also an opinion that because of disposition of cholinergic ganglion cells in the kidney gate a part of them remains safe in case of a simple (in situ) or transplantation denervation, therefore, full cholinergic denervation of the kidney does not take place [384,423]. But the normal morphologic examinations didn`t reveal strong signs of cholinergic denervation of the kidney and it doesn`t exclude the existence of reverse communication between the cathecholamines and acethylcholine secretion [309].

These data coincide with an earlier expressed opinion [287] that a pair of trophic nerves (adrenergic and cholinergic) acting in contrary directions on metabolic processes are the last distributor of nutritional resources in the organism and its various organs and tissues.

Taking into account the above mentioned considerations, it becomes clear that the investigation of nerve mediators is a principal criterion for an objective evaluation of the nervous apparatus in the transplanted kidney. Therefore this test was used in the described experiments.

They showed that in all four groups with denervation and autotransplantation of the kidney, three days after the operation, the specific luminescence of cathecholamines was stopped. The same phenomena was observed [134-139,387-390] 48 hours after the kidney autotransplantation.

The ordinary neurohistologic methods revealed irregular development of degenerative changes in renal nerves. Along with destruction there were also safe nerve fibers. But in spite of external structural safety of some nerve fibers impregnated with silver, they were defective from a functional point of view because they had lost the ability to produce cathecholamines.

In the first and third test-groups after denervation and autotransplantation of the kidneys, their condition continued up to the end of the experiment (within two years), although by four to six months a certain number of unmyelinized nerve fibers germinated along the renal blood vessels. The absence of luminescent cathecholamines testified about a loss or a sharp decrease of the ability to produce cathecholamines. Therefore these nerve fibers could not exert an effective adaptive and trophic influence on the kidney.

In the second and fourth groups of experiments, accompanied by a surgical reinnervation of the denervated and autotransplanted kidneys, the adrenergic nervous nets didn`t function for the first two months as well, but later (by four to six months and up to two years) the content of cathecholamines in regenerated nerve fibers was recovered gradually and adrenergic nerve terminals with specific luminescence were detected in the field of the kidney glomerulas, tubules, juxtaglomerular apparatus, the walls of the calices and the pyelon.

In spite of the fact that adrenergic nerve fibers were observed in the kidney parenchyma, somewhat rarely compared to intact cases, the character and intensity of their luminescence didn`t actually differ from the standard. Taking into account that the kidney cells are usually able to accept a trophic influence on adrenergic nerve fibers, not only by their direct contact with nerve terminals but also through diffusion of cathecholamines [373-375], it can be supposed that by a four to six month term, most of the kidney parenchyma began to receive a sufficient amount of cathecholamines. This means that the kidney entered in an intermediate stage of development, which was very important for normal function.

If, in respect to adrenergic nerve fibers, it was possible to observe the above described staging in the neuroregeneration dynamics, the same could not be said about the cholinergic nerve fibers. In all four groups of experiments, after denervation and autotransplantation of the kidney with and without surgical reinnervation and both in the near and remote postoperative periods, the single cholinergic nerve fibers along the big renal arteries and in the field of pyelon were seen. The fact is that in groups with surgical reinnervation such nerve fibers were found somewhat more often, but their presence in the rest of the groups (without surgical reinnervation) testified that kidney denervation and autotransplantation occurred only with partial (not full) cholinergic denervation. This phenomenon coincides with data of authors [384] explaining it using the availability of cholinergic ganglion cells located profoundly in the autotransplanted kidney gate; they play the role of an organ with autonomous cholinergic innervation. Thus, these are all reasons to conclude that the denervation and autotransplantation of the kidney caused mainly adrenergic denervation with partial preservation of cholinergic innervation. In the groups without surgical reinnervation this state was maintained up to the end of the experiments (two years), in the groups with surgical reinnervation it was maintained for no more than four months. The interesting questions arise from here: to what degree is this temporary (in second and fourth groups) or steadfast (in first and third groups) discoordination of adrenergic and cholinergic innervation affected by the kidney structural organization? Whether the partially safe cholinergic innervation compensates to some degree for a weakened trophic influence on the organ?

Comparison of general morphologic data with results of a differentiated examination of adrenergic and cholinergic nervous mediators it is not difficult to see an obvious correlation.

In all four groups of experiments for the first two months after the operation, the period of full adrenergic denervation and partially maintained cholinergic innervation, the general morphologic structure of the kidney was the same on the whole, independent of the use of surgical reinnervation or not. In all these groups the blood stagnation, lymphoid infiltration, and various degrees of dystrophic upsettings were observed. A number of the typical ultrastructural signs of these dystrophic changes had been found such as a widening of endoplasmatic net cisterns, swelling of mitochondrias with enlightenment of their matrix and destruction of cristas. The same changes were observed by other authors, also examinating the autotransplanted kidneys [248]) and denervated skin [418].

The authors didn`t confirm categorically that the described dystrophic changes were specific for denervation because the same alterations were observed by dystrophy evoked by other causes. Nevertheless they [418] expressed an interesting opinion that various pathologic factors affecting the given tissue damage its nerve elements, which somehow change the character of the metabolism in the system neuro-tissue. It means that these neuro-tissue metabolic relations are decisive in the intricate range of pathologic manifestations.

Our data permits the confirmation this opinion. Thus, in the first and third groups of experiments made without surgical reinnervation of denervated and autotransplanted kidneys for two years, the regeneration of full value adrenergic nerve fibers able to produce the luminescent cathecholamines was not detected. Dystrophic changes advanced gradually and were finished with the local and diffusive sclerosis and atrophy of a considerable part of the kidney. In this respect our data coincide with known literature completely [215,366,369,370,373].

In the second and fourth groups of experiments, made with additional surgical reinnervation of the kidney by four to six months after the operation, the regeneration of a nervous apparatus producing cathecholamines was complete. Simultaneously a normalization of the kidney general structural condition was observed.

In these cases the mentioned electron microscopic signs of dystrophy disappeared as well.

Taking into account that after the operation the animals were in identical conditions without any additional pathologic influences, the difference in the dynamics and character of the kidney structural organization can be explained by the only criterion – did the recovery of a full value adrenergic reinnervation of the kidney happen or not?

Our data allows us to express an opinion also, are the partially safe cholinergic nerve fibers able to exert any perceptible trophic influence on the kidney by absent cathecholamines or not. The results of our experiments testify that only cholinergic nerve fibers were unable to prevent the vascular and dystrophic changes which were seen with atrophy and sclerosis of the organ. In our opinion, the possible causes of this phenomenon could be noted as follows: either the cholinergic nervous apparatus of the kidney was represented so scantily that it was unable to exert an independent trophic influence on the kidney, or the cholinergic nerve fibers because of inactivity of adrenergic fibers, created a disbalance between the nervous mediators, causing a perversion in the character of kidney innervations and therefore promoted its dystrophy. These data testify that for the normal work and trophic mechanisms of the kidney it requires mainly an adrenergic innervation. This fact coincides with known literary data [369,370].

Thus, summarizing the above described morphologic investigation it can be concluded that, by the use of the mentioned method of surgical reinnervation of denervated and autotransplanted kidneys over four to six months, an anatomic and functional recovery of full value nerve fibers occurred. They contained the specific nervous mediators which took part in the regulation of the renal tissue self-renovation, promoted the maintenance of its parenchyma stable structure and prevented the atrophy and sclerosis of the organ, observed in groups with denervation and autotransplantation of the kidneys without surgical reinnervation.

Chapter VI

THE SURGICAL REINNERVATION OF THE TRANSPLANTED KIDNEY: IS IT NEEDED?

As we can see the kidney decentralization, both at the denervation in situ and in connection with kidney autotransplantation, caused certain functional and morphological disturbances; their severity and stability was dependent on the decisive degree of whether the organ surgical reinnervation was performed or not. In this respect, two principal stages may be singled out in the postoperative period, 2 months before and after the operation.

In the first stage the experimental results in all test-groups were mainly of the same kind. During this period a 15-20% decrease of vascularization, filtration, secretion, reabsorption, excretion and renographic index on both denervated and autotransplanted kidneys was observed. From a morphological point of view blood stasis, lymphoid infiltration and various degrees of dystrophy were revealed in the parenchyma. In the nephron proximal and distal segments dilation of endoplasmatic net cisterns, mitochondria swelling with cristas destruction and vacuolization were observed.

In the second stage, i. e. 2 months after the operation, a distinct difference between the results in individual groups was seen. In the 1st and 3rd groups, where kidney denervation and autotransplantation were performed without surgical reinnervation, a tendency for slight improvement in blood circulation, filtration and secretory renal functions was initially observed. However, 4 to 6 months after the operation, the functional indicies began to worsen progressively, and by the end of the 2-year period, they constituted 60-70% of the norm. From a morphological point of view, the dystrophy increase in the proximal and distal segments of the nephrons, and the phenomena of local and diffusive sclerosis, and kidney atrophy were observed after a 4 to 6 month period.

In the 2nd and 4th test-groups, where kidney denervation and autotransplantation were carried out with surgical reinnervation, a different pattern was observed.

By 4 to 6 months, progressive normalization of the functional indicators had taken place: first, the renal blood circulation was restored (within 1-2 months); then the secretory and reabsorption functions (within 2-4 months), and lastly, excretory, motor and evacuation functions (within 4 to 6 months). Subsequently, prior to completion of the experiments (up to 2 years), no functional asymmetry between the operated and intact kidneys was found. These data are in accordance with the morphological pattern.

How can one explain the difference between the results in these test-groups? Since the nature of the operation in these groups differed only in the additional surgical reinnervation of the kidneys, it seems that the answer should be sought in the renal nervous system.

Impregnational neurohistological investigations have shown that during a 1 month postoperative period, in all test-groups both with and without kidney reinnervation, a progressive degeneration of the major part of the intraorganous nervous system had taken place. However, within 2 months these investigations revealed a distinct dissociation in the character of changes in individual groups after kidney denervation and autotransplantation without reinnervation; the intergrowth of solitary nonmyelinated nerve fibers along the large blood vessels was noticed; however, these fibers ended within the connective tissue without reaching the nephrons. Furthermore, these nerve fibers have proven to be incapable of secreting nervous mediators (catecholamines) into the parenchyma; they could not absorb the horseradish peroxidase from the kidney parenchyma and transport it to the spinal ganglia. The threshold of renal nerve stump excitation exceeded the norm 10 times, and enhancement of the electrical irritation of the nerve did not lead to a substantial increase in the response potential. During the 2 years of observation, the renal nerve stump capability of spontaneous impulsation was not restored.

In the 2nd and 4th test-groups, 2 months after kidney denervation and autotransplantation with their subsequent surgical reinnervation, an intensive regeneration of nerve fibers was histologically observed along blood vessels; by 4 to 6 months these fibers reached the coils, ductules, as well as the walls of the kidney pelvis. The nerve-endings were capable of secreting specific nervous mediators such as catecholamines and acetylcholine. The intrarenal nerve terminals were capable of absorbing the horseradish peroxidase and transporting it to the spinal ganglia. This means that direct evidence of anatomical and functional restoration of the whole postganglion nervous apparatus of the kidney had been obtained. On the other hand, this fact testifies about sufficient saturation of the parenchyma with active nerve terminals.

2 months after the operation, the exitation threshold of the renal nerve was 3 times lower than that of the preciding groups. The response potential was increased (by 50-70%) with electric stimulation enhancement. 4 months after the operation, the background spontaneous impulsation from the renal nerve, specifically changing with the intravenous injection of adrenalin (disappearance of impulsation) became detectable. Thus, they testified to the adequacy of the renal nervous system and its full value.

It should be specially noted that the functional ability of the sole non-reinnervated transplanted kidney, even during the most favorable period of activity (between the 2nd and 6th months of the postoperative period), considerably lagged behind the sole surgically reinnervated transplanted kidney and the sole intact kidney under the functional (water) loading and with the adrenalin test. After a 6 month period, this lag increased and could be seen not only with functional loading, but also under ordinary regimes of kidney working.

Were these favorable results after the transplanted kidney surgical reinnervation accidental or natural phenomena? In our opinion, they were fully natural for the following reasons.

It is well known from neurophysiology and plastic neurosurgery that successful reinnervation of an organ requires the observance of certain conditions: 1) The anatomical junction of nerve endings; 2) The homogenous character of the nerve anastomosis, which means the junction of motor, vegetative, adrenergic, and cholinergic nerves with the corresponding nerves; 3) The adequate representation of a donor-nerve in the central nervous system.

The emploid method of surgical reinnervation [189] satisfied these demands fully.

1. By anatomical investigations [130,189,198] was established that the epifascial spaces around the large blood vessels are very rich with vegetative nervous nets. Therefore the sewing of fascial shreds around the renal and iliacal blood vessels created conditions very close to the nerve junction "end to end". It has to be emphasized also that the nerve growth had taken place by the natural phylogenetic way, through the kidney gate.
2. By special neurohistologic investigations [247] it was established that the dense vegetative plexus going along the iliacal blood vessels has an adrenergic nature. Taking into account that the kidney is in need of mainly just adrenergic innervation, the mentioned source of reinnervation corresponded to the natural demands of the transplanted kidney fully.
3. By anatomical investigations [369] it was established that the vegetative nervous plexus along the iliacal blood vessels takes branches from the abdominal aortic plexus and the latter, even in natural conditions, takes part in the kidney innervation. Consequently the source of kidney surgical reinnervation has an adequate representation in the central nervous system.

Thus, the mentioned method for surgical reinnervation had all the necessary anatomical and physiological grounds for effective reinnervation of the kidney. The novelty consisted in the use by experimental autotransplantation in the iliac fossa, which means in conditions very close to clinic conditions.

What is the practical value of the described data and is it expedient to carry out the surgical reinnervation of the kidney by its transplantation in clinics?

Our complex investigations showed that 2 years after the autotransplantation of the kidney without surgical reinnervation, its common functional and structural potential was 60-70% of the standard. Such a kidney, even being the sole kidney, was able to ensure homeostasis and survival during a certain period, maybe over a long time. But even in the most healthy period (between 2 and 6 months after the operation) this kidney essentially lagged behind the autotransplanted and surgically reinnervated kidney by functional loading. The non-reinnervated sole kidney worked to a limit, which was exhausted gradually.

On the other hand, in the case of the transplanted kidney surgical reinnervation, after 6 months and up to 2 years, there were not observed reliable functional or structural disturbances from the norm. Taking into account the 2 year life duration of a dog, which corresponds approximately to a 10 year life duration of a man, it can be stated that the surgical reinnervation can prevent the degenerative damage of a kidney transplant and ensure its normal and safe function during quite a long period. All this testifies in favor of its application in clinics. Furthermore, the mentioned method is technically simple, doesn`t require any special experience or device, and doesn`t extend the duration of the kidney ischemia or the whole operation.

The possible fields of its clinical application would be the auto- and allotransplantation of a kidney.

As with our experimental goals, the influence of surgical reinnervation in pure conditions without specific immunologic factors means that the model of kidney autotransplantation and the obtained results confirmed expected results fully, its use in clinical kidney autotransplantation can be considered as utterly expedient.

The question is, is the surgical reinnervation needed by the kidney allotransplantation? On the one hand, it is known that one of the important immunosuppressive substances Cyclosporin A (CsS) used by the kidney allotransplantation exerts a nephrotoxic influence, which is seen through activation of renal afferent and efferent nerves which, in their turn, cause the vasoconstriction, ischemia, sodium retention and increase of free radicals in the kidney [93,103,161,166,174,196,207,240,254,349]. Therefore some of these authors even deliberately recommend to leave the kidney allotransplant in the state of denervation.

But on the other hand, many works testify that the administration of dietary glycine (5%) can totally block these phenomena [160,399,434,435]; Vitamin E, a lipid scavenger can inhibit the malondialdehyde increase and reduce the CsA-induced renal damage [420]. Some alternative immunosuppressive substances were elaborated (rapamycin, tacrolimus, mycophenolate) for the option.

Taking into account the above mentioned considerations, the prospects of surgical reinnervation in the case of kidney allotransplantation can also be estimated positively, because there are reasons to suppose that under the proper and harmless immunosuppressive protection, the regenerated nervous apparatus of an allotransplanted kidney will function and exert favorable regulative and trophic influence on the organ, exactly as the kidney itself under immunosuppressive protection can ensure satisfactory homeostasis in the organism. What`s more, one can hope that the surgical reinnervation will essentially improve the general and remote clinical results.

Taking into account that modern science gradually, but inevitably, approaches the final decision of the problem of immune incompatibility and at the same time approaches our results to conditions of kidney allotransplantation, and the recommendations mentioned above can be estimated not only from todays point of view but also of the future. Moreover, our firm conviction is that they can be extrapolated on other transplanted organs too.

REFERENCES NO. 1

[1] Aars H., Akre S. Reflex changes in sympathetic activity and arterial blood pressure evoked by afferent stimulation of the renal nerve. - *Acta physiol.Scand.,* 1970; 78 (1): 184-188.

[2] Abdasimov T.D. A spinal sensitivity of the kidney innervation. - *Med.J.Uzbekistan,* 1961; 10 (7): 43-46.

[3] Abraham A. Morphologische Grundlagen der Nevralen Nierenregulation. - In: Nierenfunktion und Nervensystem/ Hrsg. v. H.Dutz. - Berlin: *Volk und Gesundheit.* - 1959; S. 3-44.

[4] Abramova N.M., Anisimova V.F., Gutovskaja A.V. The role of cardial dynamic nerves in regulation of trophic in the myocard. *Bulletin of Exp.Biol.Med.,* 1957; 44 (7): 50-54.

[5] Akhmeteli L.I., Gsirishvili G.A. Micromorphologic changes in kidneys after bilateral vagotomy. *Reports of Academy of Sciencies of Georgia,* 1956; 17 (5): 451-454.

[6] Adunz G.T., Oganesjan A.S. The Influence of the wandering nerve cut on diuresis and kidney filtration. - *News of Acad. of Sciences of Armenian,* 1954; 7 (10): 65-71.

[7] Alekseeva V.S. Surgical treatment of peripheric paralysis of the facial nerve after the radical removal of a neurinom. *Questions of neurosurgery,* 1960; 3: 52-54.

[8] Almgard J.E., Ljunggvist A., Ungerstedt U. The reaction of the intrarenal sympathetic nervous system to renal transplantation. - *Scand.J.Urol.Nephrol.,* 1971; 5: 65-70.

[9] Angelakos E.T. The formaldehyde condensation method for the histochemical demonstration for tissue monoamines. - *J.Histochem.Cytochem.,* 1964; 12 (11): 929-931.

[10] Andreev S.V., Kobkova I.D. The role of cathecholamins in the healthy and ill organism, Moscow, *Medicine,* 1970, -296 p.

[11] Anikin G.D. The character and mechanism of stomach functional changes by experimental renal colic. *Candidate dissertation,* Ivanovo, 1959, -12 p.

[12] Antelava A.V., Gsirishvili G.A. Some biochemistry indices of the urine before and after the vagotomy. *Works of Institute of exper. and clinical hematology.* Georgian Academy of Sciencies, Tbilisi, 1953; 4: 136-136.

[13] Antoine B., Ducrot H. Les problemes de la transplantation renale. *J.Urol.Med. et chir., 1954; 60 (5): 289-329.*

[14] Asfoury Z.M.El. Sympathectomy and the innervation of the kidney. - *Brit.Med.J.,* 1951; 4743: 1304-1306.

[15] Asfoury Z.M.El. *Sympathectomy and the innervation of the kidney.* - London: Butterworth, 1971. -255 p.

[16] Asico L.D., Eisner G.M., Jose P.A. Renal nerves and D1 - dopamine receptor - mediated natriuresis. *Clin. Exp. Hypertens.*, 1998 Feb; 20 (2): 259-271.

[17] Asratjan E.A. The influence of the wandering nerve on the kidney function. *Bulletin exper. med.,* 1940; 9 (4): 255-258.

[18] Asratjan E.A. Compensatory adaptation from the point of view of I.P. Pavlov`s doctrine. - *Successes of the modern biology,* 1953; 3: 357-381.

[19] Astrom A., Crafwood J. Afferent activity recorded in the kidney nerves of rats. - *Acta Physiol.Scand.,* 1967; 70: 10-15.

[20] Astrom A., Crafwood J. Afferent and efferent activity in the renal nerves of cats. - *Acta Physiol.Scand.,* 1968; 74: 69-78.

[21] Avakjan O.M. *Sympathetic-adrenalin system.* - Leningrad, Nauka, 1977, -183 p.

[22] Babmindra V.P., Valberg F. Sources of afferent ways of motor cortex of the cat brain revealed by means of peroxidase method. *Archives AHE,* 1978; 74 (5): 13-18.

[23] Balakshina V.L. A mechanism of the kidney conditionally - reflectory activity. *Works of physiology Institute AGU,* 1936; 17: 61-108.

[24] Balakshina V.L. Functional characteristic of urinary tract by pathology of the high nervous activity. *Works of I.P. Pavlov Physiology Institue,* 1954; 3: 463-474.

[25] Balakschina V.L. Zur der nevralen Regulation der Nierentätigkeit. - In: *Nierenfunction und Nervensystem / Hrag. von H. Dutz. - Berlin: Volk und Gesundheit,* 1959, S. 213-218.

[26] Ballantyne B. The neurohistology of the mammalian kidney. - *Univ. of Leeds Med.J.,* 1959; 8 (2): 50-59.

[27] Barajas L., Gatta H. A three-dimensional study of the juxtaglomerular apparatus in the rat. - *Labor.Invest.*, 1963; 12 (3): 257-269.

[28] Barajas L., Gatta H. The juxtaglomerular apparatus in adrenalectomized rats. - *labor. Invest.,* 1963; 12 (11): 1046-1059.

[29] Barajas L., Silverman A.J., Muller J. Ultrastructural localization of acetylcholinesterase in the renal nerves. - *J.Ultrastr.Res.*, 1974; 49 (3): 297-311.

[30] Bekauri N.V. The role of sensitive innervation in the course of some trophic processes. *Medic Doctor dissertation,* Leningrad, 1965, -29 p.

[31] Beljaeva N.N. The influence of an innervation upsettings on regeneratory processes in the kidney in experiments on rabbits. *Works of Scientific Society of Kasakhstan, Alma-Ata,* 1960, p. 271-274.

[32] Beljansky V.A. The role of antagonistic innervation of kidney pyelon, major and minor calices. *Works of Kuibyshev Medical Institute,* 1948; 1: 191-206.

[33] Bello-Reuss E., Colindress R.E., Pastoriza-Munoz E., Mueller R.A., Gottschalk C.W. Effects of acute unilateral renal denervation in the rat. *J.Clin.Invest.,* 1975 Jul; 56 (1): 208-217.

[34] Belokurenko S.P. Nerves of a human kidney fibrous capsule and some mammalian animals: *Medic. Cand. Dissertation,* Donetzk, 1965, -16 p.

[35] Bencsath P., Szalay L., Demeczky L. Effect of chlorothiazide and furosemide on sodium and water excretion after unilateral splanchnicotomy in the dog. - *Nephron,* 1971; 8: 329-343.

[36] Bencsath P., Takacs L. Intrarenal distribution of blood flow and cortico-medullary sodium gradient after unilateral splanchnicotomy in the dog. - *J.Physiol.,* 1971; 212 (3): 629-640.

[37] Beritov I.S. *The general physiology of nervous and muscular systems,* Moscow, Medgis, 1959, -600 p.

[38] Bernard C.L. *Lecons sur ler propietes physiologiques des liquides de l'organisme.* - Paris, 1959, -325 p.

[39] Berne R.M. Hemodynamics and Sodium excretion of denervated kidney in anaesthetized and unanaesthetized dog. - *Amer.J.Physiol.,* 1952; 171 (10): 148-156.

[40] Berne R.M., Hoffman W.K., Kagan A. Response of the normal and denervated kidney to l'epinephrine and l'norepinephrine. - *Amer.J.Physiol.*, 1952; 171 (3): 564-571.

[41] Bessmertnyi B.S. The influence of a kidney denervation on its function. *First Congress of Russian urologists,* Moscow, 1927, 42-44.

[42] Blake W.D. Denervation diuresis. - *Amer.J.Physiology,* 1962; 202 (1): 778-780.

[43] Blake W.D., Jurf A.N. Renal sodium reabsorption after acute renal denervation in the rabbit. - *J.Physiol.* /Lond/, 1968; 168: p. 65-73.

[44] Bonjour J.PH., Churchill P.C., Malvin R.L. Change of tubular reabsorption of Sodium and Water after renal denervation in the dog. - *J.Physiol.,* 1969; 204 (3): 571-582.

[45] Borovsky M.L. *A nerve regeneration and trophic,* Moscow, USSR Academy of Medical Sciences, 1952, -224 p.

[46] Borst J.G. The maintenance of an adequate cardiac output by the regulating of the urinary excretion of water and salt. - *Acta med.Scand.,* 1948, Suppl. 207: 130-149.

[47] Brandsburg B.B. Pathologic changes in heart muscle after a sympatectomy. *XVII Congress of Russian surgeons*, Leningrad, 1926, p. 105-105.

[48] Bricker N.S., Guild W.R., Reardan J.B. Studies of the functional capacity of a denervated homotransplanted kidney in an identical twin with parallel observations in the donor. - *J.Clin.Invest.,* 1956; 35 (12): 1364-1380.

[49] Bricker N.S., Straffon R.A., Mahoney E.P. The functional capacity of the kidney denervated by autotransplantation in the dog. - *J.Clin.Invest.,* 1958; 37 (2): 185-193.

[50] Brjusova S.S. Fire-arm wounds of cranial nerves. In the book: *Sovjet Medicine Experience in the Great Patriotic War 1941-1945,* Moscow, 1952; 20: 158-167.

[51] Bykow K.M. Die afferente impulsation der Nierennerven. - In: Nierenfunktion und Nervensystem / Hrag. von H. Dutz. - Berlin: *Volk und Gesundheit*, 1959, S. 46-49.

[52] Bykova H.A. Morphological display of a tissue incompatibility by kidney allotransplantation. *Medic Doctor Dissertation,* Moscow, 1969, -32.

[53] Bykova N.A., Perov L.D., Grobysheva V.S., Kirpatovsky I.D. Histo-fermentary activity of a dog kidney in the norm and by transplantation. *Archiv pathology,* Moscow, 1969; 6: 23-31.

[54] Buchman A.A., Slutzkin I.M. Local hypothermia in operations on the kidney. *Urology a. Nephrology,* Moscow, 1968; 5: 14-17.

[55] Bukin I.V. Morphology of abdominal part of wandering nerves. *Works of Navy medical Academy,* Leningrad, 1944; 3 (2): 125-136.

[56] Bunatjan G.Ch., Oganesjan A.S. Influence of the adrenaline on some aspects of work of an intact and denervated kidney. *News of Armenian Academy of Sciences,* 1958; 11 (6): 3-11.

[57] Bunatjan G.Ch., Oganesjan A.S. Influence of insuline and adrenaline on some aspects of work of a denervated kidney. *News of Armenian Academy of Sciences,* 1959; 12 (1): 7-15.

[58] Buresh J., Petran M., Sachar I. *Electrophysiological methods of investigation,* Moscow, IL, 1962, -456 p.

[59] Cherkasova M.E. Auto- and homotransplantation of the kidney in experiments. *Medical Candidate Dissertation,* Moscow, 1966. -19 p.

[60] Cherkasova M.E. Comparative evaluation of the kidney transplantation in the pelvis and to the neck. In the book: *Works of P. Lumumba Peoples Friendship University,* Moscow, 1967; 25 (2): 191-196.

[61] Cherkasova M.E., Bykova N.A. Clinical and morphological characteristics of the sole autotransplanted and the sole intact kidneys. In the book: *Pathology and surgical correction of blood circulation and gas exchange*, Novosibirsk, 1965, p. 26-28.

[62] Chernigovsky V.N. Investigation of internal organ receptors. *Medical Doctor Dissertation,* Leningrad, 1940, -395 p.

[63] Chernigovsky V.N. Interoceptors, Moscow, *Medgis,* 1966, -659 p.

[64] Christensen K., Lewis E. a. Kuntz A. Innervation of the renal blood vessels in the cat. - *J.Compar.Neurol.,* 1951; 95 (3): 373-385.

[65] Christy I.J., Denton K.M., Anderson W.P. Renal denervation potentials the natriuretic and diuretic effects of atrial natriuretic peptide in anaesthetized rabbits. *Clin.Exp.Pharmacol.Physiol.,* 1994 Jan; 21 (1): 41-48.

[66] Chukhrienko D.P., Ljulko A.N. Atlas of operations on organs of the urogenital system, Moscow, *Medicine,* 1972, -375 p.

[67] Ciccone C.D., Zambraski E.J. Effects of acute renal denervation on kidney function in deoxycorticosterone acetate - *hypertensive swine, Hypertension,* 1986; 8: 925-931.

[68] Circella M.G., Pellegrini P., Di Cagno N. Ricerebe sperimentali in tema di resezione renale: influenza della decapsulazione sulla funzione del parenchyma renale residuo. - *Arch.ital.urol.*, 1957; 30 (4): 279-298.

[69] Correl J.W., Adipose tissue: Ability to respond to nerve stimulation in vitro. - *Acience,* 1963; 140: 387-388.

[70] Corrodi H., Hillarp N.A. Fluoreszenzmetoden zur histochemischen Sichtbarmachung von Monoaminen. - *Helvetica Chimica Acta,* 1964; 47: 911-917.

[71] Corrodi H., Hillarp N.A., Jonsson C. Fluorescence method for the histochemical demonstration of monoamines. 3. Sodium borohydride reduction of the fluorescent compounds as a specificity test. - *J.Histochem.Cytochem.*, 964; 12 (7): 582-586.

[72] Couch N.P., McBride R.A., Dammin C.J. Observations on the nature of the enlargement, the regeneration of the nerves and the function of the canine renal autograft. - *Brit.J.Exp.Path.,* 1961; 42 (2): 106-113.

[73] Dalimov Sh.S. Some data about histochemical examination of a denervated kidney. In the book: Questions of biology and endemic medicine, Tashkent, 1963; 4: 399-403.

[74] Dalimov Sh.S. Histochemical investigation of polysakharides and lipides contents in the kidney by its denervation. In the book: *Questions of anatomy and histology,* Tashkent, 1966, vol. 2, p. 226-227.

[75] Daricheva A.V. Kidney function by experimental hypertonia. *Medical Candidate Dissertation*, Ivanovo, 1954, -20 p.

[76] Daricheva A.V. Morphological changes in dog autotransplanted kidneys. *Archiv pathologic*, Moscow, 1963; 25 (12): 56-61.

[77] Delectersky V.V., Sheklakov N.D., Shadyev H.K. Ultrastructure of M. Canis in the culture and injured hair. *Herald of Dermatology,* Moscow, 1975; 6: 10-13.

[78] Devjatjarov L.A. Experimental ground of the kidney autotransplantation to renal vessels. *Medical Candidate Dissertation,* Omsk, 1965, -16 p.

[79] Dempster W.J., Joekes. Functional studies of the kidney autotransplanted to the neck of dog. *Acta med. Scand.*, 1953; 147 (3): 99-118.

[80] Di Bona G.F. The kidney in the pathogenesis of hypertension: The role of renal nerves. *Am.J.Kidney Dis.,* 1985; 5: A 27-A 31.

[81] Di Bona G.F. Sympathetic nervous system influences on the kidney. Role in hypertension. *Am.J.Hypertens.,* 1989; 2, Suppl.: 119 S-124 S.

[82] Di Bona G.F. Neural control of renal function: Cardio vascular implications. *Hypertension,* 1989; 13: 539-548.

[83] Di Bona G.F. Jones S.Y., Sawin L.L. Renal sympathetic neural mechanisms as intermediate phenotype in spontaneously hypertensive rats. *Hypertension,* 1996; 27: 626-630.

[84] Di Bona G.F., Kopp U.C. Neural control of renal function. *Physiol. Rev.,* 1997; 77: 75-197.

[85] Dogiel A.S. Zur Kentniss der Nerven der Ureteren. - *Arch.mikr.Anat.,* 1978; 15: 64-64.

[86] Dolezel S. Vazivova kostra ledviny psa a jeji vztah k cavam a nervum. - *Ceskoslov.Morfol.*, 1957; 5 (1): 16-20.

[87] Dolezel S. Histochemische Untersuchung der Niereninnervation mittels der Reaction auf Cholinesterasen. - *Janrb. Morphol. u. Microskop.Anat.,* 1958; 63 (4): 599-608.

[88] Dolezel S. Uber die Innervation der Niere einiger Saugetiere. - In: Nierenfunktion und Nervensystem / Hrag. von H.Dutz. - Berlin: *Volk und Gesundbeit,* 1959, S. 45-59.

[89] Dolezel S. Blutkörperchenföllung der Glomerula nach der Anästhesie des Nierenplexus bei der Ratte. - *Z.Mikr. Anat.Forach.*, 1962; (1): 132-132.

[90] Dowling G.J., Harris P.J., Skinner S.L. Effects of renal denervation and atrial natriuretic factor on tubular reabsorption in anaesthetized rats. *Clin.Exp.Pharmacol.Physiol.,* 1989; Oct., 16 (10): 773-782.

[91] Eliseeva A.M. Influence of some urinogenic remedies on the function of autotransplanted and intact kidneys. *Pharmacology a. Toxicology,* Moscow, 1958; 21 (2): 56-61.

[92] Engelhorn R. Der Einfluss von Adrenalin und Nor-Adrenalin auf die Aktionspotentiale der Nierennerven. - In: Nierenfunktion und Nervensystem / Hrag. von H.Dutz. - Berlin: *Volk und Gesundheit,* 1959, S. 140-145.

[93] English J., Evan A., Houghton D.C., Bennett W.M. Cyclosporine-induced acute renal dysfunction in the rat. *Transplantation,* 1987; 44: 135-141.

[94] Eraslan S., Hardy J.D., Elliott R.L. Lung reimplantation, respiratory reflexes, vagal integrity and lung function in chronic dogs. - *J.Surg.Res.,* 1960; 6 (9): 383-388.

[95] Ericsson J., Mostofi F., Weibel J. Ultrastructure of proximal convoluted tubules: endoplasmic reticulum, Golgi apparatus and single membrane limited bodies. - *Anat. Rec.*, 1963; 145 (2): 227-227.

[96] Ericsson J.L.E., Trump B.F., Weibel J. Electron microscopic studies of the proximal tubule of the rat kidney. II. Cytosegresomes and cytosomes: their relationship to each other and to the lysosome concept. - *lab.Invest.,* 1965; 14 (7): 1341-1365.

[97] Ermakov M.V., Voronoy U.U. Excretory function of the kidney in early period after its transplantation. *Medical Journal, Kiev,* 1953; 23 (3): 35-42.

[98] Euler U.S. A specific sympathomimetic ergone in adrenergic nerve fibers (sympathin) and its relation to adrenaline and noradrenaline. - *Acta physiol.Scand.,* 1946; 12 (1): 73-97.

[99] Faarup P. On the morphology of the juxtaglomerular apparatus. - *Acta. Anat.*, 1965; 60 (1): 20-38.

[100] Falck B. Observations on the possibilities of the cellular localization of monoamines by a fluroescence method. - *Acta physiol.Scand.,* 1962; 56, Supple. 197: 1-25.

[101] Falck B., Hillarp N.A., Thieme G., Torp A. Fluorescence of cathecholamines and related compounds condensed with formaldehyde. *J. Histochem.Cytochem.,* 1962; 2 (10): 348-354.

[102] Falck B., Owman C. A detailed methodological description of the fluorescence method for cellular demonstration of biogenic monoamines. - *Acta Univers.Lundensis.,* 1965, Section II (7): 4-23.

[103] Farthing M.J.G., Clark M.L. Nature of the toxicity of cyclosporine A in the rat. *Biochem.Pharmacol.,* 1981; 24: 3311-3316.

[104] Faulkner J.W., Scheridan P.H., Macdermott G.A. The role of renal counterbalance in autogenous renal transplants. - *J.Urol.,* 1960; 84 (2): 273-277.

[105] Faure J.L. Traitment chirurgical de la paralysie faciale par l`anastomose spino-faciale. - *Rev.Chir.*, 1928; 18: 1098-1099.

[106] Fedrushkova U.N., Dosorova A.D. Influence of irritation of a sole autotransplanted kidney on its function and level of arterial pressure. In the book: *Materials of 35 Scientific Conference of Kuibyshev State Medical Institute,* 1967, p. 16-17.

[107] Feldina L., Katunsky A.Ya., Khayutin V.M. Responces or renal sympathetic nerves to stimulation of afferent A and C fibers of tibial and mesenterial nerves. *Acta Physiol.. Hung.,* 1966; 2 (29): 157-176.

[108] Fewell J.E., Bond G.C. Renal denervation eliminates the renal response to continuous positive-pressure ventilation. *Proc.Soc.Exp.Biol.Med.,* 1979; 161: 574-578.

[109] Filonova K.S. Nerves of the human kidney. In the book: *Macro- and microscopy of the vegetative nervous system, glands of mucosal membranes and skin,* Moscow, 1948, p. 83-120.

[110] Finberg J.P.M., Peart W.S. Function of smooth muscle of the rat renal pelvis-response of the isolated pelvis muscle to angiotensin and some other substances. - *Brit.J.Pharmac.,* 1970; 39: 373-381.

[111] Fischer A., Takacs L., Verga S. Glomerulusfiltrat und Natriumausscheidung der denervierten Niere. - *A.Ges. exp.med.,* 1957; 129 (1): 33-44.

[112] Fladerer H., Aubock L. Zur Ultrastruktur der obliterierenden Arterio-Arteriolopathie beim Nierentransplant. - *Vehr.Dtsch.Ges.Path.,* 1974; 58: 488-488.

[113] Fourman J.M. The adrenergic innervation of the efferent arterioles and the vasa recta in the mammalian kidney. - *Experientia,* 1970; 26: 239-294.

[114] Frazier Ch.H. The treatment of paralysis of the recurrent laryngeal nerve by nerve anastomosis. - *Ann.Surg.*, 1924; 79 (2): 161-171.

[115] Furchgott R.F., Lee K.S. High energy phosphates and the force of contraction of cardiac muscle. - *Circulation,* 1961; 24 (2): 416-428.

[116] Fuxe K., Johnsson G. The histological fluorescence method for the demonstration of cathecholamines. Theory, practice and application. - *J.Histochem.Cytochem.,* 1973; 21 (4): 293-311.

[117] Gachechiladze G.A. *Influence of a kidney full denervation on its function.* Scientific News of P. Lesgaft Institute, Leningrad, 1928; 14 (1-2): 83-112.

[118] Gant H., Baker F.W., Livingston A. Hormonal factors in conditional reflex diuresis. - In: Abst. of papers 23 int. *Congress physiol. Sciences,* Tokyo, 1965, p. 26-26.

[119] Gazdar A.F., Dammin G.J. Neural degeneration and regeneration in human renal transplants. *N.Engl.J.Med.,* 1970; 283: 222-224.

[120] Ginetzinsky A.G., Lichnitskaja I.I., Semjenova E.P. Influence of denervation on newborn animal kidneys. *Bulletin of experimental biology and medicine,* Moscow, 1952; 34 (8): 6-11.

[121] Ginetzinsky A.G. New data about a kidney work regulation. In the book: Materials of *8th Allunion Congress in physiology, Biochemistry and Pharmacology,* Moscow, 1955, p. 170-172.

[122] Ginetzinsky A.G., Lebedinsky A.V. *Course of normal physiology,* Moscow, Medgis, 1956, -535 p.

[123] Ginetzinsky A.G., Vasiljeva V.F. Efferent innervation of kidney tubules. *Reports of USSR Academy of Sciences,* 1956, vol 10, N6, p. 1382-1384.

[124] Ginetzinsky A.G., Vasiljeva V.P., Sax M.G. Importance of efferent nerves in kidney function. In the book: *Problem of evolutionary physiology,* Moscow-Leningrad, 1958, p. 17-37.

[125] Ginetzinsky A.G., Sax M.G., Titova L.K. Mechanism of action of an antidiuretic hormone. *Reports of USSR Academy of Sciences,* 1958; 120 (1): 216-218.

[126] Ginetzinsky A.G. Physiological mechanisms of the water-saline balance, Moscow-Leningrad, *Nauka,* 1964, -427 p.

[127] Ginetzinsky A.G., Sax M.G., Ivanova A.N. Mechanism of action of an antidiuretic hormone. In the book: *Materials of 9th Allunion Congress in physiology, biochemistry and pharmacology,* Minsk, 1959, p. 151-152.

[128] Ginn H.E., Unger A.M., Hume D.M. Human renal transplantation an investigation of the functional status of the denervated kidney after successful homotransplantations in identical twins. - *J.Lab. a. Clin.Med.,* 1960; 56 (1): 1-13.

[129] Gollan F. In: Inhibitors of ferments and metabolism, Moscow, *Mir,* 1966, -325 p.

[130] Golub D.M. Formation of new nervous and vascular ways in minory pelvis organs. *Minsk, Science and Techniques,* 1964, -200 p.

[131] Golub D.M., Heinman F.B. Experimental data in transplantation of nervous ganglions in the bladder wall. In the book: Reinnervation and revascularization of internal organs by means of organopexy, Minsk, *Science and Techniques,* 1969, p. 27-35.

[132] Golub D.I., Heiman F.B., Novikoff I.I. Reinnervation of internal organs and vessels by means of neuropexy. Archive AGE, Moscow, 1979; 4: 5-16.

[133] Gomba S.Z., Soltesz M.B., Endes P. Studies of the granulated cells of the juxtaglomerular apparatus. - *Acta Morphol. Acad. Sci. Hung.,* 1964; 13: 19-24.

[134] Gombos A. Transplantacia obliciek. - *Kandidatska dizertacna praca.* - Kosice, 1962. - 232 p.

[135] Gombos A., Stopek D., Gombosova M. Intrarenalna adrenerinervacia. - In: *Ved. konferencia LF UPJS,* Kosice, 1970, suhrny prac p. 3-4.

[136] Gombos A., Stopek D., Gombosova M. Monoaminergna inervacia oblicky u psa. - In. *Zbornik Lek. Fakulty UPJS,* Kosice, 1972; 14 (29): 197-208.

[137] Gombos A. Inervacia transplantovanej oblicky. - *Doktorska disertacna praca.* - Kosice, 1974, -275 p.

[138] Gombos A., Stopek D., Jacina J. Is it worth preserving the nerves in a transplanted kidney? - *Folia Morphol.,* 1975; 23 (4): 320-322.

[139] Gombosh A., Stopek D., Jasina J., Syrotjakova. Possibilities of keeping of innervation in transplanted kidneys of dogs. *Archiv AGE,* Moscow, 1978; 7: 5-11.

[140] Gosling J.A. Observation on the distribution of intrarenal nervous tissue. - *Anat.Record,* 1969; 163 (1): 81-88.

[141] Gosteeva M.N. Distribution of nerve fibers in the kidney of a human embrio. News of USSR Academy of Sciences. *Ser. Biology,* 1949; 4: 519-526.

[142] Govyrin V.A. The role of adrenalin and noradrenalin in adaptory-trophic function of the nervous system in warm-blood and cold-blood animals. In the book: *Functional evolution of the nervous system. Moscow*-Leningrad, 1965, p. 115-123.

[143] Govyrin V.A. *About an absence of sympathetic innervation in skeleton muscles.* Report of USSR Academy of Sciences, 1965; 160 (5): 1179-1181.

[144] Govyrin V.A. Trophic function of sympathetic nerves of the heart and skeleton muscles, Leningrad, *Nauka,* 1967, -131 p.

[145] Graham R.C., Karnovsky M.J. The early stages of an absorption of injected horseradish peroxidase in the proximal tubules of the mouse kidney. Ultrastructural cytochemistry by a new technique. - *J.Histochem. Cytochem.,* 1966; 14: 291-302.

[146] Grebenjuk V.I. Treatment of firm paralyses of facial muscles by means of sewing of facial and diaphragmal nerves. *Medic. Candidate Dissertation,* Leningrad, 1960, -16 p.

[147] Grigorovich K.A. Recovery operations by large nerve defects, *Surgery,* Moscow, 1968; 8: 118-122.

[148] Grigorovich K.A. Nerve surgery, Leningrad, *Nauka,* 1969, -447 p.

[149] Grigorjeva T.A. About the cause of trophic upsettings in organism parts with deprivated sensitivity. *Reports of USSR Academy of Sciences, M*oscow, 1951; 78 (2): 387-390.

[150] Grigorjeva T.A. About specific peculiarities in dystrophic processes by organ sensitive and motor denervation. In the book: *Problems of a nervous trophic in the medicine theory and practice,* Moscow, 1963, p. 98-102.

[151] Gritzman U.Ja., Masina F.V. Examination of urine excretory function of autotransplanted kidney. Report 1. *Bulletin of experimental biology and medicine,* 1952; 34 (12): 10-14.

[152] Haebler H. Über die nervosen Versörgung der Nierenkelche. - *Z.Urol.,* 1922, 16: 377-384.

[153] Hainman F.B. Structure of the kidney abdominal-aortic plexus. *Medical Candidate Dissertation,* Minsk, 1952, -18 p.

[154] Haiman F.B. Some results of investigation of the urinary tract innervation and bladder reinnervation. In the book: Reinnervation and revascularization of internal organs by means of an organopexy. *Journal Science and Techniques,* Minsk, 1969, p. 105-118.

[155] Hamitov H.S., Shvalev V.N. Histo-physiologic analysis of heart and kidney microstructures in experiments. In the book: *Materials of the 2nd Povolje Conference in physiology,* Kazan, 1961, p. 525-526.

[156] Hansen J.M., Abildaary U., Fogh-Andersen N., Kanstrup I.L., Bratholm P., Plum I., Strandgaard. The transplanted human kidney does not achieve functional reinenrvation. *Clin. Sci.,* 1994; 87: 13-20.

[157] Haritonov I.F. Nervous reflectory regulation of ureter motor function. *Medical Candidate Dissertation,* Kazan, 1958, -23 p.

[158] Haritonov U.F. Role of the sympathetic and parasympathetic nervous system in the ureter motor function. In the book: *Materials of the 2nd Povolje Conference in physiology*, Kazan, 1961, p. 529-530.

[159] Heller J. Die Veränderungen der Nierentätigkeit bei Emotionszustanden und bei der bedingtreflektorischen Wasserdiurese. - In: *Nierenfunktion und Nervensystem / Hrag. von H.Dutz.* - Berlin: Volk u. Gesundheit, 1959, S. 236-239.

[160] Heyman S.N., Brezis M., Epstein F.H., Spokes K., Rosen S. Effects of glycine and hypertrophy on renal outer medullary hypoxic injury in ischemia reflow and contrast nephropathy: *Am.J.Kidney Dis.;* 1992; 19: 578-586.

[161] Hirakawa A., Corcoran A.C. J131-o-iodohipporate excretion and a quantitative formulation of the radioisotope renogram as indices of bilateral and unilateral renal functions. - *J.Lab.a.Clin.Med.*, 1963; 63 (5): 795-807.

[162] Hitrov F.M. Demonstration of a patient after the anastomosing of a facial nerve with dyaphragmal. *Surgery,* Moscow, 1951; (2): 85-85.

[163] Hogestatt E.D., Johansson O., Andersson K.E., Kullerndorf C.M. Influence of renal denervation on vascular responsiveness of isolated rat intrarenal arteries. *Acta Physiol. Scand.,* 1988; 132: 59-66.

[164] Hume D.M. Kidney transplantation. - In: *Human transplantation.* - New York - London, 1968, p. 110-151.

[165] Hume D.M., Merril J.P., Miller B.F. Experiences with renal homotransplantations in the human: report of nine cases. *J.Clin.Invest.,* 1955; 34: 327-332.

[166] Inselmann G., Hannemann J., Baumann K. Cyclosporin A-induced lipid peroxidation and influence on glucose-6-phosphatase in rat hepatic and renal microsomes. *Res. Common Chem. Pathol. Pharmacol.*, 1990; 68: 189-203.

[167] Ivanov H.M. Innervation of human and experimental animals, *Medical Candidate Dissertation,* Kazan, 1964, -18 p.

[168] Jabotinsky U.M. Normal and pathologic morphology of vegetative ganglions, Moscow, *USSR Medical Academy of Sciences,* 1965, p. 166-167.

[169] Jabotinsky U.M. Normal and pathologic morphology of the neuron, Leningrad, *Medicine,* 1965, -323 p.

[170] Jansky M. Renalni nervosa platen a sousedni pletene u krysy. - *Ceskoslov.morfol.*, 1954; II (2): 96-109.

[171] Jeejebhoy H.F. Spontaneous reversal of homograft rejection. - *Transplantation,* 1965; 3 (2): 257-259.

[172] Jirka J. Wirkung der Nierendenervierung auf die Nierenhemodynamik bei Muskelarbeit. - In: Nierenfunktion und Nervensystem / Hrsg. von H.Dutz. - Berlin. *Volk u. Gesundheit,* 1959, S. 157-159.

[173] Jnoue H., Suzuki A., Sato S. Renal transplantation: experimental study and clinical experience. - *Urol.Internat.*, 1957; 5 (5): 253-273.

[174] Jung K., Pergande M. Influence of cyclosporine A on the respiration of isolated rat kidney mitochondria. *FEBS Lett,* 1985; 183: 167-171.

[175] Jutanov S.I. Remote results of lung autotransplantation in experiments. In the book: *Pathology a. surgical correction of the blood circulation and gas exchange,* Novosibirsk, 1965, p. 13-14.

[176] Jutanov S.I. Plasty of nerve trunks by lung transplantation in experiments. In the book: *Transplantation of organs and tissues,* Moscow, 1966, p. 60-62.

[177] Kalinina T.V. Kidney transplantation. *J. Urology,* Moscow, 1955; (1): 43-49.

[178] Kamm D.E., Levinsky M.C. The mechanism of denervation natriuresis. - *J. Clin. invest.,* 1965; 44 (1): p. 93-102.

[179] Kaplan S.A., Rapoport S. Urinary excretion of sodium and chloride after splanchnicotomy: Effect on the proximal tubule. - *Amer.J.Physiol.,* 1951; 164 (1): 175-181.

[180] Karnovsky M.J., Roots L. A "Direct-Coloring" Thiocholine method for cholinesterase. - *J.Histochem.,* 1964; 12 (3): 219-221.

[181] Karupu V.J. Role of innervation in the kidney trophic. *Physiologic Journal of Ukraine* Academy of Sciences, 1960; 6 (6): 795-800.

[182] Kaverina V.V. Nerve regeneration by neuroplastic operations, Leningrad, *Medicine,* 1975, -200 p.

[183] Kelemen J., Miskolozy D. Die intraorganischen Nervenfasern und das mikroganglionssistem der Niere beim Menschen und bei einigen Saugetieren (Beitrage zum Problem der mikroskopischen Innervation der Niere). - *Acta biologica, Acta Univer. Szegediensis,* 1963; 9: 137-151.

[184] Kennon V., Rosenbluth A. Increase of sensitivity in denervated structures: A rule of denervation, Moscow, *Mir,* 1951, -462 p.

[185] Kerdivarenko N.V. Intramural nervous apparatus of the kidney fibrous capsule. *Archiv AGE,* Moscow, 1960; 39 (9): 78-85.

[186] Kerdivarenko N.V. Morphology of the kidney fibrous capsule nervous apparatus in experiments. In the book: *Works of Kishinjev State Medical Institute, Kishinjev,* 1964; 23: 53-57.

[187] Kerr W.K., Kyle V.N., Keresteci A.G. Renal hypothermia. - *J.Urol.,* 1960; 84 (2): 236-242.

[188] Kibjakov A.V. Chemical transference of a nervous excitement, Moscow-Leningrad, *Nauka,* 1964, -208 p.

[189] Kirpatovsky I.D. Techniques of a surgical reinnervation of the kidney transplant. In the book: Questions of renal insufficiency and kidney transplantation. *Works of P. Lumamba Peoples Friendship University,* Moscow, 1969; 62 (5): 111-114.

[190] Kirpatovsky I.D., Bykova N.A. Kidney transplantation, Moscow, *Medicine,* 1969, -232 p.

[191] Kirpatovsky I.D., Cherkasova M.E. Kidney transplantation. In the book: *Selected lectures in transplantology,* Moscow, 1969, p. 60-80.

[192] Kirpatovsky I.D. Unspecific factors of transplantation. In the book: *Materials of Jubilee Conference of P. Lumumba People Friendship University,* Moscow, 1970, p. 68-74.

[193] Kirpatovsky I.D., Bykova N. Surgical ways for improvement of the state of transplanted organs. - *Europ. Surg. Research,* 1970; 2 (1): 119.

[194] Kline R.L., Mercer P.F. Functional reinnervation and development of supersensitivity to NE after renal denervation in rats. *Am.J.Physiol.*, 1980; 238: R 353-R 358.

[195] Kompanovska-Jezierska E., Walkowska A., Johns E.J., Sadowsky J. Early effects of renal denervation in the anaesthetized rat: natriuresis and increased cortical blood flow. *J.Physiol.,* 2001; 531 (2): 527-534.

[196] Kon V., Sugiura M., Inagami T., Harvie B.P., Ichikawa I., Hoover R.L. Role of endothelin in cyclosporine-induced glomerular dysfunction. *Kidney Int.,* 1990; 37: 1487-1491.

[197] Korenevsky L.I., Levtchuk G.A., Shvedova-Roshe T.S. Kideny autotransplantation. *Newspaper Medicine affairs,* 1956; (3): 277-280.

[198] Kovanov V.V. From theory to practice. *Medical paper,* 1978; 36 (3754), 5 May, p. 3.

[199] Kravacich J., Kline R.L., Mercer P.F. Supersensitivity to norepinephrine in chronically denervated kidneys: evidence for a postsynaptic effect. *Can.J.Physiol.Pharmacol.,* 1987 Nov.; 65 (11): 2219-2224.

[200] Kravtchinsky K.D. Physiology of water-saline exchange in the body liquids. Leningrad, *Medgis,* 1963, -311 p.

[201] Kriss J.P., Futcher P.H., Goldman L.L. Unilateral adrenalectomy, unilateral splanchnic nerve resection and homolateral renal function. - *Amer.J.Physiol.,* 1948; 154 (2): 229-240.

[202] Kristensson K., Olsson Y. Uptake and retrograde axonal transport of peroxidase by hypoglossal neurons. - *Acta Neuropath.* (Berl.), 1971; 19: 1-9.

[203] Kubicek K.W., Harvey R., Kottke F. The adrenaline sensitivity of the denervated kidney. - *Federat.proc.,* 1948; 7: 68-68.

[204] Kulagina V.P. Peculiarities of efferent impulsation in postganglion nervous ways of n. splanchnicus by vasoconstrictory and vasodilatatory reactions in abdominal organs. *Bulletin of Experimental Biology and Medicine,* 1964; 57 (3): 6-10.

[205] Kulik V.P., Maximenkova A.N. Function and morphology of a transplanted intestine, Moscow, *Nauka,* 1974, -159 p.

[206] Lackner L.H., Mckay M. Observation into mechanism of denervation natriuresis. - *Invest.Urol.,* 1971; 9 (1): 44-46.

[207] Lanese D.M., Conger J.D. Effects of endothelin receptor antagonist on cyclosporine-induced vasoconstriction in isolated rat renal arterioles. *J.Clin.Invest,* 1993; 91: 2144-2149.

[208] Lang R., Michels J., Becker-Berke R., Lukowski K., Vlaho V., Grundmann R. Die sympathische Aktivität bei terminaler Niereninsuffizienz und Nierentransplantation. *Klinische Wochenschrift,* 1984; 62: 1025-1031.

[209] Lapchinsky A.G. Remote results of extremities and kidney transplantation in dogs. *Pathological Physiology and Experimental Therapy,* 1960; 4 (6): 17-23.

[210] Lebedev A.A., Sevastjanova L.V. Conditional reflectory changes of diuresis in dogs with an intact, transplanted and denervated kidney. In the book: *Second Allunion Student Conference of Medical, Pharmacological,* Stomatologic Institutes, Moscow, 1952, p. 59-60.

[211] Lebedev A.A., Sevastjanova L.V. Conditional-reflectory changes of diuresis in dogs with a transplanted kidney. *USSR Physiological Journal,* 1954; 60 (4): 441-444.

[212] Lebedev A.A. Influence of adrenalin on the function of a transplanted reinnervated kidney. *USSR Physiological Journal,* 1961; 47 97): 892-899.

[213] Lebedev A.A. Efferent nerves of a transplanted reinnervated kidney. *Bulletin of Experimental Biology and Medicine,* 1961; 51 (4): 8-12.
[214] Lebedev A.A. Vicarious hypertrophy of a transplanted reinnervated kidney. *Bulletin of Experimental Biology amd Medicine, 1*962; 54 (8): 41-43.
[215] Lebedev A.A. Function of a transplanted reinnervated kidney. *Medical Doctor Dissertation,* Leningrad, 1963, -28 p.
[216] Lebedev A.A. Method of a spleen autotransplantation and reinnervation. In the book: *Inventions in the field of medicine and biology,* Ivanovo, 1963, p. 67-68.
[217] Lebedev A.A. Kidney autotransplantation, Leningrad, Nauka, 1971, -122 p.
[218] Lebedenko V.V. Segmentary innervation of a kidney. *Urology,* (Moscow), 1928; 2 (20): 65-71.
[219] Lebedinskaja S.I. About conditions for neurogenous necroses beginning. In the book: *Current questions of general pathology and medicine,* Moscow, 1950, p. 31-39.
[220] Leibson L.G. About the nervous regulation of the kidney work. 1st report. Influence of an one-side cutting of n. splanchnici on the work of the corresponding kidney in dogs. *Russian physiologic journal,* 1926, vol. 9, N2, p. 265-310.
[221] Leibson L.G. About the nervous regulation of the kidney work. *Russian physiologic journal,* 1927; 10 (3-4): 179-182.
[222] Leranth G.S., Uncvary G.Y., Donath T. The innervation of the juxtaglomerular apparatus. - *Acta Morphol.Hung.,* 1969; 17 (2): 131-141.
[223] Liberman E.A., Chailakhjan l.M. About a nature of the potential action. *Biophysics,* 1959; 4 (5): 622-639.
[224] Ljunggvist A., Wagermark J. The adrenergic innervation of intrarenal glomerular and extra-glomerular circulatory routs. - *Nephron,* 1970; 7: 218-229.
[225] Lopuchin J.M., Kogan E.M., Karaganov J.L. Ultrastructural backgrounds of liver, kidney and heart vitality, Moscow, *Medicine,* 1977, -255 p.
[226] Lysov V.F. New data about the neuro-humoral regulation of the kidney work. In the book: *Material of 2nd Conference in physiology, biochemistry, pharmacology,* Kasan, 1961, p. 305-306.
[227] Lysov V.F. Innervation of kidney tubules. *Bulletin of experim.* biology a. medicine, 1962; 54 (10): 118-122.
[228] Lysov V.F. About a reflectory influence of the wandering nerve on the kidney function. In the book: *Physiology and pathology of cortico-visceral relations,* Ivanovo, 1965; 1: 603-606.
[229] Maichel R., Sussman H., Yamada K. Control of adipose tissue lipase activity by the sympathetic nervous system. - *Life Sci.,* 1963; 3: 210-214.
[230] Malmfors T., Sachs C.H. Direct studies on the disappiarence of the transmitter and changes in the uptake-storage mechanisms of degenerating adrenergic nerves. - *Acta physiol. Scand.,* 1965; 64 (3): 211-223.
[231] Mavrin M.I. Influence of n. splanchnicus on the kidney hemodynamics, reabsorption and electrolyt excretion. *USSR physiologic journal,* 1973, N10, p. 1602-1607.
[232] Mavrin M.I. About the mechanism of sympathetic nerves influence on the kidney function. *Bulletin of experim. biology a. medicine,* 1976; 8: 910-911.
[233] Mavrin M.I. Nervous regulation of glucose, Na and K transport in kidneys. *USSR Physiologic journal,* 1978; 3: 364-367.

[234] Mavrin M.I. Role of wandering nerves in regulation of tubulary processes in the kidneys. *USSR Physiological journal,* 1979; 5: 764-768.
[235] Maunsbach A.S. The influence of different fixatives and fixation methods on the ultrastructure of rat kidney tubule cells. 1. Comparison of different perfusion fixation methods and of glutaraldehyde, formaldehyde and osmium tetroxide fixatives. - *J.Ultrastruct. Res.*, 1966, vol. 15, p. 242-260.
[236] Maysjuck A.P., Gritzman Ju.ja. Morphologic changes in auto- and homoplastic transplanted kidneys. *Experimental surgery a. anaesthesiology,* 1962; 7 (4): 36-40.
[237] Maximenkova A.N. Role of reinnervation in restoration of thin intestine function by its autotransplantation. *Medical Candidate Dissertation,* Moscow, 1970, -21 p.
[238] McKenna o.C., Angelakos E.T. Adrenergic innervation of the canine kidney. - *Circul. Res.,* 1968; 22 (3): 345-354.
[239] McKenna o.C., Angelakos E.T. Acetilcholinesterase-containing nerve fibers in the canine kidney. - *Circul. Res.,* 1968; 23 (5): 645-651.
[240] Mehring N., Neumann K.H., Rahn K.H., Zidek W. Mechanisms of cyclosporine induced vasoconstriction in the isolated perfused rat kidney. *Nephron,* 1992; 60: 477-481.
[241] Mendez R.E., Lopez R., Lopez G., Marti M.S., Martinez-Maldanodo M. Effects of dopamine-receptor antagonists and renal denervation on amino acid-induced hyperfiltration. *Am.J.Physiol.,* 1991; 261: 70-75.
[242] Merill J.P., Murray J.E., Harrison J.H. Successful homotransplantations of the human kidney between identical twins. - *J.A.M.A.,* 1956; 160 (4): 277-282.
[243] Merill J.P., Harrison J.H., Murray J.E. Successful transplantation of the kidney between nonidentical twins. - *New Engl. J. Med.,* 1960; 262 (25): 1251-1260.
[244] Mesulam M.M. The blue reaction product in horse radish peroxidase neurohistochemistry: incubation, parameters and visibility. - *J.Histochem.Cytochem.,* 1976; 24 (12): 1273-1280.
[245] Mikhailova I.A. Kidney function after its denervation. *Pathologic physiology a. experimental therapy,* Moscow, 1957; 1 (4): 43-49.
[246] Mikhelson A.A. *Comparative examination of normal and denervated kidneys function.* News of P. Lesgaft scientific Institute, Leningrad, 1934; 17-18: 183-220.
[247] Mingasova I.B., Shvalev V.N. About the adrenergic innervation of the abdominal aorta and kidney, *Archiv AGE,* 1970; 8: 77-82.
[248] Mitin K.S., Bykova N.A. Electron microscopic examination of the kidneys by their autotransplantation in dogs. In the book: *Ultrastructure of cells tissues and organs in the norm and pathology,* Moscow, 1970, p. 125-129.
[249] Mitchell G.A. The nerve supply of the kidneys. - *Acta Anat.,* 1950; 10 (1-2): 1-37.
[250] Mjasoedova N.A. Comparative influence of interreceptory irritations on the function of intact and transplanted kidneys. In the book: *Scientific works of Ivanovo State Medical Institute*, 1952; 8: 111-114.
[251] Mjasoedova N.A., Tjurina E.I. Changes of filtration and reabsorption in a transplanted kidney by interreceptory irritations. In the book: *Scientific works of Ivanovo State Medical Institute*, 1952; 8: 103-106.
[252] Moiseeva O.I. *Influence of kidney denervation on erythropoetic activity of rabbit blood plasma. Problems of hematology a. hemotransfusion,* Moscow, 1964; 9 (2): 8-13.

[253] Moiseeva O.I. Changes of the blood erythrocitary composition after the kidney partial denervation in rabbits. *Bulletin of experim. biology a. medicine,* 1964; 57 (3): 41-44.

[254] Moss N.G., Powell S.L., Falck R.I. Intravenous cyclosporine activates afferent and efferent renal nerves and causes sodium retention in innervated kidneys in rats. *Proc. Natl. Acad. Sci.* USA, 1985; 82: 8222-8226.

[255] Mueller P.I., O`Hagan K.P., Skogg K.A., Buckwalter J.B., Clifford P.S. In *vivo verification of renal denervation.* FASEB J., 1998; 12: A 690.

[256] Mueller P.I., O`Hagan K.P., Skogg K.A., Buckwalter J.B., Clifford P.S. Renal hemodynamic responses to dynamic exercise in rabbits. *J.Appl.Physiol.,* 1998; 85: 1605-1614.

[257] Mulbauer B., Spohr F., Schmidt R., Osswald H. Role of renal nerves and endogenous dopamine in amino acid-induced glomerular hyperfiltration. *Am.J.Physiol.*, 1997; 279: 144-149.

[258] Muller J., Barajas L. Electron microscopic and histochemical evidence for a tubular innervation in the renal cortex of the monkey. - *J.Ultrastr.Res.,* 1972; 41 (5-6); 533-549.

[259] Murray J.E., Lang S., Miller B.F. Functional status of single autotransplanted kidneys in the dog. - *Fed.Proc.*, 1954; 13 (1): 268-268.

[260] Murray J.E., Lang S., Miller B.F. Prolonged functional survival of renal autotransplants in the dog. - *Surg.Gynec.Obst.,* 1956; 103 (1): 15-22.

[261] Murray B.M., Paller M.S., Ferris T.F. Effect of cyclosporine administration on renal hemodynamics in conscious rats. *Kidney int.,* 1985; 28: 767-774.

[262] Murvanidze D.D. *The kidney,* Tbilisi, Mezniereba (science), 1975; 1: -388 p.

[263] Muylder C.D. The *"Neurility" of the kidney. A monograph on nerve supply to the kidney.* - Oxford: Blackwell, 1952, -195 p.

[264] Nadelsson F.E. Influence *a kidney of denervation on its basic excretory functions. Pathologic physiology a. experim. therapy,* Moscow, 1958; 2 (1): 53-54.

[265] Nadelsson F.E. *Influence of a kidney denervation on its basic excretory functions. Medical Candidate Dissertation,* Perm, 1961, -16 p.

[266] Nadelsson F.E. *Influence of a kidney denervation on its basic excretory functions. Experim. surgery a. anaesthesiology,* Moscow, 1966; (5): 10-11.

[267] Nasarishvili G.I. *Three versions of formation of two-chamber bladder for separate collection of the urine from kidneys.* In the book: Works of Urology Institute, Tbilisi, 1967; 4: 177-184.

[268] Nemes Z., Bodolay E., Pecze R. Morphological examination of the juxtaglomerular apparatus following the fluorescence microscopic demonstration of sympathetic nerves. - *Acta morph. Acad. Sci. Hung.*, 1975; 23 (1): 71-82.

[269] Niculescu L.T., Hagi-Paraschiv A., Enachescu A. Contributie la studiul terminatiilor nervoase din ripichi. - *Morfologia Normale si Patologia,* 1958; 3 (3): 203-212.

[270] Niederhausern W. La question du parasympathic renal. Recherches sur la limite inferieur du domaine du nerf vague. - *J.Urol.,* 1953; 59 (9-10): 565-577.

[271] Nikitina I.P. *About a receptory function of the kidney. Medical Candidate Dissertation,* Leningrad, 1947, -19 p.

[272] Nikitina I.P. Influence of a neurotic state and some factors on a water-excretory function of kidneys. *USSR Physiology Journal,* 1956; 42: 119-124.

[273] Nilsson O. *The adrenergic innervation of the kidney.* - *Lab.Invest.,* 1965; 14 (7): 1392-1395.

[274] Nomura G., Kibe Y., Arai S., Uno D., Takaechi J. Distribution of intrarenal blood flow after renal denervation in the dog. *Nephron,* 1976; 16: 126-133.

[275] Norvell J.E., Weitsen H.A., Dwyer J.J. Degeneration and Regeneration of adrenergic nerves in the autotransplanted kidney. - *Transplantation,* 1969; 7 (3): 218-220.

[276] Norvell J.E., Weitsen H.A., Sheppek C.G. The intrinsic innervation of human renal homotransplants. - *Transplantation,* 1970; 9 (2): 168-176.

[277] Oganesjan A.S. Influence of a cold irritation on the reabsorption of phosphates and chlorides in kidneys. *News of Armenian Academy of Sciences,* Erevan, 1956; 9 (9): 33-38.

[278] O`Hagan K.P., Bell L.B., Mittelstadt S.W., Clifford P.S. Effect of dynamic exercise on renal sympathetic nerve activity in conscious rabbits. *J.Apple.Physiol.,* 1993; 74: 2099-2104.

[279] Orbeli L.A. *Separate taking out of ureters as a method for examination of kidney functions.* News of P. Lesgaft Scientific Institute, Leningrad, 1924; 8: 375-380.

[280] Orbeli L.A. *About the physiologic surgery of the kidney. Herald of surgery,* Moscow, 1927; 9 (25): 42-49.

[281] Orbeli L.A. *New data in the doctrine about the autonomous nervous system. Selected works, 2nd edition.* USSR Academy of Sciences, Moscow-Leningrad, 1962, p. 67-71.

[282] Orbeli L.A. *Physiology of vegetative nervous system. Selected works,* 2nd edition, USSR Academy of Sciences, Moscow-Leningrad, 1962, p. 95-137.

[283] Orbeli L.A. *Theory of adaptive-trophic influence of the nervous system.* Selected works, 2nd edition, USSR Academy of Sciences, Moscow-Leningrad, 1962, p. 227-234.

[284] Osinskaja V.O. Examinations of adrenalin and noradrenalin exchange in the animal organism tissues. *Biochemistry,* 1957; 22 (3): 537-545.

[285] Pachmurnyi B.A. Filtration-reabsorption function of a denervated kidney in usual conditions and after influence of some neurotrophic substances. *Bulletin of exper. biology a. medicine,* Moscow, 1962, 53 (5): 84-89.

[286] Page E.B., Baxter C.F., Reem G.H. Effect of unilateral splanchnic nerve resection on the renal excretion of sodium. - *Amer.J.Physiol.,* 1954; 177: 194-300.

[287] Pavlov I.P. *About the trophic innervation. Full collection of works.* USSR Academy of Sciences, Moscow-Leningrad, 1951, p. 577-582.

[288] Pavlovskaja A.A. About the work of a denervated kidney. *Bulletin of exper. biology a. medicine,* Moscow, 1951; 31 (5): 305-308.

[289] Pernow J., Lundberg J.M. Release and vasoconstrictor effects of neuropeptide Y in relation to non-adrenergic sympathetic control of renal blood flow in the pig. *Acta Physiol. Scand.,* 1989; 136: 507-517.

[290] Perret G. Results of phrenicofacial nerve anastomosis for facial paralysis. - *Arch.Surg.,* 1967; 94: 505-508.

[291] Petersen J.S., Dibona G.F. Reflex control of renal sympathetic nerve activity during furosemide diuresis in rats. *Am.J.Physiol.,* 1994; 266: 537-545.

[292] Petrovsky B.V., Perelman M.I., Rabinovich J.J. Lung transplantation in experiments, Moscow, *Nauka,* 1975, -351 p.

[293] Pickford M. The inhibitory effect of acethylcholine on water diuresis in the dog and its pituitary transmission. - *J.Physiol.,* 1939; 95 (1): 226-238.

[294] Pines J.L. Electrophysiologic characteristics of afferent and efferent impulsation in kidney nerves. *Medical Candidate Dissertation,* Leningrad, 1952, -21 p.

[295] Pines J.L. Electrophysiologic examination of vascular mechanoreceptors in the kidneys. *USSR Physiologic Journal,* 1959; 65 (11): 1339-1347.

[296] Pines J.L. About an adaptation of kidney receptors. *USSR physiologic Journal,* 1965; 51 (9): 1116-1122.

[297] Pines J.L. Afferent impulsation of kidney nerves by influence of some chemical substances. In the book: *Works of I.P. Pavlov Institute of Physiology,* Leningrad, 1965, 11: 143-147.

[298] Pines J.L. About the tiredness of kidney receptors. *Bulletin of experim. biology a. medicine,* 1966; 62 (12): 16-21.

[299] Pines J.L. Afferent impulsation in kidney nerves by experimental ischemia. Reports of USSR Academy of Sciences, Moscow, 1967; 173 (3): 725-729.

[300] Pines J.L. Electrophysiologic investigation of influence of urine chemical substances on kidney receptors. *Bulletin of experim. biology a. medicine,* 1969; 67 (4): 3-7.

[301] Podkopajev N.A. Influence of extracardial nerves on the dog heart weight loss by the absolute hunger. *USSR Physiologic Journal,* 1936; 20: 277-279.

[302] Podshibjakin A.K. About a trophic function of the nervous system, Kiev, *Ukrainian Academy of Sciences,* 1964, -63 p.

[303] Polycar A. Boo Sh. Submicroscopic structure of cells and tissues in the norm and pathology, Leningrad, *Medgis,* 1962, -471 p.

[304] Polycarpova G.A. Sensitive innervation of renal vessels. In the book: Questions of sensitive innervation morphology, *Kazan,* 1958, p. 100-105.

[305] Pollock D.M., Arendshorst W.J. Effect of acute renal denervation and ANF on renal function in adult spontaneously hypertensive rats. *Am.J.Physiol.,* 1991, Oct; 261 (4 Pt 2): R 835-841.

[306] Pomeranz B.H., Birtch A.G., Barger A.C. Neural control of intrarenal blood flow. - *Amer.J.Physiol.,* 1968; 215 (5): 1067-1081.

[307] Protopopov S.J. Materials to anatomy and physiology of ureters. *Medical Doctor Dissertation,* Kazan, 1996, -227 p.

[308] Pytel J.A. Intramural nervous apparatus of the human upper urinary tract. *Medical Candidate Dissertation,* Moscow, 1960, -13 p.

[309] Raab W. The adrenergic-cholinergic control of cardiac metabolism and function: physiological and clinical aspects. - *Fortschr.Cardiol., Basel,* 1956; 1 (6): 65-152.

[310] Rabinovich J.J., Kulik A.M., Denisov-Nikolsky J.I. Lung autotransplantation in experiments and Gering-Braier reflex. *Journ.Experim.* surgery a. anaesthesiology, Moscow, 1975; 4: 31-35.

[311] Radostina T.N. Some questions of innervation and vascularization of digestive tract. *Medical Doctor Dissertation,* Moscow, 1954, -26 p.

[312] Rahmouni K., Barthelmebs M., Grima M., Imbs J.L., De Jong W. Brain Mineralocorticoid Receptor Control of Blood Pressure and Kidney Function in Normotensive Rats. *Hypertension,* 1999; 33: 1201-1206.

[313] Raiskina M.E. Energetic processes in the heart muscle and electrocardiogram under the influence of adrenalin and acetilcholin. *Journ.Pharmacology a. Toxicology,* 1951; 14 (1): 31-33.
[314] Raiskina M.E. Examination of phosphor compounds metabolism in the heart by means of radioactive phosphor. Report II. *Bulletin of exper. biology a. medicine,* 1956; 41 (5): 44-47.
[315] Raiskina M.E. Biochemistry of the heart nervous regulation, Moscow, *Medgis,* 1962, - 319 p.
[316] Ramchandra R., Barret C.J., Guild S.J., Malpas S. Is the chronically denervated kidney supersensitive to catecholamines? *Am.J.Physiol.Regul.Intergr.Comp.Physiol.*, 2002; 282: 603-610.
[317] Ratner M.J. About the role of a renal factor in the pathogenesis of hypertonic disease. *Therapy Archive,* Moscow, 1956; 28 (8): 9-18.
[318] Rawa A.L. Über das Zusammenwachsen der Nerven verschiedener Bestimmungen und verschiedener Funktionen. - *Arch.Physiol.*, 1985, S. 296-354.
[319] Rehn N.O. Effect of decentralization on the control of cathecholamines in the spleen and kidney of the cat. - *Acta Physiol.Scand.,* 1958; 42: 309-312.
[320] Renner O. Die Innervation der Niere. - In: *Müller, Die Gebensnerven.* - Berlin: Springer, 1924. - 196 S.
[321] Retzius G. Zur Kentniss der Nerven der Milz und der Niere. - *Biol.Unters. N.F.,* 1892; 3: 53-56.
[322] Rhodin J.A.G. Electron microscopy of the kidney. - *Amer.J.Med.,* 1958; 24: 661-675.
[323] Roads C.P., Van Slyke D.D., Hiller A. The effects of novocainization and total section of the nerves of the renal pedicle on renal blood flow and function. - *Amer.J.Physiol.,* 1934; 110: 392-398.
[324] Rohle L., Ritz E., Ziegler M. Zum derzeitigen Stand der Nierentransplantation. - *Urologe,* 1971; 10: 1-10.
[325] Rosovskaja E.S. Changes of chemical composition in the heart muscle under the influence of vegetative toxins (adrenalin, acetylcholine). In the book: Experimental investigations in the heart pharmacology, Ukrainian Institute of Experim. *Medicine,* Charkov, 1941, p. 67-78.
[326] Rosybakijev M.A. Function of dog intact and denervated kidneys by their overheating. Bulletin of experim. biology a. *medicine,* 1948; 25 (4): 283-285.
[327] Rudd M.A., Grippo R.S., Arendshorst W.S. Acute renal denervation produces diuresis and natriuresis in young SHR but not WKY rats. *Am.J.Physiol.,* 1986 Oct., 251 (4 Pt 2): F 655-661.
[328] Ryjov E.V. About the reinnervation and additional vascularization of a transplanted kidney by means of ileo-renopexy. In the book: Embryogenesis and reinnervation of internal organs. Scientific a. *Techniques,* Minsk, 1971, p. 150-156.
[329] Sadowski J., Gellert R., Kurkus J., Portalaska E. Denervated and intact kidney responses to exercise in the dog. *J.Appl.Physiol.*, 1981, Dec; 51 (6): 1618-1624.
[330] Samarina L.A. Conditionally reflectory changes of diuresis in dogs with an autotransplanted kidney. In the book: *Reports of 35th Scientific Conference of Kuibyshev State Medical Institute.*, 1967, p. 15-16.
[331] Samsonidze G.G. Morphophysiologic analysis of a kidney regeneration process. Tbilisi, *Sabtchota Sakartvelo* (Sovjet Georgia), 1958, -112 p.

[332] Sarry-Levi G.M. Intraorganic innervation of the kidney. In the book: Scientific reports of Odessa section of Allunion Scientific Society of Anatoms, Histologists a. Embriologists. *Odessa,* 1958; 1: 81-87.

[333] Sartorius O.W., Burlington H. Acute effects of denervation on kidney function in the dog. - *Amer.J.physiol.,* 1956; 185 (2): 407-412.

[334] Savtchenko N.E., Mochort V.A. Experimental and clinical data about the reinnervation of bladder by mixion neurogenous disorders. In the book: Reinnervation and revascularization of internal organs by means of organopexy. *Scientific a. Techniques,* Minsk, 1969; p. 120-132.

[335] Scalia F., Coleman D.R. Aspects of the central projection of the optic nerve in the frog as revealed by anterograde migration of horseradish peroxidase. - *Brain Res.,* 1974; 79: 496-504.

[336] Schram L.P., Adair J.R., Stribling J.M. Preganglionic innervation of the adrenal gland of the rat: a study using horseradish peroxidase. - *Exp.Neurol.,* 1975; 42 (2): 540-553.

[337] Schram L.P., Stribling J.M., Adair J.R. Developmental reorientation of sympathetic proganglionic neurons in the rat. - *Brain.Res.,* 1976; 106 (1): 166-171.

[338] Schwalew W.N. Innervation des Nephrons. - *Z.mikr. - anat. Forsch.*, 1963; 70 (4): 517-531.

[339] Schwalew W.N. Zur Morphologie des gangliosen Nerveapparatus der Niere und seine afferenten Innervation. - *Z.mikr. - anat. Forsch.*, 1964; 72 91): 81-96.

[340] Sechenov I.M. *Physiology of the nervous system,* 1966, -506 p.

[341] Seddon H.J. Nerve grafting and other unusual forms of nerve repair. - In: *Peripherial Nerve injuries* / Ed.H.J. Seddon, - London, 1954; p. 389-417.

[342] Selye H. Acguisition de resistance a la nephrocalcinose au cours de l`adaptation au froid. - *J.Physiol.,* 1957; 49 (5): 1021-1023.

[343] Sennikoff V.M. About the function of transplanted and intact kidney. Bulletin of experim. biology a. *medicine*, 1952; 34 (8): 11-13.

[344] Sennikoff V.M. Function of transplanted and intact kidneys in conditions of a sleeping braking. *Journ. Medical Affair,* 1953; 10: 887-890.

[345] Sent-Djerdy A. *Introduction in submolecular biology,* Moscow, Mir, 1964, -358 p.

[346] Sergievsky V.S., Devjatjarov O.A., Didenko V.I. Experimental materials in kidney autotransplantation. In the book: *2nd final scientific session in pathology and surgical correction of blood circulation.* Novosibirsk, 1964, p. 23-26.

[347] Serjanina N.A. Innervation of kidney calices and pyelon. In the book: *Works of Voronej State Medical Institute,* 1963; 52: 55-57.

[348] Serov V.V. Ultramicroscopical structure of the nephon and its significance in the pathology. *Journ. Archiv of pathology*, 1962; 10: 3-18.

[349] Serov V.V., Sorokina M.J. Morphology of the human kidney homotransplant in conditions of immunosuppressive therapy. In the book: Transplantation of organs and tissues. *Materials of 4th Allunion Conference in organs and tissues transplantation problem,* Moscow, 1966, p. 27-29.

[350] Sharkey R.A., Mulloy E.M.T., Long M., O`Neil. The effect of continous positive airway pressure (CPAP) on renal vascular resistance: the influence of renal denervation. *Critical Care,* 1999; 3: 33-37.

[351] Shioshvili T.J., Gurova E.V. About a kidney functional asymmetry in men. In the book: *State of the recipient and transplant after extremities auto- and homotransplantations,* Tzelinograd, 1968; 1: 154-161.

[352] Shioshvili T.J. Radiologic evaluation of the functional state of a denervated kidney and a kidney transplant after their surgical reinnervation. In the book: Questions of clinical a. experim. *urology*, Tbilisi, 1977; 12: 146-153.

[353] Shioshvili T.J. Functional state of a sole transplanted kidney in conditions of spontaneous and surgical reinnervation. In the book: *Questions of clinical a. experim. urology*, Tbilisi, 1977; 12: 140-145.

[354] Shioshvili T.J. Apparatus for local renal hypothermia. *USSR Author`s certificate N340327, 1972; USA Patent N3738372, 1972; UK Patent N1331002, 1973; Norway Patent N130751,* 1974.

[355] Shioshvili T.J. Reinnervation of an autotransplanted kidney and its functional state. In the book: *Materials of the 10th Conference of Moscow society of the nature testers.* Kutaisi, 1978, p. 52-53.

[356] Shioshvili T.J. Bioelectric potentials of nerves of denervated and autotransplanted dog kidneys by natural and surgical reinnervation. *Pathol. Phyiol. Exper. Therapy,* Moscow, 1986; 2: 46-49.

[357] Shioshvili T.J. Denervation and reinnervation of the transplanted kidney. Survey of literature. *J.Urol.Nephrol.,* Moscow, 1988, 5: 60-65.

[358] Shioshvili T.J. Surgical reinnervation of the transplanted kidney: *Is it needed? Europ. Urol.,* 1988; 14 (1): 56-61.

[359] Shioshvili T.J. The influence of a surgical reinnervation on the morpho-functional state of a transplanted kidney. In the book: *Modern problems of neurobiology,* Saransk, Russia, 2001, 142-143.

[360] Shlykov I.P. Changes in the kidneys after their denervation. *Medical Candidate Dissertatiuon*, Moscow, 1956, -16 p.

[361] Shlykov I.P. *About changes in the kidney after its sensitive denervation Archiv* AGE, 1959; 36 (1): 52-54.

[362] Shlykov I.P. Changes in kidneys after their denervation. Bulletin of Moscow Society of the nature testers, Moscow, 1960; 65: 56-56.

[363] Shpuga G.M. Urine excretory function of a transplanted kidney as compared with an intact one. In the book: Materials of 7th Congress of Caucasian physiologists, biochemists and pharmacologists, Krasnodar, 1937, p. 101-103.

[364] Shpuga G.M. About the function of a transplanted kidney. In the book: problems of sovjet physiology, biochemistry a. pharmacology, Moscow, 1949; 1: 535-543.

[365] Shpuga G.M., Lebedev A.A. About the function of a transplanted and reinnervated kidney. *Journ.Experim. surgery a. anaesthesiol.,* 1956; 4: 59-64.

[366] Shpuga G.M. About the function of a transplanted kidney. Medical Doctor Dissertation, Ivanovo, 1957, -22 p.

[367] Shvalev V.N. Experimental-morphologic examination of a receptory innervation of the pyelon and some sections of the kidney. *Medical Candidate Dissertation,* Kazan, 1956, -13 p.

[368] Shvalev V.N. *About the morphological character of kidney innervation.* - Ceskoslov. Morphol., 1964; 12 (4): 418-429.

[369] Shvalev V.N. Kidney innervation, Moscow-Leningrad, *Nauka* (Science), 1965, -179 p.

[370] Shvalev V.N. Afferent innervation of the kidney. *Medical Doctor Dissertation,* Leningrad, 1965, -35 p.

[371] Shvalev V.N. *Kidney innervation in the norm and pathology. In the book: Questions of morphology and geographic pathology of nephrolithiasis,* Moscow, 1966, p. 14-18.

[372] Shvalev V.N. Examination of nervous elements in transplanted kidneys and their urinary tract. In the book: *Materials of Conference dedicated to 100 year jubilee of the histology department of the S.M. Kirov Military Medical Academy,* Leningrad, 1968, p. 247-249.

[373] Shvalev V.N., Bykova N.A., Kirpatovsky I.D. State of the nervous apparatus in the kidney autotransplant. In the book: *Questions of renal insufficiency and kidney transplantation. Works of P. Lumumba People`s Friendship University,* Moscow, 1969; 62 (5): 114-121.

[374] Shvalev V.N. Some morphologic grounds of the doctrine about the nervous system trophic function. *Archiv AGE,* Moscow, 1971; 61 (8): 8-29.

[375] Shvalev V.N., Reidler R.M., Mingasova I.V. Stages of the vegetative nervous system formation in connection with development of its principal mediators in the process of embryogenesis. Prenathal formation of cholin- and adrenergic nervous elements in men and rabbits. *Archiv AGE,* Moscow, 1972; 8: 48-66.

[376] Shvalev V.N. Pathology of urinary organs by head brain injuries. In the book: Visceral pathology by central nervous system injuries, Leningrad, *Medicine,* 1975, p. 166-203.

[377] Shvalev V.N., Shioshvili T.J. Influence of a reinnervation on the state of a transplanted kidney in dogs, *Archiv AGE,* Moscow, 1978; 74 (2): 42-50.

[378] Shvalev V.N., Stropus R.A. Mediatory stage of vegetative nervous system functioning in the pre- and postnathal ontogeneses and the significance of its investigation for clinics. *Archiv AGE,* Moscow, 1979; 5: 5-20.

[379] Shvalev V.N., Juchkova N.I. A simple method for revealing of adrenergic nervous structures in human and animal tissues with application of the glioxil acid. *Archiv AGE,* Moscow, 1979; 6: 114-117.

[380] Sidorenko P.I. Influence of a decapsulation on the kidney function. In the book: *Works of 2nd Congress of Russian Urologists,* Moscow, 1928, p. 36-37.

[381] Siljutin V.G. Intraorganeous nervous system of the kidney. In the book: *Works of Kuibyshev section of pathologic anatomists society*, Kuibyshev, 1957, p. 103-112.

[382] Simonsen M., Buemann J., Cammeltoft A. Biological incompatibility in kidney transplantation in dogs. - *Acta path.Microbiol.Scand.,* 1953; 32 (1): 1-35.

[383] Sinelnikoff R.D. Atlas of the human anatomy, Moscow, *Medicine,* 1963, -452 p.

[384] Sirotjakova M., Stopek D., Gombos A. "Short" cholinergic neurons of the kidney. - *Folia Morphol.,* 1975; 25 (4): 323-325.

[385] Smirnow A.E. Über die Nervenendigungen in den Nieren der Saugetiere. - *Anat.Anseiger,* 1901; 19: 347-359.

[386] Stancic-Rokotov M.F. La combination de l`anastomose spinofaciale et de l`ablation du ganglion sympathique cervical superieur dans le traitement des paralysis facials. - *Neurochirurgie,* 1971; 17 (1): 71-75.

[387] Stopek D. Adrenergicka charvacia normalnej a transplantovanej oblicky u psov. - Kandidatska dizertacia. - *Kosice,* 1972, -186 p.

[388] Stopek D., Gombos A., Gombosova M. Prispevok k problematike adrenergnej inervacie eferentnych arteriol a mikricirkulacie krvi v oblicke u psov. - In: *Zbornik Lek.Fakulty,* Kosice, 1972; 14 (28): 209-217.

[389] Stopek D., Gombos A. Adrenergic denervation and reinnervation possibilities of autotransplanted kidneys in dogs. - F*olia Morphol,* (Prague), 1973; 21: 361-363.

[390] Stopek D., Gombosh A., Sirotjakova M. Adrenergic and cholinergic innervation of the kidney in some mammalia. *Archiv AGE,* 1978; 75 (9): 37-43.

[391] Strelkoff R.B. Method for calculation of the standard error and intervals of reliability in mean arithmetic value by means of tables, *Suchumi*, Alashara, 1966, -41 p.

[392] Sunahara F.A., Bogriand T., Chappel C.J. Pharmacology of vasodepressor material of renal medullary origin. - In: Abst. of papers 23 internat. *Congress physiol. sciences,* Tokyo, 1965, p. 511-511.

[393] Surtshin A., Hoeltzenbein J. Effect of chronic denervation on response of renal vessels to epinephrine. - *Amer.J.Physiol.,* 1952; 171 (1): 169-173.

[394] Surtshin A., Mueller C.N., White H.L. Effect of acute changes in glomerular filtration rate on water and electrolyte excretion: mechanism of denervation diuresis. - *Amer.J.Physiol*., 1952; 169 (1): p. 159-173.

[395] Takacs L., Benesath P., Demeczky L. Renal sodium and water excretion after unilateral splanchnicotomy in the dog. - *Acta Physiol. Acad.Scient.Hung.,* 1971; 39 (4): 283-291.

[396] Takaechi J., Uchida E., Nakayama A. Experimental studies on the nervous control of the renal circulation. Effect of the electrical stimulation of splanchnic, vagal and other somatic nerves and the occlusion carotids arteries on the renal circulation. - *Jap.heart.L.*, 1961; 2 (1): 65-76.

[397] Takeuchi J., Ohya N., Sakai S. Nervous control of the renal tubular function. - *Jap.Heart J.,* 1968; 9: 564-572.

[398] Ter-Kasparova M.R. Influence of the denervation on amiloidose formation in kidneys. Journ. of experim. a. *clinical medicine,* 1969; 9 (4): 8-12.

[399] Thurman R.G., Zhong Z., Frankenberg M.V., Stachlevitz R.F., Bunzendahl H. Prevention of cyclosporine-induced nephrotoxicity with dietary glycine. *Transplantation,* 1997; 63: 1661-1667.

[400] Tisher C.C., Bulger R.E., Trump B.F. Human renal ultrastructure. I. Proximal tubule of health individuals. - *Lab.Investig.,* 1966; 15 (8): 1357-1394.

[401] Tishler V., Iacina J., Gombosh A. Investigation of transplanted kidneys function in dogs. *USSR physiologic journal,* 1962; 48 (12): 1488-1493.

[402] Tjurina E.I. Excretion of urine in dogs with a transplanted kidney under the influence of the saline loading. Journ. of Pharmacology a. *Toxicology,* 1951; 14 (5): 46-47.

[403] Tjurina E.I. Excretion of urine in dogs with a transplanted and intact kidney under the influence of loading with coffein. In the book: *Scientific works of Ivanovo State Medical Institute,* 1952; 8: 107-110.

[404] Troshanova E.S. Biochemical peculiarities of the heart muscle in intact and vagotomied animals and their changes under the influence of training, *Ukrainian biochemical Journal,* 1952; 24 (3): 312-326.

[405] Tucek S., a. VLK. The effect of vagotomy on the acetylcholine content and cholinesterase activity in various regions of the rat heart atria. - *Physiol.Bohemoslov.,* 1962; II (4): 319-328.

[406] Utevsky A.M. Investigation of adrenalin and noradrenalin changes in the nervous tissue and effectory organs. In the book: Questions of the nervous system biochemistry, Ukrainian Academy of Sciences, *Kiev,* 1957, p. 131-141.

[407] Utevsky A.M. About the functional significance of adrenalin and adrenalin like substances exchange for nervous mediation and trophic. In the book: *Neuro-humoral and endocrine factors in the work of the nervous system in the norm and pathology.* USSR Academy of Sciences, Moscow-Leningrad, 1959, p. 40-47.

[408] Utevsky A.M. Exchange of catecholamines and its functional significance. In the book: *Adrenalin and noradrenalin,* Moscow, 1964, p. 8-18.

[409] Valeeva H.G. Comparative morphologic examination of human and vertebrates kidney nervous apparatus, *Medic. Doctor Dissertation,* Kazan, 1968, -25 p.

[410] Valishin E.S. Influence of denervation on the kidney parenchyma and intraorganic vascular system. In the book: *Works of Kasan Medical Institute,* 1966; 18: 355-364.

[411] Vander A.J. Effect of cathecholamines and the renal nerves on renin secretion in anaesthetized dogs. - *Amer.J.Physiol.,* 1966; 209 (3): 659-692.

[412] Vasilenko V.A. Function of an autotransplanted (denervated) kidney by compensatory hypertrophy. In the book: Materials of scientific conference: "*Physiology and pathology of cortico-visceral relations and functional systems in the organism*". Ivanovo, 1965; 1: 228-230.

[413] Vasilenko V.A. Mechanism of regulation of the kidney function in the process of compensatory hypertrophy. In the book: *Kidney and electrolytes.* Works of Kuibyshev Medical Institute, 1967; 43: 157-164.

[414] Vasiljeva V.F. Influence of efferent nerves on of kidney function. *Medic. Candidate Dissertation,* Novosibirsk, 1953, -12 p.

[415] Vasiljeva V.F. Influence of denervation on the kidney function. *Physiology J. of USSR,* 1958; 44 (3): 236-242.

[416] Vasiljeva V.F. Influence of adrenalin of the kidney function. I. Setchenov *J. Physiology,* 1958; 44 (5): 450-458.

[417] Villareal D., Freeman R.H., Johson R.A., Simmons J.C. Effects of renal denervation on postprandial sodium excretion in experimental heart failure. *Am.J.Physiol.,* 1994; 226: R 1559-R 1604.

[418] Volkova O.V. Morphological meaning of a nervous apparatus in the viability of organs and tissues. In the book: *Nervous regulation of tissue processes. Scientific works of the second Medical Institute,* Moscow, 1970, p. 7-22.

[419] Waleewa C.G. Vergleichend-anatomische Untersuchungen uber die Mikromorphologie des Nervenapparaten der Niere. - *Anat.Anz.,* 1963; (112): 165-171.

[420] Wang C., Salahudeen A.K. Lipid peroxidation accompanies cyclosporine nephrotoxicity: Effects of Vitamin E, *Kidney Int.,* 1995; 47: 927-934.

[421] Warr W.B. Olivocochlear and vestibular efferent neurons of the feline brain stem. Their location, morphology and nimber determined by retrograde axonal transport and acetylcholinesterase histochemistry. - *J.comp.Neural.,* 1975; 161: 159-182.

[422] Wassink W.F. *Over Peristaltick van het Nierenbekken.* - Nederl. Tijdschr. V. Genesk., 1921; 66: 29-31.

[423] Weitsen H.A., Norvell J.E. Cholinergic innervation of the autotransplanted canine kidney. - *Circ.Res.,* 1969; 25 (5): 535-541.

[424] Wogermark J., Ungerstedt U., Ljunggvist A. Simpathetic innervation of the juxtaglomerular cells of the kidney. - *Circul.Res.*, 1968; 22 (2): 149-153.

[425] Woodcock E.A., Morris M.J., Me Leod J.K., Johnston C.I. Specific increase in renal alpha-adrenergic receptors following unilateral renal denervation, *J. Receptor Res.*, 1985; 5: 133-146.

[426] Woodruff M.F., Robson J.S., Ross J.A. Transplantation of a kidney from an identical twin. - *Lancet,* 1961; I: 1245-1249.

[427] Yamada E. The fine structure of the renal glomerulus of the mouse. - *J.Biophysic and Biochem.Cytol.,* 1955; I (6): 554-566.

[428] Zachary R.B. Results of nerve suture. - In: *Peripheral nerve injuries* / Ed. E.J.Seddon. - London, 1954, p. 354-388.

[429] Zayko N.N. Nervous trophic. *Journal Nealth,* Moscow, 1964; 12: 3-5.

[430] Zayko N.N. Nervous trophic and distrophic process, Kiev, *Zdorovja,* 1969, -139 p.

[431] Zayko N.N. Some new data about the essence of neurogenic dystrophies. In the book: Pathophysiological aspects of the nervous trophic, Kiev, *Zdorovja,* 1974, p. 43-46.

[432] Zaretzky I.I., Mikhailova I.A., Rosanova N.S. Functional significance of the kidney efferent innervation. *USSR Physiological Journal, Moscow,* 1960; 46 (5): 593-601.

[433] Zaretzky I.I. Clinical physiology and methods of kidney functional diagnostics, Moscow, *Medgis,* 1963, -280 p.

[434] Zhong Z., Arteel G.E., Connor H., Yin M., Frankenberg M.V., Stachlewits R.F., Raleigh J.A., Mason R.P., Thurman R.G. Cyclosporin A increases hypoxia and free radical production in the rat kidney: Prevention by dietary glycine. *Am.J.Physiol.,* 1998; 275: 595-604.

[435] Zhong Z., Connor H.D., Yin M., Moss N., Mason R.P., Bunzendahl H., Forman D.T., Thurman R.G. Dietary Glycine and Renal Denervation Prevents Cyclosporine-A-induced Hydroxyl Radical Production in Rat Kidney. *Am.J.Physiol.,* 1999; 56: 455-463.

[436] Zimmermann H.D. Einige feinstrukturelle Veränderungen in den intrarenalen Nerven bei Verschiedenen Nierenerkrankungen. - *Verch.Dtsch.Ges.Path.,* 1974; 58: 487-490.

[437] Zincke H., Ott N.T., Woods J.E., Wilson D.M. The role of denervation in renal transplantation on renal function in the dog. *Invest. Urol.,* 1976, Nov.; 14 (3): 210-212.

[438] Zlotnik E.I. Some questions of acoustic nerve neurinome surgery. *Questions of Neurosurgery, Moscow,* 1972; 6: 25-29.

[439] Zufarov K.A., Rassulev N.I. Histochemical investigations of nucleine acids and glycogen in the kidney after its deafferentation. In the book: Questions of physiology of endemic pathology, *Tashkent,* 1960, p. 13-16.

[440] Zufarov K.A. Influence of kidney deafferentation on its morphological condition and excretory function. In the book: Works of Endemic and Experimental Medicine Institute, *Tashkent,* 1961, p. 142-149.

[441] Zufarov K.A., Tarakulov J.H. Some data about histochemical and biochemical examination of kidneys by their deafferentation. In the book: Works of Endemic and Experimental Medicine, *Tashkent,* 1961; 2: 150-156.

[442] Zufarov K.A. Cytological and histochemical analysis of changes in the deafferentated kidney. Medical Doctor Dissertation, Tashkent, 1962, -26 p.

[443] Zufarov K.A., Gontmacher V.M. Electron microscopy of the kidney. Atlas, *Tashkent, Medicine,* 1969, -102 p.

Chapter VII

THE KIDNEY TEMPORARY ISCHEMIA AND ITS RENDERING HARMLESS

One of the significant nonspecific damaging factors inevitably accompanying a kidney transplantation is its ischemia. This problem has a particular importance because along with the heart and liver, the kidney is in need of extremely intensive blood circulation and reacts to hypoxia very sensitively [15-19,82,133,166,184,185]. Therefore the research of such an intricate and high differentiated system as the nervous apparatus in connection with transplantation is impossible without consideration of ischemic damage of the transplanted kidney. Therefore, the investigation of consequences of a blocade of the renal blood circulation, elaboration of measures for their prevention and preservation of the kidney survival, as very important segments of theoretical and clinical transplantology, also became subjects of our research.

7.1. THE INFLUENCE OF AN ISCHEMIA ON THE KIDNEY: SURVEY OF LITERATURE

The experiments with a blocade of the kidney blood circulation showed its high sensitivity to anoxia and were accompanied with serious functional and morphologic disturbances.

[48,181,182] observed the kidney functional depression 5-15 minutes after the occlusion of its vascular pedicle.

[105,142] found that a 1-3 minute duration ischemia didn`t produce reliable functional disorders, but the lengthening of ischemia duration to 12, 30, 45 and 90 minutes caused an oliguria, an increase of creatinine, urea and chloride level in the plasma.

[9,43,45,59,63,65,67,68,72,107,108,171,183,187] stated that 1-2 hour long ischemia with small fluctuations is top-limit duration for kidney admitting followed its recovery. But 3-hour and longer ischemia of a sole kidney or bilateral ischemia caused a progressive uremia and death of animals in all cases [42-44,75,102,152,176,183].

For the research of a physiological background of an anoxic injury [174], the kidney blood circulation was blocked for 20 minutes and then examined its diuresis. Within the first 5-50 minutes the authors observed an anuria and then an oliguria. Because of the two-phase change of diuresis the authors concluded that the blockade of blood circulation was due to two factors acting on the kidney, firstly the anoxia itself and then the postischemic circulatory upsettings.

The experiments of [97-99] with the use of clearance-tests confirmed the above mentioned opinion. Furthermore, it was stated that the short-term anoxia mainly damaged the renal circulation and tubular reabsorption, at the same time the changes of a glomerular filtration were expressed considerably less.

In order to determine the minimal duration of ischemia causing morphologic changes in the kidneys, [199] subjected them to 10-150 minutes of normothermal ischemia. It was stated that a 20-minute ischemia was accompanied with local necroses in the nephron proximal segment epithelium. The lengthening of ischemia caused more extended necroses which spread on other segments of the nephron as well as on the arteriole walls.

Special investigations [25,43,56] stated that after the influence of ischemia on the kidney and then of its blood recirculation, a certain period of time has to be passed in order to reveal some of the morphological changes in the organ. So, after a 60-minute normothermal ischemia and restoration of the blood circulation, the kidney was examined in the dynamics from 15 minutes to 5 weeks. The most expressed structural changes were observed on the 3rd day after ischemia. After the 4th day the signs of regeneration were revealed [199].

For evaluation of the dying process in the ischemized kidney [166] 3 periods were established. The first period of reliably reversible changes lasting up to 20 minutes of ischemia. It is the period of mobilization of energetic resources or the period of a so-called cellular agony.

The second, transitory period lasting from 20 to 40 minutes of ischemia. It is the period of beginning and developing of cellular death, which is characterized with a sharp depression of energetic and diffusive processes in cells.

The third is the period of relatively reversible changes which have taken place after 40-60 minute long ischemia for a dog kidney and 90-100 minute long ischemia for a human kidney. It is the period of expressed autolytic changes in the kidney.

After the authors [166] definition, a specific peculiarity of a living cell is the ability to maintain homeostasis by means of a permanent exchange of substance and energy with the surrounding environment. This exchange is realized through cellular membranes which, on the one hand, carry out an integration of the cellular composition at the expense of a selective permeability to certain ions and molecules and, on the other hand, ensure the proper relations with cellular organelles. In these relations an intracellular bound water has a very important role. Thanks to anisotropic properties, the bound water stipulates the rupture of intracellular moleculas and the creation of free radicals having a very high reactive ability.

Thus, the mechanism of cellular death can be imagined in the following way. The hypoxia first causes a brake in the transport of electrons and hydrogenic ions, then the oxidation-restoration balance is deplaced by the accumulation of restorated forms. It is accompanied with a stipulation of an anaerobic glycolyse, but its energetic efficacy is only 25% of aerobic respiration. It results, on the one hand, in accumulation of partially oxidized metabolic substances in the cell, such as milk, vinegar acids, and free radicals and on the other hand, it creates a deficit of energy which is needed for the maintenance of the ion-balance across cellular membranes. All this damages their specific function, increases their permeability and results in desintergration of cellular metabolism: the ferments go out in the cytoplasma, evoke a hydrolytic splitting of proteins, nuclein acides, polysaccharides, and phosphatides; Na-ions and water moleculas from the extracellular space enter the cell and block synthetic processes and elimination of harmful products of disintegration. By the end of the first hour the common influence of a metabolic injury, autolyse and protein denaturation lead to the irreversible destruction of the cell [96,166-169].

For much time the question of what segments of the nephron are most sensitive to anoxia was disputed. [4,5,56,75,82,115,116,127,133,135,177,178,184,185,187] found more expressed changes in proximal tubules. [9] mentioned a deterioration in the distal tubule epithelium. [199] observed approximately equal injury to proximal and distal segments of the nephron.

Along with common morphologic investigations of kidney ischemia consequences, the works were performed with the use of more sensitive histochemical and electron microscopic methods. The content of oxidation-restoration and hydrolytic ferments in dog intact kidneys was examined by [93,171], which observed the most fermentation activity in the proximal and distal segments of the nephron.

After 15-19 and 120-minute long ischemia [123,186] found that a considerable depression of phosphatase activity and [46] the activity of succinatdehydrogenase.

[52] revealed that after 15-minutes of ischemia there was already swelling of mitochondria in the epithelial cells of proximal tubules, an expressed depression of fermentative activity and various upsettings of intracellular metabolism.

25-minute ischemia of rat kidneys caused marked damage in the proximal tubules seen by electron microscope, with dilatation and widespread loss of proximal brush border. The lumen of this segment was filled with cytoplasmic blebs and necrotic cell debris. There was also pronounced vascular congestion of the capillary plexus in the inner stripe of the outer medulla [82].

The same (25 minute) duration ischemia caused, in rat kidneys, the death and exfoliation of S3 cells in the proximal tubule. The majority of brush border microvilli underwent coalescence by membrane fusion and thus, were internalized into the cytoplasma of the proximal tubule cells [184,185].

By special histoensimatic investigation of the rat, renal brush border microvilli, after 25-minutes of normothermic ischemia, it was shown that the activities of alkaline phosphatase, gamma-glutamyl transpeptidase and alpha-glucosidase were decreased to 50% of the standard [93,133,171].

By electron microscopy of the kidney after a 60-minute long ischemia [106,177,178], swelling of the mitochondria, especially in the nephron proximal segment and an increase of permeability of the basal membrane were observed.

After a 180-minute long ischemia [148] more expressed intracellular disturbances like the vacuolization of endothelial cells in glomerular capillaries, irregular fenestration of endothelium, and shortening or lengthening of podocyte pediculas were observed. In the epithelial cells of the nephron proximal segment the decrease of cytoplasma density, compression of cells and their nuclei and destruction of intracellular organells were mentioned.

The high sensitivity of the kidney to anoxia was also confirmed with clinical data. On the basis of the clinical experience [140] it is recommended to not exceed the duration of ischemia for more than 8-10 minutes by operations on a sole kidney.

[153-157] who performed 15 partial resections of the sole kidney in conditions of the blocked blood circulation and was obliged to exceed the mentioned period of time because of

the clinical need, noticed the direct dependence between the ischemia duration and death of the kidney functional depression: after 11-minute ischemia they observed a light reaction with oliguria within 3 days and hyperasothemia to 70 mg%; afterward 18-minute ischemia - a moderate reaction with oliguria within 13 days and hyperasothemia to 150 mg%; after 60-minute ischemia with a subsequent oliguria and hyperasothemia up to 400 mg%.

Some authors [85,88,90] observed the functioning of kidney allotransplants after 82- and 120-minute normothermic ischemia. But such examples of high resistance to ischemia are rare exceptions. Therefore the majority of surgeons making such operations [57,129-132,140,153-157] warn against blocking the kidney blood circulation in normothermic conditions for more than 15-20 minutes. Because this period of time in most clinical cases is insufficient for the radical carrying out of a complicated operation on the kidney, moreover for its transplantation, many attempts were undertaken in order to increase the tolerance of the kidney to anoxia.

Some authors [41,151,198] restored the kidney blood circulation after every 30 minutes of ischemia. The authors explained the positive effect of this procedure firstly as a recovery of energetic potential in the kidney tissue and secondly by removal of toxic metabolic products from the kidney. But in real clinical situations, for example by large nephrotomy or kidney transplantation such a method is connected with massive bloodloss. Therefore this method didn`t receive widespread practical application.

For prevention of bad consequences of anoxia some authors tried to use the chemical combinations having certain antitoxic properties like ethyluretan, octyluretan [65], chlortetracycline, lowmolecular dextran [63] Euro-Collins or HTK-solution of Bretschneider [6,34,71-73]. But their efficacy towards the ischemized kidney was unfortunately insufficient.

Thus, the experimental and clinical observations showed that surgical and chemical methods of protection of the kidney against normothermic ischemia were insecure. Therefore the trials of investigators were continued in other direction, such as in the field of decrease of metabolic intensity at the expense of ischemized kidney cooling.

7.2. The Cooling of a Kidney in Experiments and Clinics

On the background of the Arrenius rule about the exponential dependence between the temperature and speed of the chemical reaction, [15] firstly in the medical practice a hypothermia for protection of such important organs as heart, lungs and head brain from anoxia was used.

In accordance with their data the cooling of the body by every 1°C decreased the need for oxygen by 5%. For example, at the body temperature +28°C the need for oxygen was 50%, and the temperature +20°C was only 15-18%.

These works founded a new prospective direction in theoretical and practical medicine. They became the beginning of the widespread application of hypothermia in regard to the whole body as well as its separate organs. The most widespread object of cooling became the kidney. It was determined due to the higher occurrence of transplantation as compared with other organs.

By selective renal hypothermia the needs of the kidney tissues for oxygen were changeable and had the same conformity to natural laws as the body in general to hypothermia: by the temperature +29°C the need for oxygen was 50%, by +20°C-21% [156]: - 16% [81], by +10°C - 5% [81], by +5°C - less than 5% of the standard [26]. And what`s more, the utilization of oxygen with the kidney tissue decreased more sharply by cooling to +20°C, more slowly by further cooling to +10°C and had almost no change by cooling below +3°C [114].

The reduction of organ temperature stopped the formation of hydrogen ions and decreased the tissues needs for oxygen. Thanks to this the cells were able to maintain their vitality through the lower membraneous potential [22,30,81,107,126].

In order to achieve the safest protection of the kidney from anoxia the authors aspired initially to use deep hypothermia. So, [20,21,152] observed the survival of dogs after 7.5-8 hour-long ischemia of the sole kidney by local hypothermia +2+4°C. At the same time in the control test-group of animals 2-hour long normothermal ischemia of the sole kidney caused irreversible changes and the death of animals.

The investigation of the kidney tissue by means of a Varburg apparatus stated that the cooling to 0°C preserved the respiratory activity of the organ through a 34-hour long ischemia [143].

[11-14] demonstrated the possibility of successful conservation of kidneys within 24-72 hours by means of extracorporal perfusion and cooling to +8+12°C. The kidney vitality was confirmed by their following autotransplantation and removal of opposite intact kidneys.

[3] combined the deep hypothermia +2+6°C with hyperbaric oxygenation and could maintain the capacity for work within 24-48 hours.

The temperature in ranges +5+15°C preserved the normal activity of alkaline and sour phosphatase by 2-hour ischemia. In comparison, the normothermal ischemia of the same duration caused a sharp depression of these ferments [186].

In similar experiments [123] the decrease of alkaline and sour phosphatase activity was already observed in 15-19 minute long ischemia. In parallel groups with cooling of the ischemized kidneys to +6+15°C, the fermentative activity remained normal.

By 2-hour ischemia in conditions of normothermia (+37°C) and hypothermia (+16°C) the morphologic structure of the kidney in the second test-group was more preserved [4].

The investigations mentioned above convincingly showed that the deep hypothermia through a decrease of the metabolism intensity considerably softend the harm consequences of anoxia. But at the same time it was found that the deep hypothermia caused circulatory upsettings resulting in prolonged secondary postoperative ischemia of the organ [115,116,144-147].

The electron microscopic examination of the kidney after ischemia and deep hypothermia (0+5°C) revealed the degenerative changes in the arterial walls, hemostasis, and blood vessel throbosis. In the authors [111-113,148,159] opinion, these phenomena could cause local kidney infarctions in the following period.

The harmful influence of the deep hypothermia consisted of a disbalance in separate systems of the tissue metabolism: the speed of a resynthesis and delivery of energy to tissues was decreased more than the speed of its utilization. Because of discoordination between the release and utilization of energy the cellular transmembrane gradients became gradually even, which resulted in the swelling and destruction of cells. Thus, the deep hypothermia evoked a predisposition of tissues to intracellular swelling. In such conditions even a short-time perfusion could aggravate the hyperhydration of the cell and accelerate its death. It was concerned especially about nonbalanced isotonic perfusates injected into the kidney under a high pressure [170].

The cooling of the kidney by means of ice sometimes caused cortical necroses [21,119,124].

Therefore, surgeons warned [55,92,116,193] that in an attempt to lengthen the permissible limit of ischemia, the negative influence of hypothermia has to be taken into account.

In order to determine the optimal level of an ischemized kidney hypothermia, a number of experiments were undertaken on animals with a sole kidney.

[75] compared the protective effect of various levels of hypothermia (0+5°C, +10+15°C, +20+25°C) in 6-hour long ischemia of a sole kidney. In the test-group with 0+5°C hypothermia 100% of the animals survived; in the group with hypothermia +10+15°C the survival rate was 80%; by cooling to +20+25°C the rate was 30%.

[115,116] subjected the kidney to 2-hour ischemia with cooling to +20°C, +10°C and +5°C. The experiments showed that hypothermia over +20°C rendered insufficient protection from anoxia. At the same time the cooling below +10°C caused considerable circulatory disturbances. In the author`s opinion, the best temperature is +10+20°C.

In contrast with these data, [69] observed the survival of animals after 8-hour long ischemia of the sole kidney cooled to +20°C. The cooling to +20°C increased the resistance of the kidney to anoxia more than 3 times.

These data were confirmed with results of other experimental and clinical works [36,191,194-196]. Their opinion is that by hypothermia of +20°C the ischemia duration of 80-90 minutes has minimal risk.

[56] investigated the influence of hypothermia on the kidney. It was cooled to 0+5°C, +10+20°C and +25°C. The duration of ischemia was 5 minutes. In the test-group with kidney cooling to 0+5°C the highest mortality from uremia was observed. Morphologically, local necroses and haemorrhages were found. In the test-group with kidney cooling to +10°C the necrobiotic, necrotic changes, and blood stagnation in the juxtamedullar zone were observed. After the hypothermia of +20+25°C, there were noticed minimal dystrophic and circulatory upsettings.

After preservation of blood within 24 hours at temperatures of 37°C, 22°C, 15°C, 8°C and 3°C [170] it was found that a hypothermal optimum, where the used energy is balanced with diffusive processes in cells, is located at a range of +18+24°C. It means that this temperature maintained the energetic equilibrium, metabolic systems were able to ensure their biologic pumps with energy and prevention of cellular swelling. By the further decrease of temperature, exactly to +6+8°C, in spite of lowering of cellular needs for oxygen, the transmembrane ion gradients became even and the cellular swelling was aggravated further. Nevertheless, because of a relatively high level of metabolism at a temperature of +18+24°C, the authors recommended making a compromise to keep the organs at a temperature of +10+12°C. Their opinion was that this range ensures the most longterm conservation with the maintenance of a minimal energoproduction in cells.

It has to be noted that using biophysical methods of investigation (calorimetric evaluation of energetic needs, level of oxidation-restoration potentials, state of Na-ions diffusion in the conservated organ) the same authors were able to calculate mathematically and confirm in experiments and clinics the optimal duration of kidney vitality by different levels of hypothermia. So, by the temperature +10°C a permissible duration of storage was 3-4 hours, by the temperature +2+4°C it was 11 hours.

In other authors [58,176] opinion, the hypothermia range 0+10°C can prolong the dying time up to 6-7 hours.

Some authors [18,51] observed the survival of a kidney kept within 12 hours by 0+4°C and transplanted to the same dog simultaneously with removal of its opposite kidney.

The next authors [40,73,80] noticed the vitality of a kidney after keeping within 24-48 hours by 0+2°C.

Although the method of kidney hypothermic conservation was still not fully perfected, the protective effect of hypothermia was so convincing and impressed so much optimism, that many surgeons risked using it and continue to use it at present in clinics, before making more precise interpretations of various important aspects.

The hypothermia is now considered the most effective method of conservation and respects an obligatory stage by allo- and autotransplantation of the kidney in clinics and is applied separately as well as in combination with perfusion, hyperbaric oxygenation, pharmacologic remedies and so on [8,11-14,32,33,37,76,86,88,100,101,139, 166-168,179]. The majority of surgeons use deep hypothermia in the ranges of 0+12°C.

Widespread is the selective hypothermia of the kidney by removal of staghorn and multiple stones by temporarily blocking blood circulation [1,7,24,49,56,60,87,110,129-132,135,154,173,180,188,189,196,197]. The level of hypothermia by such operations fluctuated by various authors in wide ranges from +2°C to +32°C [27,28,135].

Most recently there were first attempts in the use of selective renal hypothermia by a laparoscopic approach [54,64,121,190].

It has to be mentioned that in spite of numerous experimental and clinical observations even today there is not a common, generally accepted opinion about the optimal method of kidney conservation, particularly about the optimal level of hypothermia.

The conservation of a kidney transplant within 24-72 hours was achieved by using a temperature from 0 to +12°C [11,18]. By nephrolithotomy of a "dry" kidney, it was cooled in wide ranges from +32°C to +2°C [135]. These data testify about the discrepancy of experimental and clinical results in the field.

The complexity of the problem and necessity of a compromise between the various factors, which was impossible to generalize in one experiment, sometimes obliged the authors to deviate in their recommendations even from results of their own investigations. Characteristic in this respect is that [170] for example, even having determined the hypothermic optimum of +18+24°C for erythrocytes kept within 24 hours, they nevertheless recommended the temperature interval +10+12°C for the kidney conservation.

[75] having had 100% age survival of dogs by deep hypothermia (0+5°C) of a sole kidney ischemized within 6 hours and 30% survival by moderate hypothermia (+20+25°C) considered the best interval, not 0+5°C but, the temperature "Below +15°C".

[116] recommended the temperature range +10+20°C as an optimum based on the data that the test-group with the kidney cooling to below +5°C and over +20°C had 2 animals die, at the same time in the group with the cooling from +10°C to +20°C one animal died.

The experiments with short-time (within 5 minutes) ischemia and hypothermia [56] didn`t actually answer the question of what temperature is optimal for protection of the kidney from the long term ischemia.

Considering that "biocinetic zone" means the sphere of conformity between the metabolic and functional activity of cells for the majority of warm-blooded organisms is located in the interval from +10 to +45°C [170], furthermore in such extreme conditions as full organ ischemia this zone is evidently narrower, it seems to be urgently necessary to define more precisely the optimal level of hypothermia for an ischemized kidney.

A discrepancy of experimental data in that field can obviously be explained with different conditions of experiments. For example, the duration of kidney ischemia by various authors was from 5 minutes to 10 days. The kidney was cooled using diverse methods, external or perfusion, in combination with hyperbaric oxygenation or without it. For the perfusion different solutions were used, separately or in complex with other conservation methods, and various pharmacologic conservation remedies were applicated.

What can be considered as a principal criterion for the correct orientation in the wide stream of information in this field and for a justified decision?

All the previous experience testifies that the obligatory conditions for the objective evaluation of positive and negative aspects of different levels of hypothermia are firstly, a clear definition for what duration of ischemia is necessary to determine the optimal temperature, and secondly, for specific durations of conservation various pathophysiological aspects of anoxia and hypothermia influence need to be taken into sccount (the state of metabolism, protective and harmful properties of different levels of hypothermia) in order to achieve the most favorable compromised combination.

In other words, a universal best level of hypothermia suitable for every long ischemia does not exist. For each duration of ischemia and conservation a search of the corresponding protective temperature zone is needed.

What are the most typical durations of kidney anoxia by various operations in clinics?

Without any pretension to novelty, only on the background of known clinical experience described in the literature and theoretical reasons related to peculiarities of an ischemized kidney conservation, the following typical durations of ischemia can be distinguished: 2 hours, 3-5 hours and over 5 hours.

The ischemia to 2 hours has taken place by planned kidney transplantations, for example from living donors [109], and more rarely by transplantation of a cadaverous kidney. The duration of ischemia doesn`t exceed 2 hours by the majority of autotransplantations of the kidney in clinics [61,62,76,86] and by nephrolithotomia and partical resection of the kidney with its temporarily blocked blood circulation [23,56,87,129-132,149,160-165,180,188, 189,197].

The duration of an ischemia to 3-5 hours and over 5 hours is observed, as a rule, by transplantation of a cadaverous kidney.

Without concern for longterm conservation (over 5 hours) it has to be noticed that there is a discrepancy between the experimental and clinical data related to the proper level of hypothermia for a kidney by 2 hour-long ischemia. Single works in that field [4,36,56,116,146,147,194-196] gave contradictory results, because they didn`t embrace various ranges of hypothermia and used test-methods that were not specific enough.

As the questions mentioned above have an important theoretical and practical significance, we considered it expedient to perform our own experimental and clinical investigation for the definition of the best temperature regime in the case of 2 hour ischemia of the kidney.

7.3. Material and Methods

In accordance with the planned intention, experiments were made on 65 mongrel dogs of both sexes divided on 5 group (Table 16). In the 1st, 2nd, 3rd and 4th test-groups (at 15 animals in the each group) the left kidney underwent 2 hour ischemia at temperatures of +37C, +4+7C, +10+15C and +20+25C, respectively. The 5th group (5 dogs) was the control (only a mobilization of the kidney and its magistral blood vessels was performed).

For prevention of compensatory hypertrophy of the operated kidney and achievement of the most natural dynamics of changes, the opposite kidney of animals was preserved.

The selection of the left kidney as the object of operations was determined in order to keep the standard conditions of experiments and in connection with comfort of manipulations on the longer vascular pedicle of the left kidney.

Under general anaesthesia (30-50 ml of 1% Hexenal Solution intravenously) the left kidney was separated through transabdominal approach. After mobilization of its vascular pedicle the blood circulation was interrupted for 2 hours. It has to be noted that the existent methods for this do not require surgery. The simultaneous blocade of the whole vascular pedicle of the kidney [132] increases its internal blood pressure and causes a considerable stagnation and capillary thromboses. The blockage of only the renal artery [56,99,122] or separate clipping of firstly an artery and then a vein [197] in the first case can not ensure the full cessation of bleeding from the kidney and in the second case is connected with hazards of vessels injury.

Taking into account these considerations we have used our modification [162] for the safe blockade of the renal blood circulation. According to this method a renal artery is first digitally pressed (to the touch, after its pulsation) and 15-20 seconds later, after a sufficient unloading of blood from the kidney the whole vascular pedicle (artery and vein) is clipped together. Thanks to this method a full blockade of the renal blood circulation and a minimal danger of capillary thromboses and injury of the nervous-vascular apparatus of the kidney were ensured.

Furthermore, the "dry" kidney was cooled by means of a specially designed apparatus for external local renal hypothermia [150,158] in ranges of +20+25°C, +10+15°C and +4+7°C. The temperature of the kidney was measured by an electrothermomether with a needle gauge on the tip with limits of measure from -50 to +50°C.

The kidney was covered with the heat exchanger of this apparatus. The latter was switched on and began to ensure the circulation of the refrigerant agent between the walls of the heat exchanger. In the initial phase of cooling the temperature in the cortical substance of the kidney exceeded 2°C and in the medullar substance exceeded 4°C of the external temperature of the kidney. After 2-3 minutes the temperature in all its layers became even and was maintained in desired intervals within the whole period of ischemia (2 hours). A periodic temperature control and repeated switching of the mentioned apparatus were required for that.

In the 1st test-group the kidney with blocked blood circulation was immersed back into the wound, which is why it maintained normothermia (+37°C).

After 2 hour occlusion of the renal vascular pedicle the clips were removed. Being convinced of the restoration of blood pulsation, the kidney was returned to the wound which was tightly closed.

Before and after the operation the following examinations were made: rediorenography, kidney scintigraphy, general morphologic, histoensimatic and electron microscopic test-methods. The mentioned functional examinations were performed before and one-three, nine-ten, fifteen days, one, two, three and six months after the operation. The morphologic examinations were made before and three, ten days, one, three and six months after the operation. Intact kidneys of the same animals were examined for comparative morphologic control.

The detailed description of the technical execution and interpretation of the mentioned functional and morphologic test-methods are given in chapter 2.

The fermentary activity of succinatdehydrogenase (SDG) additionally examinated in these series of experiments was detected after the Nachlass et al. method [84], with the use of blue tetrasolium. The results were evaluated visually using a five-score system, high, sufficiently high, middle, weak and absent activity.

The best regime of hypothermic protection from ischemic injuries and designed technical equipment for the experiments were applied in clinical practice by segmentary resection and removal of large staghorne and multiple stones from the kidney with temporarily blocked blood circulation. As well as by auto- and allotransplantation of kidneys and testes from living and cadaverous donors.

Table 16. Scheme of experiments for determination of a best level of hypothermia by 2-hour ischemia of the kidney

Kinds of operations		Quantity of animals for morphologic examinations according to observation terms					
		3 days	10 days	1 month	3 months	6 months	in all
1st gr.	Normothermic (+37°C) ischemia	3	3	3	3	3	15
2nd gr.	Ischemia by +4+7°C	3	3	3	3	3	15
3rd gr.	Ischemia by +10+15°C	3	3	3	3	3	15
4th gr.	Ischemia by +20+25°C	3	3	3	3	3	15
5th gr.	Control (mobilization)	1	1	1	1	1	5
							65

Chapter VIII

ISCHEMIA AND HYPOTHERMIC PROTECTION OF THE KIDNEY

8.1. RADIOLOGIC EVALUATION OF FUNCTIONAL CHANGES IN KIDNEYS AFTER 2 HOUR ISCHEMIA IN VARIOUS TEMPERATURE REGIMES

One day after the normothermic ischemia (+37°C) the renogram was two-phase, the amplitude of the vascular segment decreased to 62.3±2.4%, secretory segment - to 16.6±3.8% of the norm ($p<0.001$), residual activity 15 minutes after the radioactive isotope injection was 125.0±4.8% ($p<0.001$), the period of semi-excretion exceeded 15 minutes, and the renographic index was 4.9±0.8 ($p<0.001$) (Figure 121.2, Tables 17-21).

On the renoscintigrams the operated kidney was represented by single touches (Figures 121.6).

Within six months the renograms remained two-phase with a considerable decrease of all indices. By the end of the experiments (to six months) touches of the operated kidney on scintigrams were very rare, in contrast, there was compensatory hypertrophy of the opposite kidney (Figures 121.3,4,7).

In the second and third test-groups, one day after the ischemia and deep hypothermia (+4+7°C and +10+15°C), the renograms were two-phase as well, the amplitudes of vascular and secretory segments were decreased (63.8±2.5%; 40.0±2.9% and 75.8±3.6%, 52.0±2.9% of the standard, respectively, $p<0.001$). The period of semi-excretion exceeded 15 minutes. RI was also reduced (9.9±0.9 and 13.9±2.8, respectively, $p<0.001$, Figures 122.2, 123.2).

On renoscintigrams, the radioactivity at the site of the operated kidneys was very low (Figures 122.7, 123.6).

In these test-groups the renograms became three-phase after 15 and 9 days, respectively. Furthermore the gradual restoration of renographic indices occurred. Particularly, the normalization of the vascular segment had taken place (two and one month, respectively) and later (three and two months, respectively) the asymmetry between the operated and intact kidneys gradually disappeared (Figures 122.3-5, 8, 9, Figures 123.3, 4, 6, Tables 17-21).

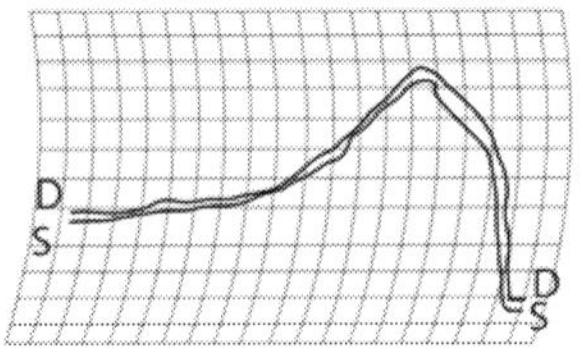

121.$_1$

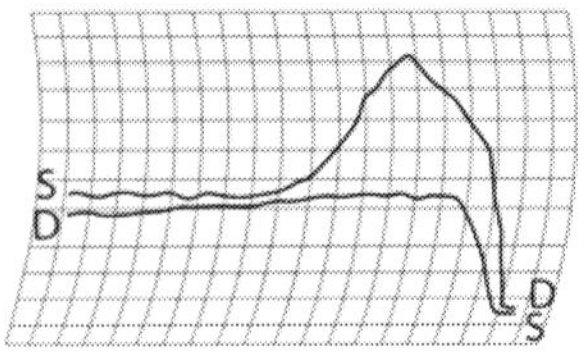

121.$_2$

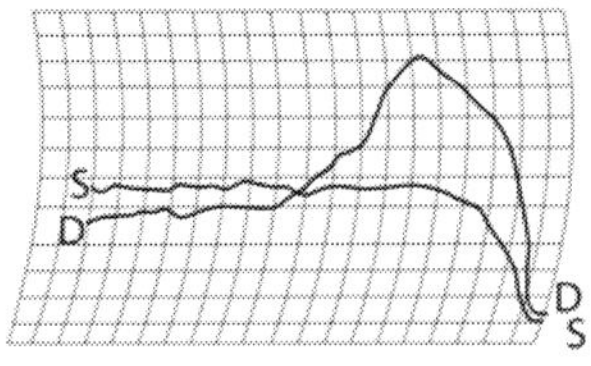

121.$_3$

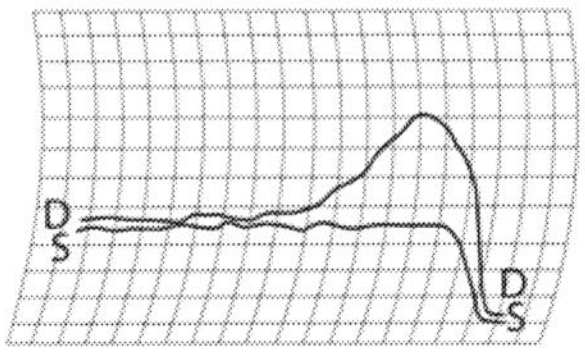

121.$_4$

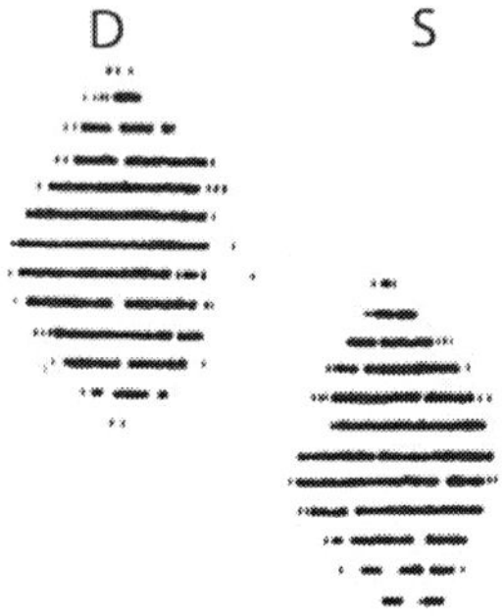

121.$_5$

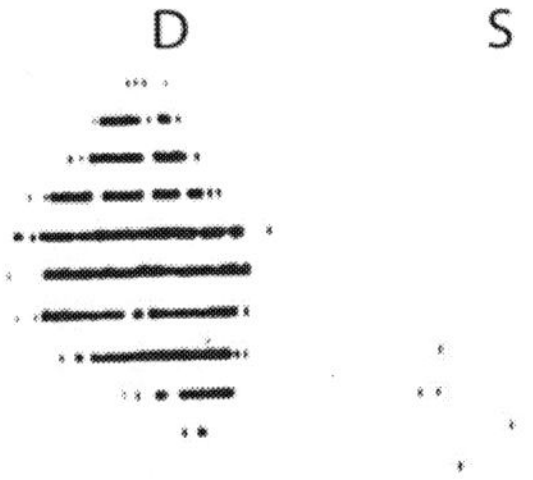

121.$_6$

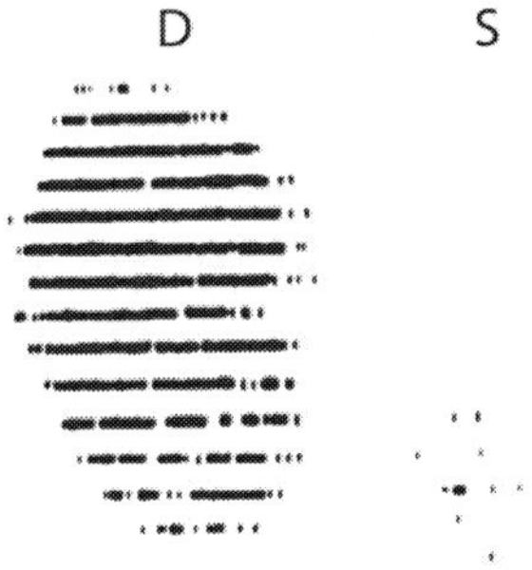

121.$_7$

Figure 121. Two-hour normothermic ischemia of the left kidney.
Radiorenograms:
121.$_1$ – before the operation; 121.$_2$ – 1 day afater the operation; 121.$_3$ – 1 month later; 121.$_4$ – 6
Renoscintigrams:
121.$_5$ – before the operation; 121.$_6$ – 3 days later; 121.$_7$ – 6 months later.

In the fourth test-group, one day after the ischemia, by middle level hypothermia (+20+25°C) the renograms kept a three-phase character. Their indices were decreased moderately, so the amplitude of the vascular segment was 68.4±2.7%, the secretory segment was 61.0±2.7% of the standard, and the period of semi-excretion exceeded 15 minutes. RI was reduced to 20.1±1.7 ($p<0,001$). The renoscintigrams were characterized with diffusive weakening of radioactivity at the site of the operated kidney (Figures 124.$_{2,6}$).

9 days after the operation the amplitude of the vascular segment became normal (97.9±1.6%, $p>0.05$) but the amplitude of the secretory segment remained slightly decreased (84.9±0.5% of the norm): the period of semi-excretion of the isotope was also prolonged (8.2±0.9 min); RI was 38.5±2.7 ($p<0.05$) (Figures 124.$_3$).

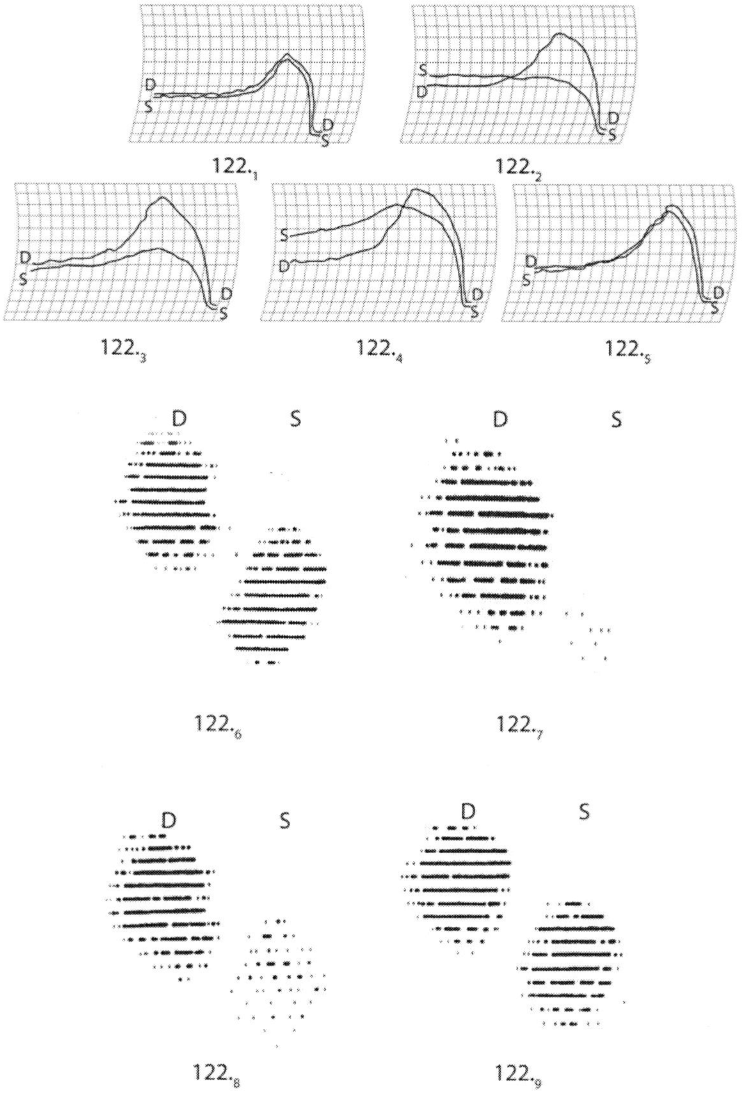

Figure 122. Two-hour ischemia of the left kidney by the temperature +4+7°C.
Radiorenograms: $122._1$ – before the operation; $122._2$ – 1 day after the operation; $122._3$ – 15 days later; $122._4$ – 2 months later; $122._5$ – 3 months later.
Renoscintigrams: $122._6$ – before the operation; $122._7$ – 3 days after the operation; $122._8$ – 1 month later; $122._9$ – 3 months later.

15 days after the operation the asymmetry between the operated and intact kidneys on the renograms and renoscintigrams disappeared. RI reached 55.5±3.0 ($p>0.05$).

Within the following period of observations (up to 6 months) the radiologic data retained normal characteristics (Figures 124.4, 7, Tables 17-21).

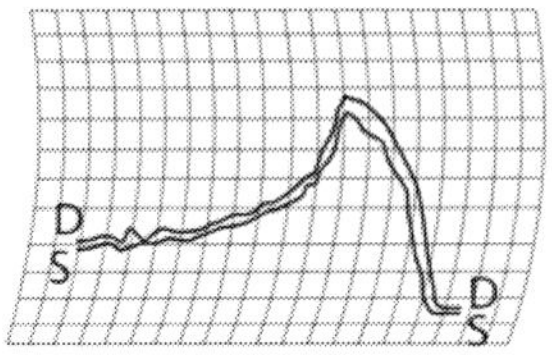

123.$_1$

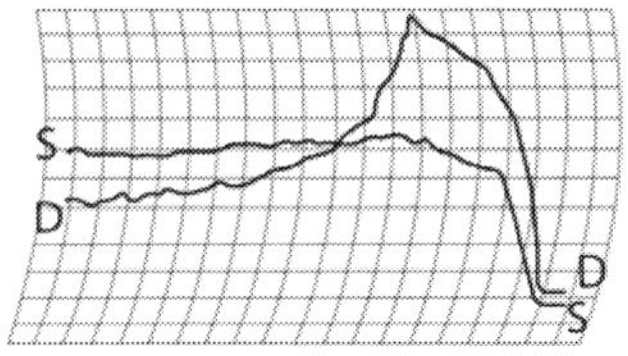

123.$_2$

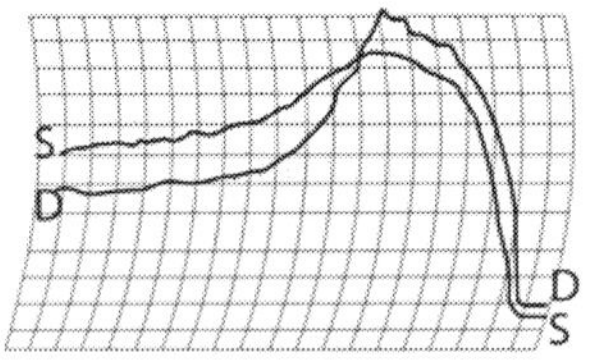

123.$_3$

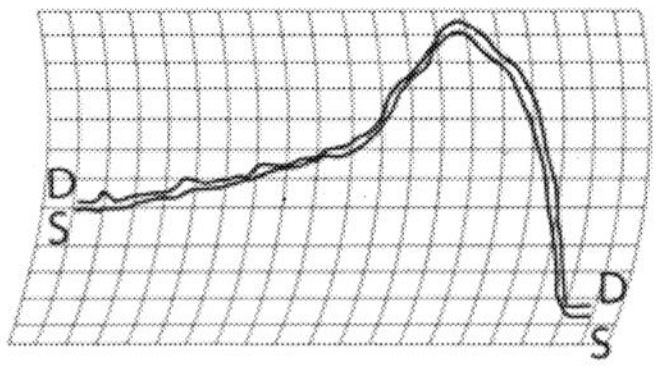

123.$_4$

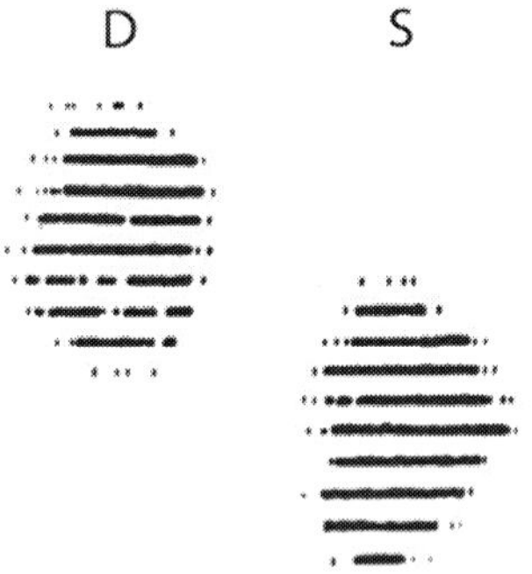

123.$_5$

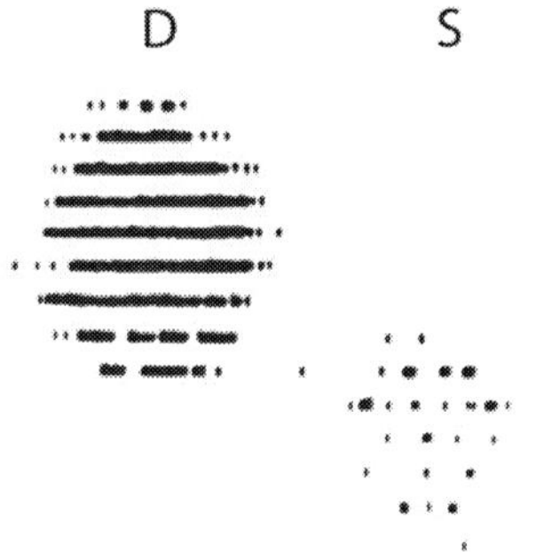

123.$_6$

123.$_7$

Figure 123. Two-hour ischemia of the left kidney by the temperature +10+15 °C.
Radiorenograms: 123.$_1$ – before the operation; 123.$_2$ – 1 day after the operation; 123.$_3$ – 1 month later; 123.$_4$ – 2 months later.
Renoscintigrams: 123.$_5$ – before the operation; 123.$_6$ – 3 days after the operation; 123.$_7$ – 2 months later.

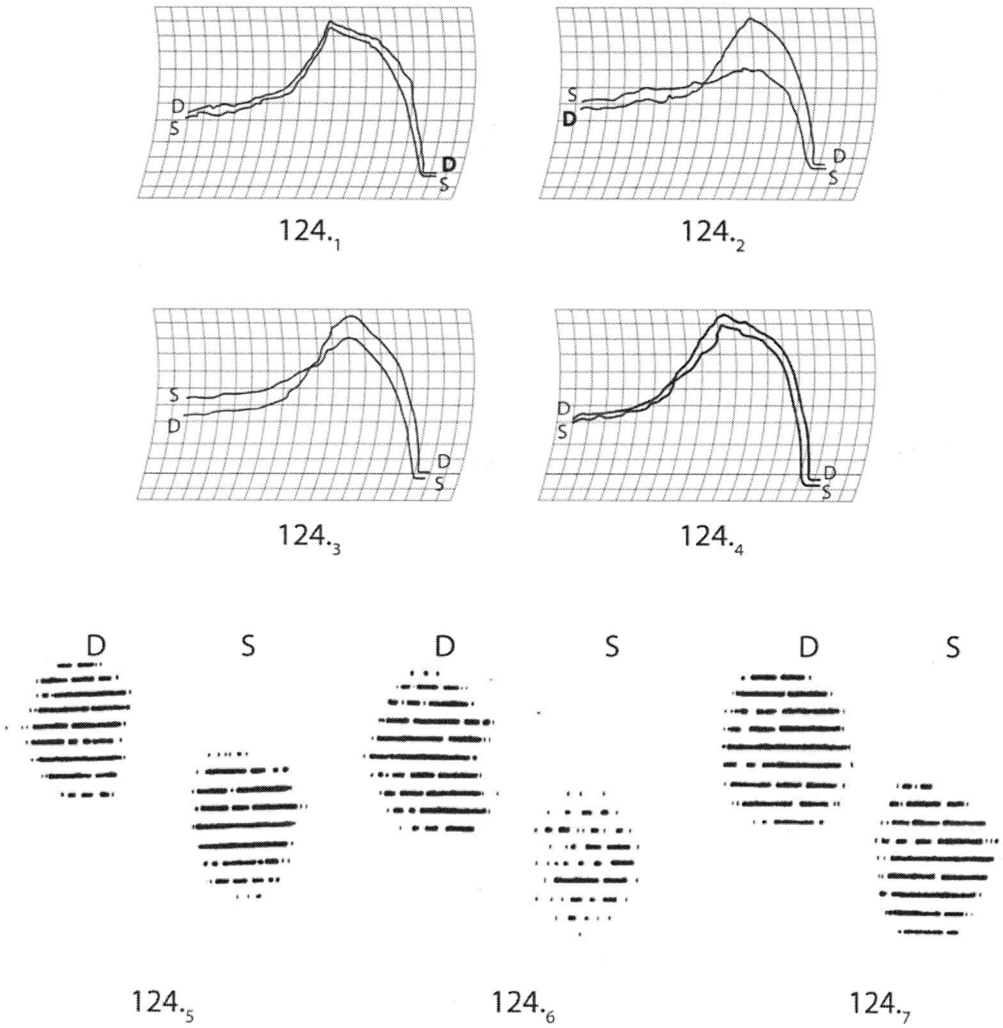

Figure 124. Two-hour ischemia of the left kidney by the temperature +20+25 °C.
Radiorenograms: $124._1$ – before the operation; $124._2$ – 1 day after the operation; $124._3$ – 9 days later; $124._4$ – 15 days later.
Renoscintigrams: $124._5$ – before the operation; $124._6$ – 3 days after the operation; $124._7$ – 1 month later.

Table 17. Two-hour kidney ischemia by different levels of the local hypothermia: Correlation of renogram vascular segment amplitudes of operated and intact kidneys (%)

Kinds of operations			Terms of observations							
			Before the operation	after 1 day	9 days	15 days	1 month	2 months	3 months	6 months
1st gr..	Normothermic (+37°C) ischemia	M±m	99,8±1,5	62,3±2,4	72,8±4,8	66,0±1,2	68,4±4,5	57,3±2,7	68,4±8,2	62,4±3,2
		n	5	9	8	5	8	7	6	3
		p		<0,001	<0,001	<0,001	<0,001	<0,001	<0,001	<0,001
2nd gr.	Ischemia by +4+7°C	M±m	99,5±0,5	63,8±2,5	77,5±2,9	71,0±5,5	80,8±3,9	96,2±3,0	97,9±3,2	98,3±2,3
		n	7	11	10	8	9	8	5	3
		p		<0,001	<0,001	<0,001	<0,01	>0,05	>0,05	>0,05
3rd gr.	Ischemia by +10+15°C	M±m	100,0±1,1	75,8±3,6	76,2±4,7	83,3±5,0	94,9±2,7	98,8±2,0	99,5±3,0	97,6±1,6
		n	5	8	7	6	7	5	5	3
		p		<0,001	<0,001	<0,01	>0,05	>0,05	>0,05	>0,05
4th gr.	Ischemia by +20+25°C	M±m	100,9±0,9	68,4±2,7	97,9±1,6	99,2±1,4	99,8±1,0	98,9±1,1	99,5±0,9	98,9±0,8
		n	5	7	7	8	7	6	6	3
		p		<0,001	>0,05	>0,05	>0,05	>0,05	>0,05	>0,05
5th gr.	Control (mobilization)	M±m	99,2±0,9	94,9±3,6	100,8±0,9	98,9±1,4	101,4±1,4	102,0±1,3	98,4±2,9	100,0
		n	5	5	4	3	3	2	2	1
		p		>0,05	>0,05	>0,05	>0,05	>0,05	>0,05	

Table 18. Two-hour kidney ischemia by different levels of the local hypothermia: Correlation of renogram secretion segment amplitudes of operated and intact kidneys (%)

Kinds of operations			Terms of observations							
			Before the operation	after 1 day	9 days	15 days	1 month	2 months	3 months	6 months
1st gr.	Normothermic (+37°C) ischemia	M±m	99,8±0,9	16,6±3,8	17,8±2,4	19,3±2,8	22,2±1,7	21,0±2,0	21,3±0,8	20,0±0,7
		n	5	9	8	5	8	7	6	3
		p	>0,05	<0,001	<0,001	<0,001	<0,001	<0,001	<0,001	<0,001
2nd gr.	Ischemia by +4+7°C	M±m	99,7±0,3	40,0±2,9	48,8±4,5	62,5±3,8	73,4±1,7	75,0±2,8	96,8±2,1	98,0±0,8
		n	7	11	10	8	9	8	5	3
		p	>0,05	<0,001	<0,001	<0,001	<0,001	<0,001	>0,05	>0,05
3rd gr.	Ischemia by +10+15°C	M±m	100,2±1,9	52,0±2,9	63,5±2,7	74,5±3,3	80,0±4,1	98,2±3,6	99,0±0,7	98,8±0,5
		n	5	8	7	6	7	5	5	3
		p	>0,05	<0,001	<0,001	<0,001	<0,01	>0,05	>0,05	>0,05
4th gr.	Ischemia by +20+25°C	M±m	99,1±0,8	61,0±2,7	84,9±0,5	97,3±1,0	99,2±0,8	98,8±1,2	99,0±1,4	98,5±1,0
		n	5	7	7	8	7	6	6	3
		p	>0,05	<0,001	<0,01	>0,05	>0,05	>0,05	>0,05	>0,05
5th gr.	Control (mobilization)	M±m	99,5±0,5	90,5±5,5	100,5±0,5	99,3±0,8	98,8±2,1	101,1±1,9	101,1±1,9	100,0
		n	5	5	4	3	3	2	2	1
		p	>0,05	<0,05	>0,05	>0,05	>0,05	>0,05	>0,05	

Table 19. Two-hour kidney ischemia by different levels of the local hypothermia: Correlation of residual activity in operated and intact kidneys

Kinds of operations			Terms of observations							
			Before the operation	after 1 day	9 days	15 days	1 month	2 months	3 months	6 months
1st gr.	Normothermic ischemia (+37°C)	M±m	101,2±1,2	125,0±4,8	135,4±3,6	133,5±3,3	130,8±4,7	132,8±0,7	130,5±3,2	128,1±1,2
		n	5	9	8	5	8	7	6	3
		p	>0,05	<0,001	<0,001	<0,001	<0,001	<0,001	<0,001	<0,001
2nd gr.	Ischemia by +4+7°C	M±m	100,7±0,7	122,2±1,8	92,2±3,8	80,0±1,8	122,5±2,7	140,0±7,5	102,5±2,4	101,3±0,7
		n	7	11	10	8	9	8	5	3
		p	>0,05	<0,001	<0,05	<0,001	<0,001	<0,001	>0,05	>0,05
3rd gr.	Ischemia by +10+15°C	M±m	102,2±1,5	140,0±4,6	136,3±5,2	134,8±2,1	133,3±3,6	102,5±4,4	101,4±0,8	99,6±0,5
		n	5	8	7	6	7	5	5	3
		p	>0,05	<0,001	<0,001	<0,001	<0,001	>0,05	>0,05	>0,05
4th gr.	Ischemia by +20+25°C	M±m	100,2±0,5	127,8±4,5	136,0±5,5	98,3±2,5	99,5±0,6	101,6±0,7	98,8±1,2	103±2,7
		n	5	7	7	8	7	6	6	3
		p	>0,05	<0,001	<0,001	>0,05	>0,05	>0,05	>0,05	>0,05
5th gr.	Control (mobilization)	M±m	101,2±1,4	104,5±3,4	101,4±1,6	101,9±1,4	102,2±2,8	103,3±3,8	97,1±3,6	100,0
		n	5	5	4	3	3	2	2	1
		p	>0,05	>0,01	>0,05	>0,05	>0,05	>0,05	>0,05	>0,05

In the fifth control test-group, after the mobilization of the kidney and its vascular pedicle, only an insignificant and unreliable depression of the secretory segment was observed the next day. Furthermore, the radiologic indices didn`t differ from preoperative indices (Tables 17-21).

Table 20. Two-hour kidney ischemia by different levels of the local hypothermia: Changes of the isotope semi excretion time in renograms (in minutes)

Kinds of operations			Terms of observations							
			Before the operation	after 1 day	9 days	15 days	1 month	2 months	3 months	6 months
1st gr.	Normothermic ischemia (+37°C)	M±m	3,9±0,5	>15	>15	>15	>15	>15	>15	>15
		n	5	9	8	5	8	7	6	3
		p	>0,05	<0,001	<0,001	<0,001	<0,001	<0,001	<0,001	<0,001
2nd gr.	Ischemia by +4+7°C	M±m	4,8±0,9	>15	>15	>15	>15	10,5±0,8	5,2±0,5	4,0±0,2
		n	7	11	10	8	9	8	5	3
		p	>0,05	<0,001	<0,001	<0,001	<0,001	<0,01	>0,05	>0,05
3rd gr.	Ischemia by +10+15°C	M±m	4,7±1,2	>15	>15	>15	9,0±0,5	5,1±0,3	4,7±0,2	4,1±0,4
		n	5	8	7	6	7	5	5	3
		p	>0,05	<0,001	<0,001	<0,001	<0,01	>0,05	>0,05	>0,05
4th gr.	Ischemia by +20+25°C	M±m	4,6±0,7	>15	8,2±0,9	6,0±0,4	5,2±0,3	4,8±0,1	4,0±0,5	4,1±0,3
		n	5	7	7	8	7	6	6	3
		p	>0,05	<0,001	<0,05	>0,05	>0,05	>0,05	>0,05	>0,05
5th gr.	Control (mobilization)	M±m	3,3±0,5	5,7±2,8	4,6±0,9	4,6±0,8	4,6±0,3	3,5±1,0	5,2±1,1	5,0
		n	5	5	4	3	3	2	2	1
		p	>0,05	>0,05	>0,05	>0,05	>0,05	>0,05	>0,05	

Table 21. Two-hour kidney ischemia by different levels of the local hypothermia: Changes of Hirakawa-Corcoran`s renographic index

Kinds of operations			Terms of observations							
			Before the operation	after 1 day	9 days	15 days	1 month	2 months	3 months	6 months
1st gr.	Normothermic ischemia (+37°C)	M±m	55,7±1,8	4,9±0,8	6,8±1,2	8,1±0,3	9,3±1,4	9,9±1,8	8,0±1,3	7,8±2,3
		n	5	9	8	5	8	7	6	3
		p	>0,05	<0,001	<0,001	<0,001	<0,001	<0,001	<0,001	<0,001
2nd gr.	Ischemia by +4+7°C	M±m	59,7±4,9	9,9±0,9	12,4±0,5	32,1±3,0	27,4±1,8	32,0±2,4	51,3±1,8	62,2±2,7
		n	7	11	10	8	9	8	5	3
		p	>0,05	<0,001	<0,001	<0,001	<0,001	<0,001	>0,05	>0,05
3rd gr.	Ischemia by +10+15°C	M±m	59,9±2,9	13,9±2,8	16,6±3,8	27,4±5,2	32,0±1,8	51,5±2,0	62,4±3,6	60,3±2,5
		n	5	8	7	6	7	5	5	3
		p	>0,05	<0,001	<0,001	<0,001	<0,001	>0,05	>0,05	>0,05
4th gr.	Ischemia by +20+25°C	M±m	59,4±3,6	20,1±1,7	38,5±2,7	55,5±3,0	59,5±4,2	57,3±4,1	60,6±2,2	62,2±3,2
		n	5	7	7	8	7	6	6	3
		p	>0,05	<0,001	<0,05	>0,05	>0,05	>0,05	>0,05	>0,05
5th gr.	Control (mobilization)	M±m	58,4±4,8	42,0±6,3	57,4±2,8	55,8±7,4	62,0±2,4	52,3±1,4	56,5±3,4	65,1
		n	5	5	4	3	3	2	2	1
		p	>0,05	>0,05	>0,05	>0,05	>0,05	>0,05	>0,05	>0,05

8.2. The Discussion of Kidney Functional Examination Results

An analysis of radiologic investigations of kidneys that underwent a 2-hour long ischemia in different temperature conditions permits us to distinguish certain types of renograms, which testify to the character and degree of pathology in operated kidneys: 1) two-phase renogram (Figure 125.1); 2) three-phase renogram with low amplitudes of the vascular and secretion segments and prolonged excretion (Figures 125.2); 3) three-phase renogram with a normal amplitude of the vascular segment, but delayed excretion (Figures 125.3); 4) normal three-phase renogram which didn`t differ from the intact kidney renogram (Figures 125.4).

The renoscintigrams can be divided in following types: 1) A complete absence of touches or single touches (Figures 125.5); 2) Rare touches and decrease of functioning parenchyma dimensions (Figures 125.6); 3) Rare touches with normal dimensions of the kidney (Figures 125.7); normal renoscintigrams which didn`t differ from the intact kidneys (Figures 125.8).

The first type of renograms (two-phase, Figures 125.1) was observed within 6 months in the test-group where the kidney was subjected to normothermic (+37°C) ischemia and in the immediate period (to 9-15 days) after ischemia and deep hypothermia (+10+15°C and +4+7°C, respectively).

The mentioned renograms corresponded with the first type of renoscintigrams with single or completely absent touches (Figures 125.5). These data testified about the most expressed functional depression in the mentioned test-groups.

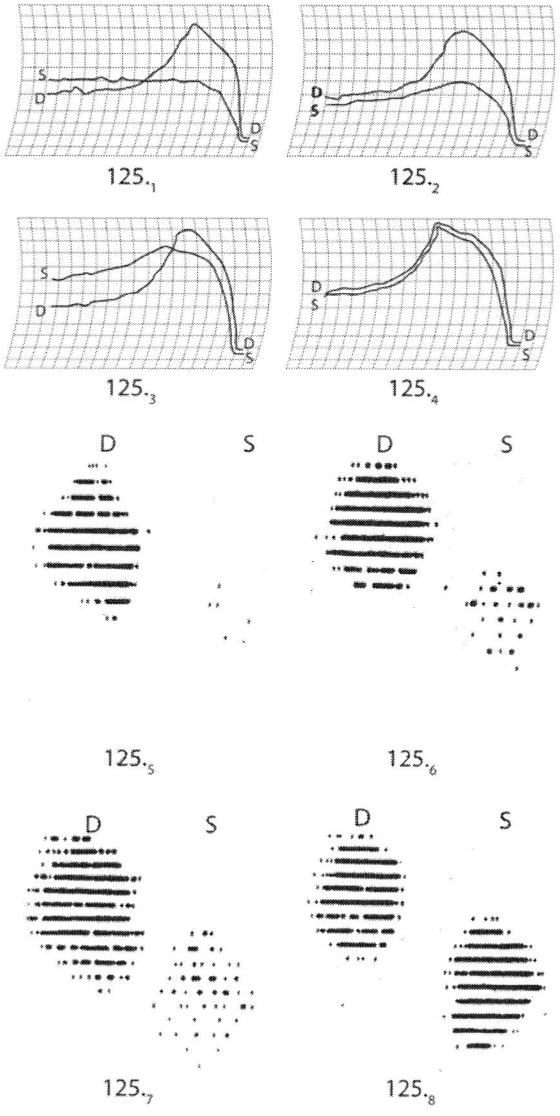

Figure 125. Types of radiorenograms and renoscintigrams after the ischemia and hypothermia of the kidney.
Radiorenograms: $125._{1}$ – 1st type; $125._{2}$ – 2nd type; $125._{3}$ – 3rd type; $125._{4}$ – 4th type. Renoscintigrams: $125._{5}$ – 1st type; $125._{6}$ – 2nd type; $125._{7}$ – 3rd type; $125._{8}$ – 4th type.

The second type of renograms (three-phase with decreased amplitudes of vascular and secretory segments and delayed excretion, Figures 125.2) were observed in the test-group after ischemia and deep hypothermia (+10+15°C and +4+7°C) in the period between 9-15 days after the operation and on the day following ischemia in conditions of moderate hypothermia (+20+25°C).

This type of renogram corresponded to the second type of renoscintigram, with rare touches and a decrease of working kidney parenchyma (Figures 125.6).

The described radiologic data, on the one hand, reflected less serious functional disturbances as compared with the above mentioned types and, on the other hand, represented the tendencies of an improvement of kidney functional state.

The third type of renogram with normal amplitude of vascular segment (Figures 125.3) and the third type of renoscintigram with diffusive rare touches but normal kidney dimensions (Figures 125.7) were observed in test-groups with ischemia and hypothermia of the kidneys. The data testified to a gradual restoration of the separate kidney functions. Particularly, after the ischemia and deep hypothermia (+4+7°C) the blood circulation was restored within 2 months, with secretory and excretory function restoration after 3 months. In the kidney subjected to ischemia by +10+15°C, the blood circulation was recovered after 1 month, followed by secretory and excretory functions after 2 months. The kidney underwent ischemia by moderate hypothermia (+20+25°C) which restored vascularisation in 9 days, ND secretory and excretory functions in 15 days.

The fourth (normal) type of renogram and renoscintigram (Figures 125.4,8) confirmed the described dynamics and further testified about the stable functional restoration of the kidney.

Thus, the radiologic investigations showed that the depth and firmness of functional changes and the character of rehabilitation in ischemized kidneys were dependent on temperature conditions.

The most serious and irreversible injuries in the kidney came after normothermic (+37°C) ischemia.

Ischemia by hypothermia caused less expressed changes which were reversible. Particularly, in a shorter period (15 days) the recovery of function of the kidney came with cooling to +20+25°C. A more deep cooling of the ischemized kidneys to +10+15°C and +4+7°C was accompanied with circulatory upsettings within 1-2 months, but the full functional rehabilitation of the kidney had taken place in the more remote period of 2 and 3 months after the operation, respectively.

Taking into account the high sensitivity of the applied radiologic test-methods, specifically their ability to give objective information about blood circulation, secretion and excretion of the kidneys, it can be asserted that the best temperature zone which ensures functional safety of the kidneys by 2 hour long ischemia is the interval of +20+25°C.

8.2. The Morphologic State of Kidneys after Two-hour Ischemia in Various Temperature Conditions

8.2.1. The Influence of a Normothermic Ischemia on the Kidney

In the first test-group, three days after the normothermic (+37C) ischemia of the kidney, stagnation of blood in the glomerulas, various degrees of dystrophic changes in the proximal and distal segments of the nephron, and necroses were observed (Figure 126). The succinatdehydrogenase (SDG) activity in these segments of the nephron was absent (Figure 127).

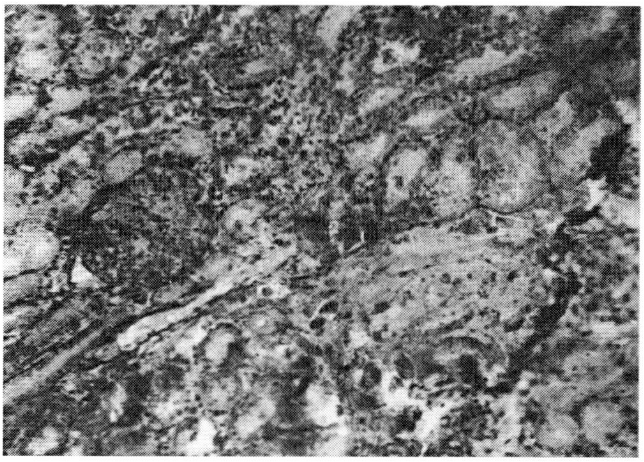

Figure 126. microphotogram of the kidney 3 days after two-hour normothermic (+37 °C) ischemia. Numerous necroses are observed in the parenchyma. Painted with hematoxilin a. eosin.x150.

By electron microscopy the endothelium (En) and basal membrane (BM) of the glomerulas were relatively preserved. In podocytes (Pd), swelling of mitochondrias (M), widening of endoplasmatic net cisterns (ENC) and the appearance of multivesicular bodies (MVB) were noticed (Figure 128).

In the epithelial cells of the proximal and distal segments of the nephron, most typical changes were of the vacuolization (V) of the nuclei (N) (Figure 129), and the appearance of spiral laminated bodies (SLB) (Figure 130) which often accompanied the full destruction of the central part of nuclei (Figure 131). The cellular cytoplasma is distinguished by low electronic density, vacuolization, and swelling of mitochondrias (Figure 130). In some mitochondrias the matrix was clear, the external membranes (M) were destroyed and the mitochondrial content increased in the cytoplasma (Figure 132). In the cytoplasma there were often autophagic vacuoles containing osmiophyl granular inclusions (OGI) and mitochondria in diverse stages of destruction. In the apical part of the cell local necroses were revealed (Figure 133).

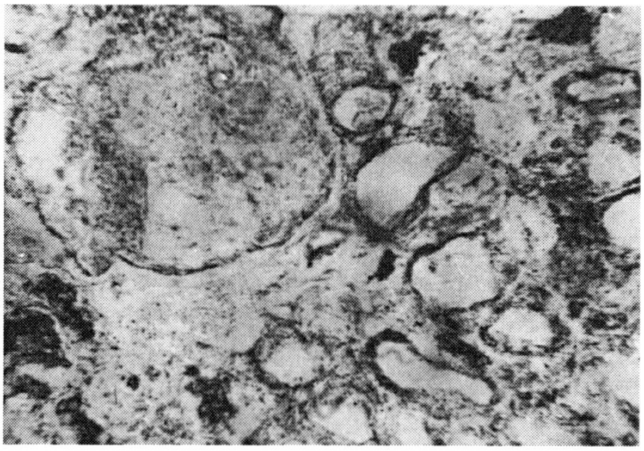

Figure 127. The same case. Succinatdehydrogenase activity in the kidney parenchyma is sharply reduced. painted with nitro-blue tetrasolium.x400.

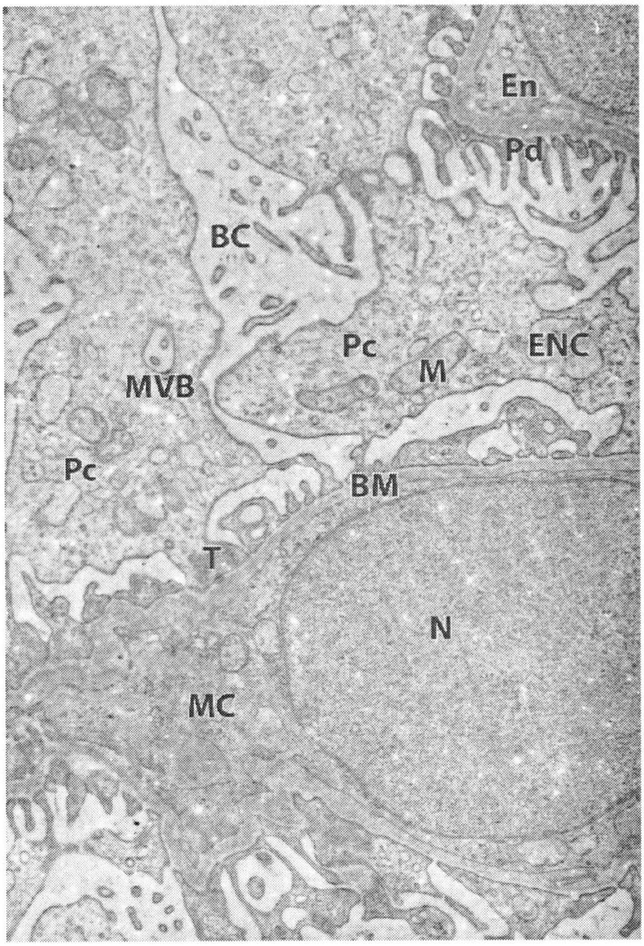

Figure 128. Electronogram of the glomerula section 3 days after the two-hour normathermic ischemia (+37 °C) of the kidney. In podocytes (Pc) widened cisterns of endoplasmatic net (ENC), swelling mitochondrias (M) and multivesicular bodies (MVB) are seen. x30.000.

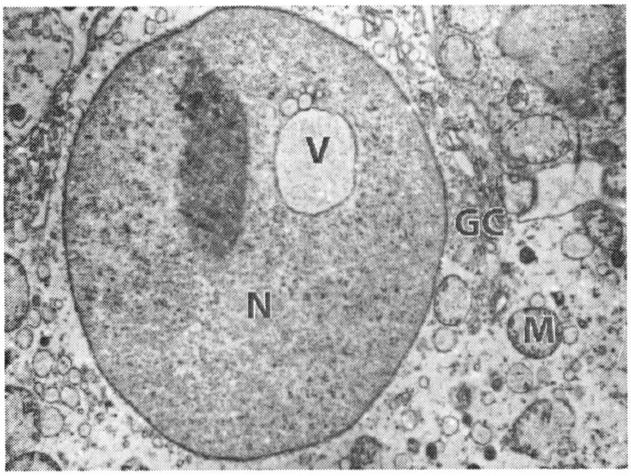

Figure 129. Ultrastructure of an epithelial cell of the nephron proximal segment 3 days after 20-hour normathermic ischemia (+37 °C). A vacuolization (V) of the cytoplasma and nucleus (N) are observed.x11.000.

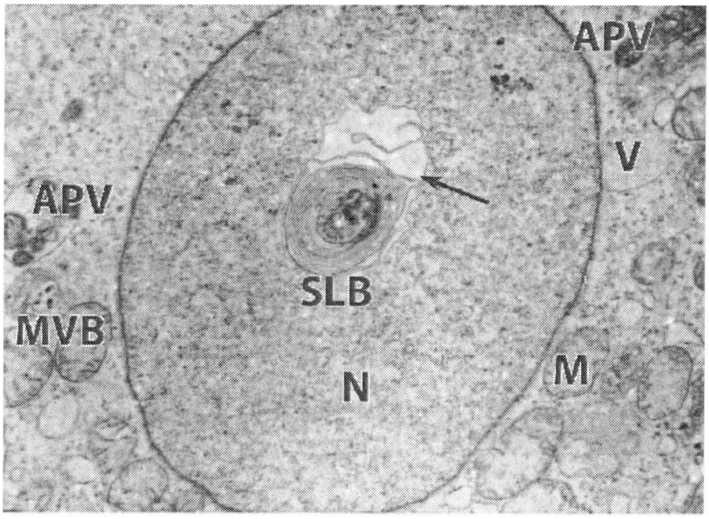

Figure 130. The same case. in the middle of nucleus (N) a spiral laminated body (SLB) is detected with formation of a cavity (indicated with an arrow).x15.000.

The epithelial cells of the thin segment of the nephron and collective tubules were distinguished by a decrease of electronic density of cellular cytoplasma and a swelling of mitochondria.

Ten days after the operation, the local necroses were found histologically in the cortical substance of the kidney. Only traces of SDG activity could be seen in various segments of the nephron.

One month after the operation a blood stagnation, local necroses, and development of connective tissue (CF) were observed in the cortical and medullar substances of the kidney. The SDG activity in all sections of the kidney parenchyma was absent.

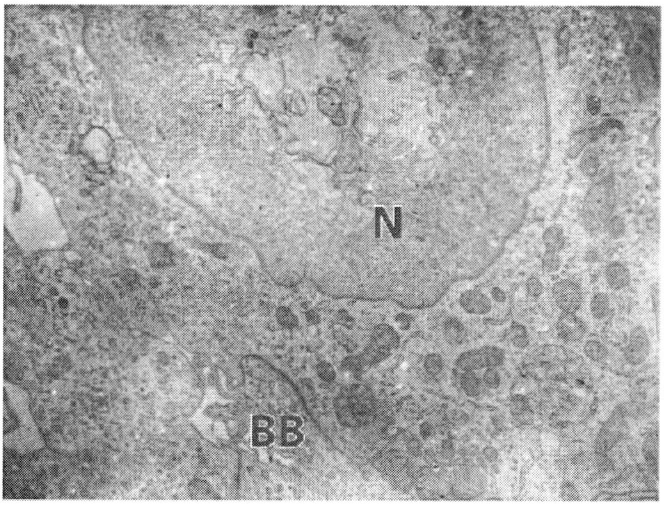

Figure 131. Electronogram of an epithelial cell of the nephron proximal segment 3 days after 2-hour normothermic(+37 °C) ischemia. Destruction of the nucleus (N) is observed.x15.000.

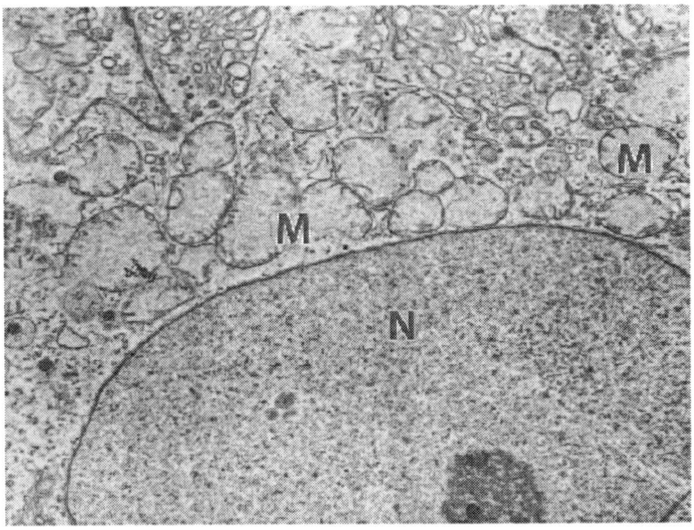

Figure 132. The same case. Destruction of mitochondrias (M) in the cytoplasma is observed.x17.000.

Three and six months later, macromorphologically, the kidney was atrophied, lagged behind the intact kidney by 50%, and had a slack consistency. Microscopically, diffusive development of rough connective tissue, atrophy of nephron epithelial cells, and desolation or obliteration of glomerulas were observed (Figure 134). SDG activity was absent in all segments of the nephron.

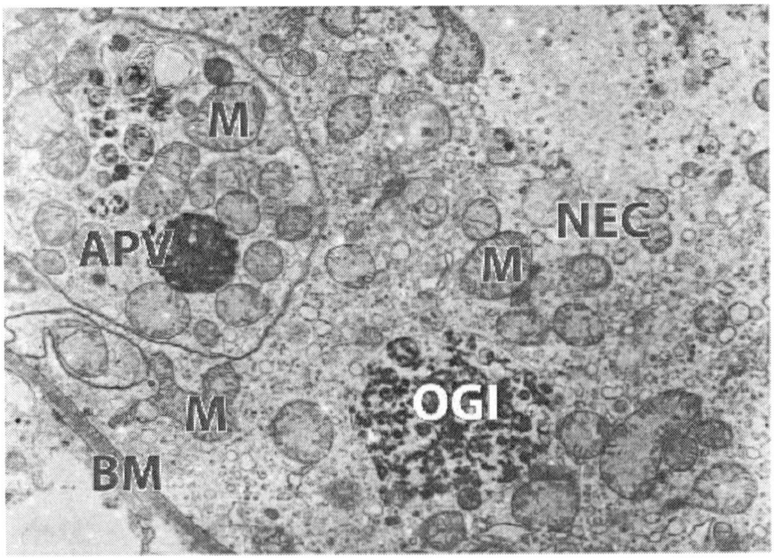

Figure 133. ultrastructu4re ofr the nephron proximal segment epithelial cell 3 days after 2-hour normothermic (+37 °C) ischemia of the kidney. In the basal part of the cell autophagocitous vacuoles (APV) with osmiophyl granular inclusions (OGI) and mitochondrias (M) in various stages of destruction are observed. In the apical part of the cell a local necrosis (NEC) is seen.x10.000.

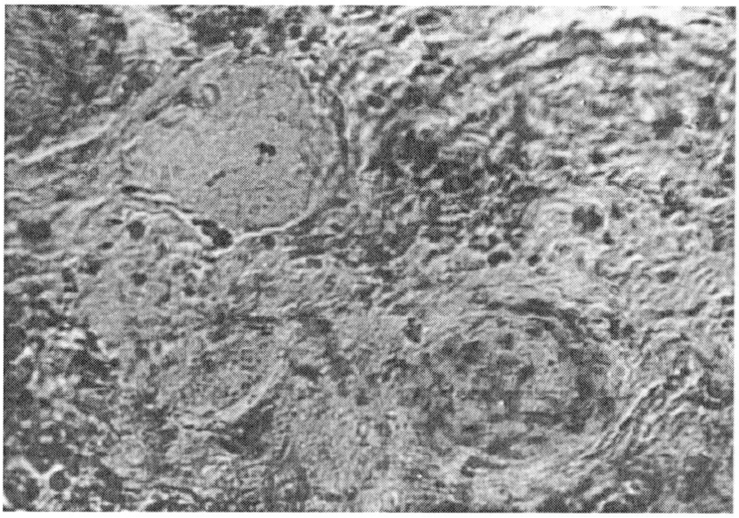

Figure 134. Microphotogram of the kidney 6 months after 2-hour normothermic (=37 °C) ischemia. Formation of a rough connective tissue in the parenchyma is observed. Painted with hematoxilin a. eosin.x200.

8.2.2. The Influence of Ischemia and Hypothermia +4+7°C on the Kidney

In the second test-group, three days after the ischemia and hypothermia of +4+7°C, blood stagnation and the appearance of hyalinous cylinders in the tubular channels of the kidney cortical substance were observed microscopically. SDG activity in the proximal nephron, thin and distal segments was moderate, and in the collective tubules was weak.

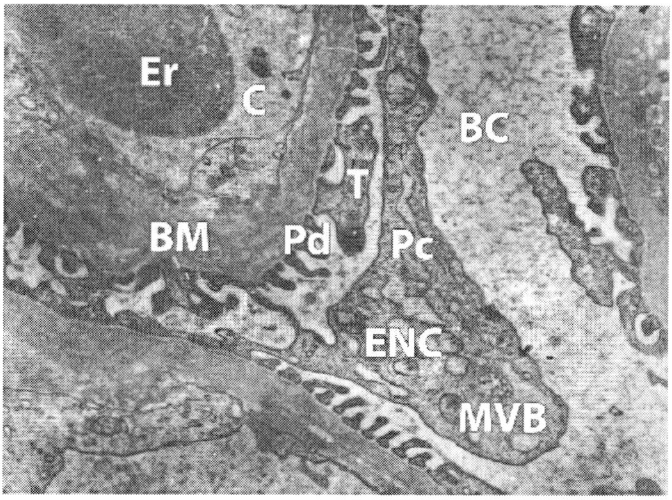

Figure 135. Ultrastructure of a glomerula 3 days after 2 hour ischemia by the temperature +4+7 °C. The basal membrane (BM) is slightly loosened. there are traced widened cisterns of the endoplasmatic net (ENC) and multivesicular bodies (MVB).x11.000.

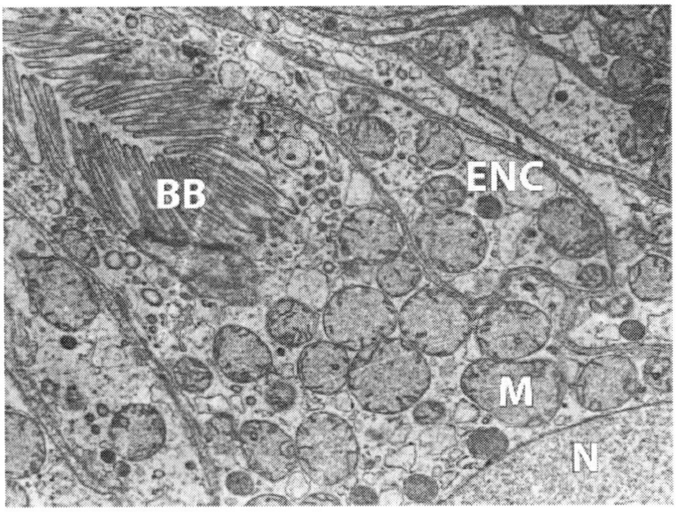

Figure 136. The same case. In the epithelial cell of the nephron proximal segment aq widening of endoplasmatic net cisterns (ENC) and swelling of mitochondrias (M) are observed.x10.500.

By electron microscopy, in glomerular podocytes, there was a vacuolization at the expense of widened cisterns of the endoplasmatic net. Furthermore, there were multivesicular bodies (Figure 135).

In the epithelial cells of the proximal segment of the nephron a swelling of the mitochondria (Figure 136), widening of cisterns of the endoplasmatic net, and accumulation of a big number of ribosomes (R) on their external membranes were observed (Figure 137). The brush border (BB) was well preserved (Figure 136). The arterioles around the tubules were sharply contracted (Figure 138), and diapedesis occurred (Figure 139). In the epithelial cells of the nephron thin and distal segments a swelling of the mitochondria was noticed. The collective tubules remained relatively intact.

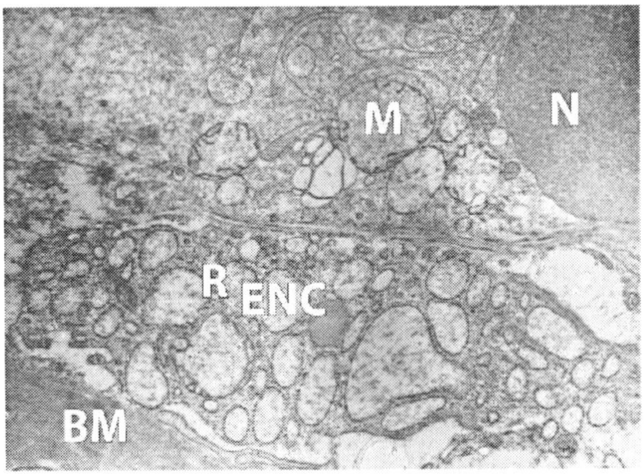

Figure 137. Section of an epithelial cell of the nephron proximal segment 3 days after 2-hour ischemia by the temperature +4+7 °C. An increase of the quantity and diameter of endoplasmatic net cisterns (ENC) is mentioned. On their external membranes chains of ribosoms (R) are located. Mitochondrias (m) are selled. x14.000.

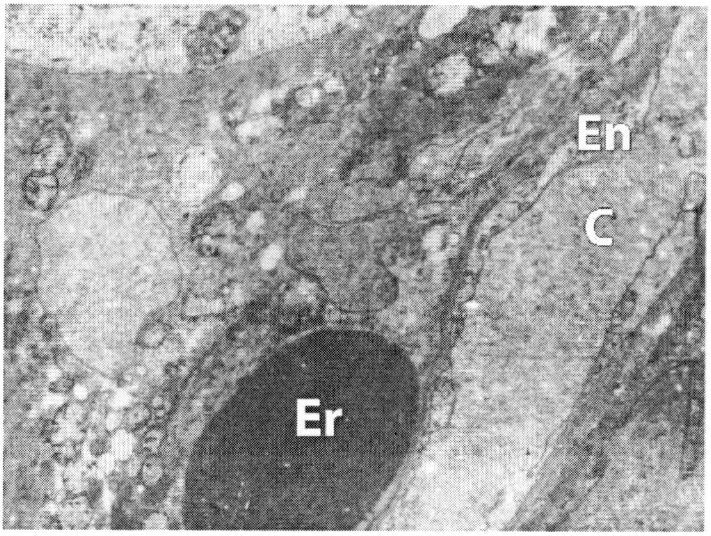

Figure 138. Arteriola in the cortical substance of the kidney 3 days after its 2-hour ischemia by the temperature +4+7 °C. Arteriola is sharply narrowed, its channel space is closed (indicated with arrows). x10.000.

Ten days after the operation, blood stagnation was noted histologically in the cortical and distal substances of the kidney. The SDG activity in the nephron's proximal, thin and distal segments was moderate, and in the collective tubules it was weak, as before.

One month later the histologic picture coincided mainly with one of the previous term. It has to be noted that there are appearances of local sclerotic changes in the interstitial tissue. The SDG activity in the nephron segments were moderate, as before.

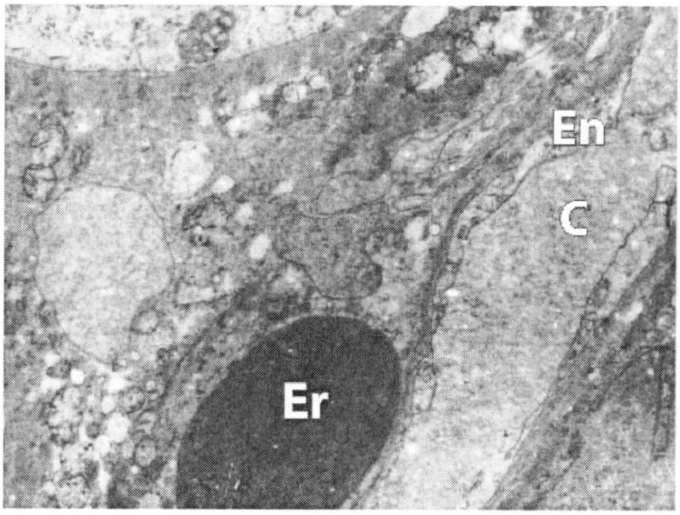

Figure 139. Section of a kidney capillary (C) 3 days after 2-hour ischemia by the temperature +4+7 °C. An erytrocyte (Er) diapedesis is observed.x10.000.

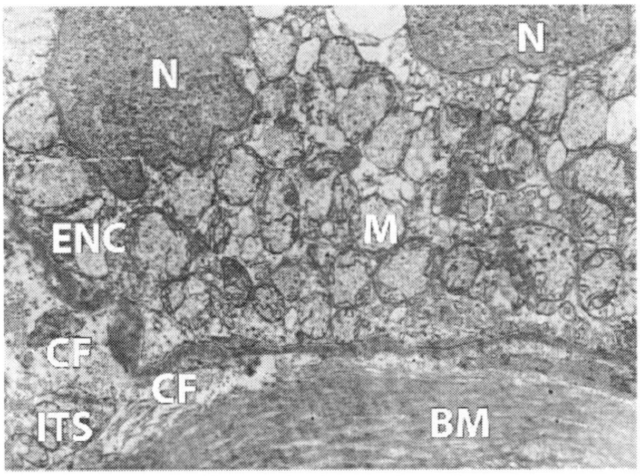

Figure 140. Section of an epithelial cell of the nephron proximal segment 1 month after 2-hour ischemia by the temperature +4+7 °C. The basal membrane (BM) is loosened, splintered and thickened. Bunshes of collagen fibers (CF) are revealed in it and in the intertubular space (ITS). In the cytoplasma mitoch9ondrias (M) are swelled, nuclei (N)-squeezed and deformed.x12.000.

By electron microscopy, a swelling of the mitochondrias of various degrees and vacuolization of the cellular cytoplasma were observed in the proximal and distal segments of the nephron. Furthermore, a thickening and loosening of the basal membrane and the appearance of collagen fibers in the intertubular spaces (ITC) could be noticed (Figure 140).

Three and six months later the general histological and electron microscopical pictures of the kidney mainly corresponded to the standard, except for a small interstitial sclerosis. Simultaneously there was a restoration of SDG activity in all segments of the nephron.

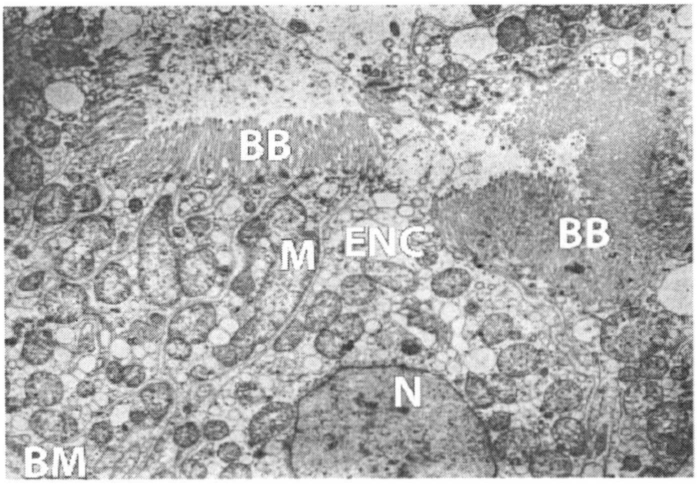

Figure 141. Section of an epithelial cell of the nephron proximal segment 3 days after 2-hour ischemia of the kidney by the temperature +10+15 Figure 140. Mitochondrias (M) are swelled, cisterns of endoplasmatic net (ENC) – widened.x10.000.

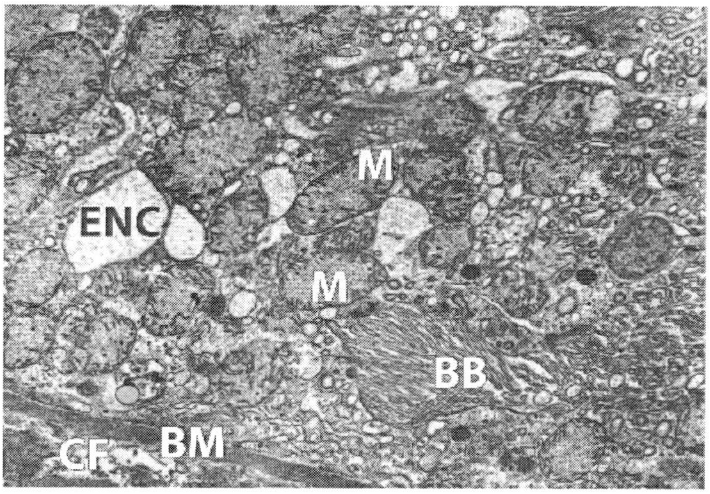

Figure 142. Section of an epithelial cell of the nephron proximal segment 1 month after 2-hour ischemia of the kidney by the temperature +10+15 °C. Mitoch9ondrias (M) are swelled, cisterns of endoplasmatic net (ENC) widened, in the intertubular space collagenous fibers (CF) are seen.x15.000.

8.2.3. The Influence of Ischemia and Hypothermia +10+15°C on the Kidney

In the third test-group, three days after the ischemia by hypothermia of +10+15°C, blood stagnation was revealed in the kidney cortical substance. The SDG activity in the nephron proximal, thin and distal segments was sufficiently high.

By electron microscopy, in the proximal and distal segments of the nephron, a swelling of the mitochondria and vacuolization in the cytoplasma were observed (Figure 141). In the thin segment and collective tubules no essential pathology was seen.

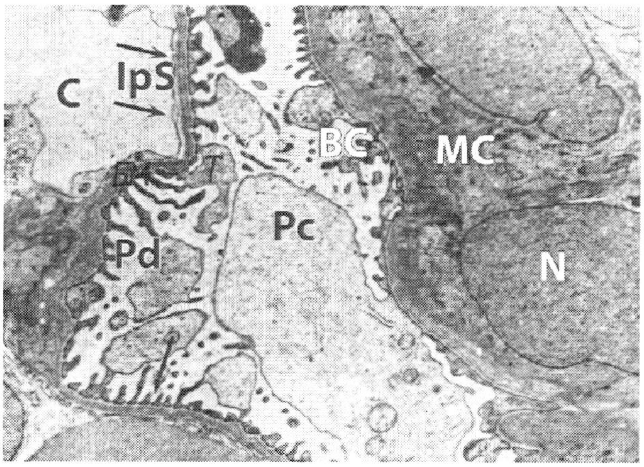

Figure 143. Section of a glomerula 3 days afater 2-hour ischemia of the kidney by the temperature +20+25 °C. The thickness and structure of the basal membrane (BM) are standard. The alternation of interpediculary splits (IpS) is clear and regular (Indicated with arrows).x10.500.

Ten days after the operation, histologically, a blood stagnation was noticed, as before, in the kidney cortical and juxtamedullar substance. At the same time, SDG activity in the proximal and distal segments of the nephron was changed to moderate.

One month later, histologically, there was no significant pathology in the kidney parenchyma. The SDG activity in the proximal and distal segments of the nephron was increased to a level of "sufficiently high". By electron microscopy, the glomerulas were quite safe. In the epithelial cells of the proximal and distal segments of the nephron, a swelling of the mitochondria and vacuolization of the cytoplasma were mentioned. In the interstitial tissue, connective tissue developed (Figure 142). At the same time the majority of epithelial cells was intact.

Three and six months after the operation the structure of the kidney on the micro- and electron microscopical levels and SDG activity didn`t differ from the standard.

8.2.4. The Influence of Ischemia and Hypothermia +20+25°C on the Kidney

In the fourth test-group, three days after the ischemia in conditions of a moderate hypothermia of +20+25°C, microscopically, a slightly expressed blood stagnation was noticed in the kidney cortical substance. SDG activity in various segments of the nephron was safe.

By electron microscopy the structure of the glomerulas was normal (Figure 143). In the epithelial cells of the proximal and distal segments of the nephron, a light swelling of some mitochondria was observed. Vacuolization of the cytoplasma had not taken place (Figure 144). The brush border had an usual structure. In the thin segment and collective tubules there was no pathology.

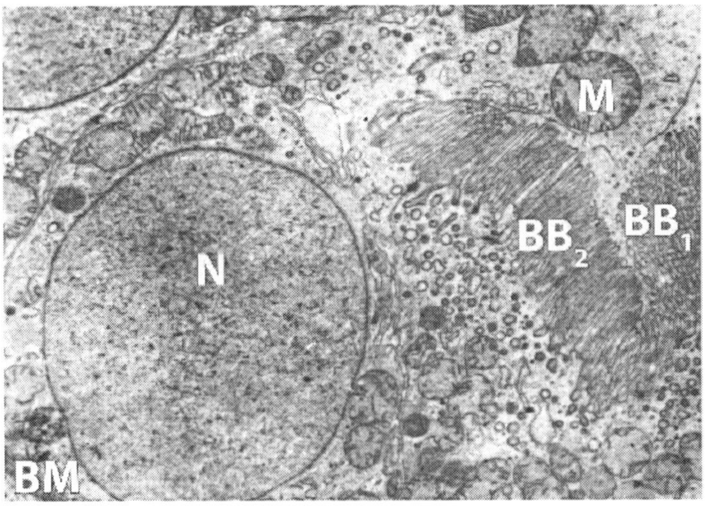

Figure 144. Section of an epithelial cell of the nephron proximal segment 3 days after 2-hour ischemia of the kidney by the temperature +20+25C. The brush border is cross (BB_1) and longitudinal (BB_2) sections is intact. Mitochondrias (M)_ are slightly swelled.x11.000.

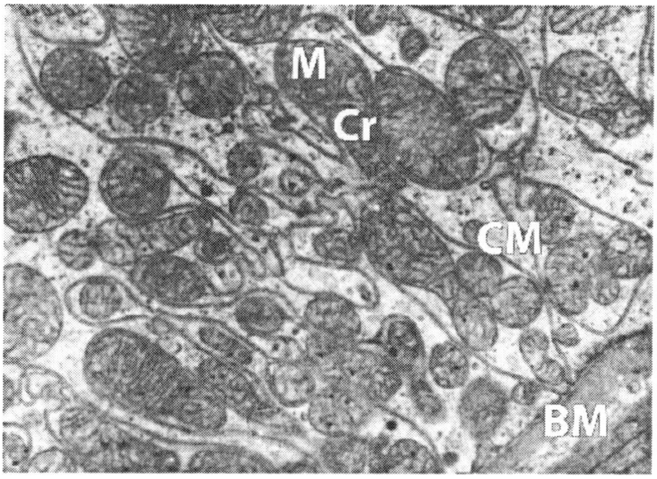

Figure 145. Epithelial cell of the nephron distal segment 1 month after 2-hour kidney ischemia by the temperature +20+25 °C. Folds of the cytoplasmatic membrane (CM) are without any pathology, mitochondrias (M) have a dense matrix and clear system of cristas.x12.000.

Ten days later the microscopical picture of the kidneys was lacking significant changes. There was only a slight decrease of SDG activity in the nephron proximal segment to the level of "sufficiently high". The electron microscopical structure of the kidneys didn`t differ from the previous term.

One month after the operation up to the completion of the experiment, the general morphologic, electron microscopic structure (Figure 145) and SDG activity (Figure 146) in the various segments of the nephron didn`t differ from the standard.

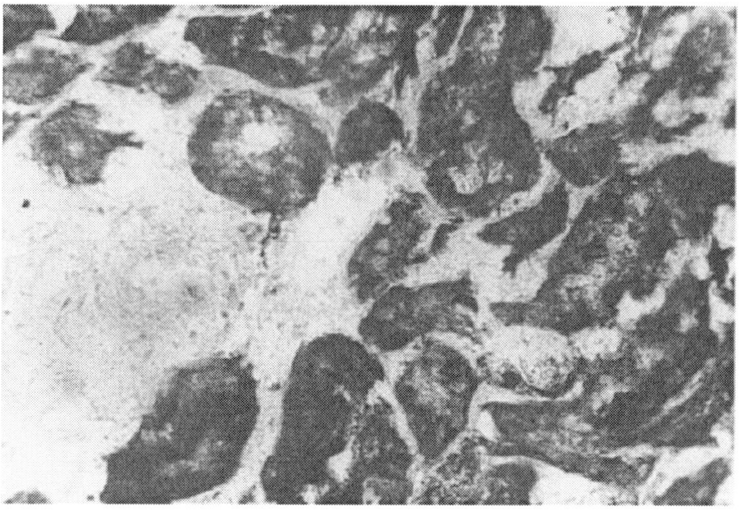

Figure 146. The same case. The succinatdehydrogenase activity in the kidney tubules is high. Painted with nitro-blue tetrazolium.x400.

8.2.5. Results of Examinations of Kidneys in the Control Animal Group

In the fifth control test-group where only kidney mobilization was performed, within six months of the operation, the histologic and electron microscopical pictures didn`t represent any deviation from the norm. The tetrasolium-reaction showed high activity of SDG in the proximal, thin and distal segments of the nephron, with moderate activity in the collective tubules. At the same time the ferment activity in the glomerulas and small blood vessels was absent. This phenomenon coincided with the known literature related to the norm [70,91,200].

8.2.6. Discussion of Kidneys Morphologic Investigation Results

The described morphologic investigations testify to the direct correlation between the applied temperature regime of an ischemized kidney and the depth of pathological changes.

The most significant vascular dystrophic injuries, including necrotic and full depression of a SDG activity, occurred in the kidneys after normothermic ischemia (+37°C). Initially, vacuolization of the nuclei and the appearance of spiral laminated bodies, often with the full destruction of the nuclei, attracted attention.

Similar formations are described in the cytoplasma and mitochondria. The authors explained their appearance with a concentration of substances inside the cells which are subject to removal. There is an opinion that myelinlike membranes of the mentioned spiral laminated bodies ensure isolation of such substances for subsequent autophagocytosis [82, 184,185,200]. In accessible literature, there was not any information concerning the appearance of these bodies in the nuclei of epithelial cells. Therefore, it is necessary to interpret this phenomenon.

It is known from the literature that a cytoplasmatic membrane is developed intensively in the proximal and distal segments of the nephron. In this way it ensures the close intra- and intercellular communications in these segments of the nephron [200]. All this testifies to an active transitory ability of the epithelial cells and a high level of metabolism in their nuclei. Therefore it is quite understandable that there is a natural high sensitivity of the cellular nuclei to anoxia and the corresponding morphologic manifestation in them, like the above mentioned spiral laminated bodies.

The high metabolism in the proximal and distal segments of the nephron and the sensitivity to anoxia can be explained by other intracellular changes such as vacuolization of cytoplasma, various degrees of swelling of mitochondria often with destruction of their cristas and external membranes, and the appearance in the cytoplasma of osmiophyle masses fenced with a partitive membrane. It has to be noted that the changes mentioned above were most expressed in the proximal segment of the nephron, which testified to its sensitivity to anoxia.

Other segments of the nephron displayed more resistance to oxygen hunger. Particularly, in the visceral epithelium of the glomerulas, mainly a vacuolization of the cytoplasma and moderate swelling of the mitochondria were noticed.

As in this test-group, within six months, the progressive destructive morphologic changes and full depression of SDG activity were observed, so it can be concluded that the two-hour long normothermic (+37°C) ischemia caused irreversible morphologic injuries in the kidneys.

It can be mentioned that in the second test-group where the kidney was subjected to ischemia in conditions of deep hypothermia (+4+7°C), certain dystrophic and circulatory upsettings were also seen such as vacuolization of glomerular podocytes, swelling of mitochondria and vacuolization in epithelial cells of the proximal segment of the nephron, a decrease of SDG activity in the proximal and distal segments, a spasm of arterioles and diapedesis. But in contrast with the previous test-group, the spiral laminated formations, autophagic vacuoles with osmiophyle granulary inclusions and local necroses in epithelial cells were not found in these cases. All this testified that the deep hypothermia (+4+7°C) to a significant degree rendered the negative influence of anoxia harmless.

At the same time, after the deep hypothermia (+4+7°C), an increase in number and a widening of cisterns of the endoplasmatic net with a high concentration of ribosomes on the external membranes, destruction of permeability and spasming in peritubular blood vessels in the epithelial cells of the proximal segment of the nephron were found. On the one hand, it obviously testified to a discoordination of intracellular metabolism, and on the other hand, evidenced that the deep hypothermia evoked a vicious circle of vascular disorders, which in turn caused a secondary porstoperative ischemia in the kidney. In favor of this opinion, there was also a gradual decrease of SDG activity in the proximal and distal segments of the nephron within one month of residual vascular disorders.

It has to be emphasized that pathological changes in test-groups with ischemia and hypothermia of +4+7°C and +10+15°C were quite reversible, and three and two months later, respectively, a normalization of the morphologic structure of the kidney occurred.

By a cooling of the ischemized kidney to +20+25°C, only minimal changes and the most rapid recovery of the morphologic picture and fermentary activity were observed, it can be asserted that this level of hypothermia efficiently ensured the morphologic safety of the kidney by its two-hour ischemia.

8.3. The Kidney Transplant Cooling

Among the other methods of kidney conservation, the local hypothermia is at present the most effective for protection against ischemic injury. But the best practical result can be achieved only through efficient realization of cooling.

There is complex equipment for the hypothermic conservation of the kidney transplant. It can be divided into 2 groups based on purpose: 1) The hypothermic means for preserving a kidney beginning from its extraction from a donor organism until the operation; 2) The means for the maintenance of renal hypothermia during the transplantation.

The equipment related to the first group is perfect from a general biologic, physiologic point of view, as well as by technical execution. Among them there are an apparatus which carries out hypothermic perfusion of the kidney with various solutions [2,6,11,12,34,39,40, 42-44,47,50,71,77,94,95,102,103,136,137,141], an apparatus and device for external non-perfusion cooling of an organ [64,66,74,121,150,167,168], and baro-chambers for hyperbaric oxygenation of the kidney transplant [8,37,83,89,90]. Retrograde cold irrigation is performed through the ureter [10,78,79]. The methods of organ conservation are used due to the virtue of their biologic perfusion by means of an isolated heart-lung preparation, artificial heart or allogen perfusion [17,90,170].

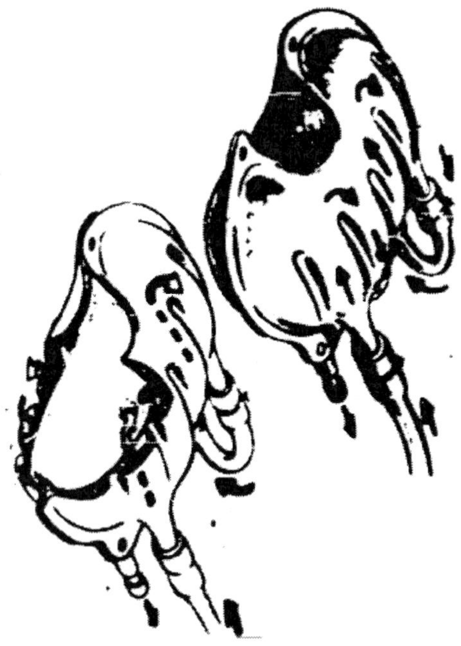

Figure 147. A tool for the kidney cooling (Moscow research and testing institute for surgical apparatus and instruments).

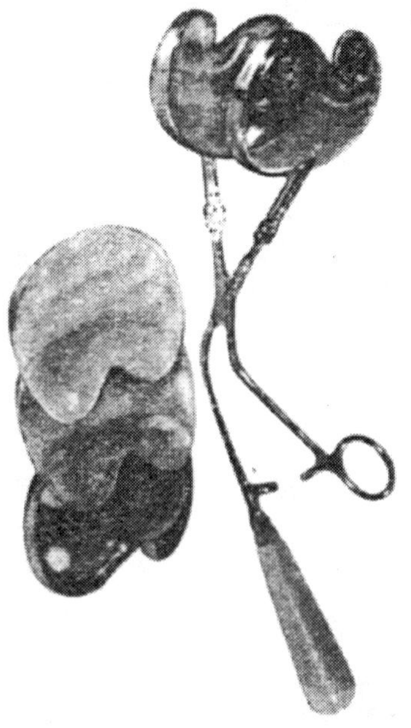

Figure 148. The heat exchanger of A.T. Cockett's apparatus for the kidney cooling.

The apparatus and devices which carry out a combination of conservation measures proved to be more effective, for example: hypothermic perfusion and hyperbaric oxygenation (ВНИИЭХАИ a. VICCERS, [170]; and external cooling and hyperbaric oxygenation [37]. The mentioned technical means permit the maintenance of transplant vitality during two-three days. Perhaps, they don`t completely solve the problem of real organ bank creation, but they are able, even at present, to make feasible the inter-town as well as international transport of organs, which is essential for the effective cooperation of transplantation centers.

But if on the stage of transplant preoperative conservation everything is satisfactory, the same can not be said about kidney hypothermic protection in the process of the operation itself. The corresponding technical means obviously need further perfection.

For the cooling of the kidney during the operation [31] suggested an apparatus with a heat exchanger made from two double wall stainless chambers having a kidney form with a circulating refrigerant agent inside (Figure 148).

There are also modified versions of this apparatus with circulation of the refrigerant agent inside the heat exchanger [88], as well as without circulation [138] (Figure 147).

The described rigid heat exchangers have such essential shortcomings that even their numerous collections are not able to ensure a sufficient contact with the variable external surfaces of the kidney. Because of low heat conduction of the kidney tissue, it results in a decrease of kidney cooling efficacy. Therefore the apparatus with rigid heat exchangers like [31] didn`t find wide application in clinics.

Existent devices and apparatus with elastic heat exchangers also proved to be insufficient.

In the apparatus of [146] the heat exchanger was represented by an elastic tube with circulating refrigerant agent inside. The tube is placed around the kidney like a ring. Ths way, the parts of the kidney poles, as well as its external border and gate don`t come into contact with the tube (Figure 149).

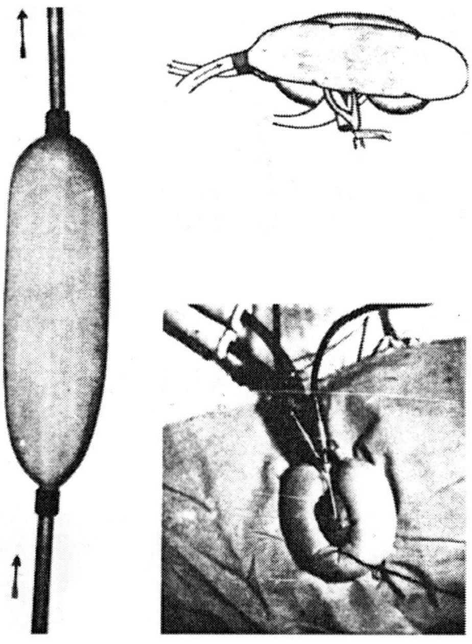

Figure 149. A. Ruffo's apparatus for the kidney cooling.

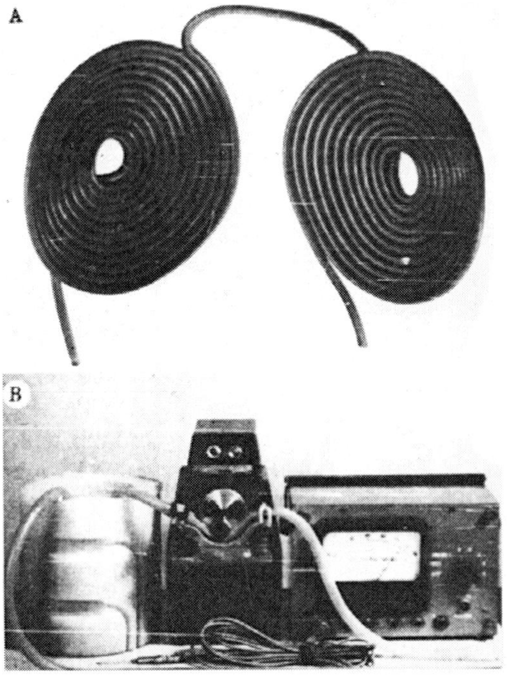

Figure 150. J. Wickham's apparatus for the kidney cooling.

In the apparatus of [195], the heat exchanger is made from a latex tube which is reeled around the neck of a bottle with the curls glued together. As a consequence the curls become the form of the cone. A liquid refrigerant agent circulates through the tube by means of a roller pump (Figure 150).

There is also a heat exchanger elaborated in the Moscow Institute of clinical and experimental surgery [170] which is represented as two hermetically sealed plastic plates having a shell form with anti-freeze inside. These heat exchangers are cooled beforehand (without refrigerant agent circulation) and ensure kidney cooling at the expense of cold stock, after warming they are substituted by other cooled heat exchangers (Figure 147).

In the recently elaborated [66], device (Figure 151) for local renal hypothermia, the kidney cooling modules are made from 4 mm copper tube serpentines joined together in the form of a square plate (4 x 4 x 0,2 cm) and mounted on the reverse surface of the kidney. The water, as a refrigerant agent, moves along the serpentines and returns by a plastic pipe with a passing temperature control. Because of the flat form and rigidity, these modules have no contact with the poles and external parts of the kidney.

Because of the discrepancy of the described elastic heat exchangers to the form and sizes of kidneys, and consequently their insufficient contact with the kidney , the mentioned apparatus and devices have low efficacy and don't have wide application.

There are also more simple methods of kidney cooling by means of covering it by bubbles with ice, ice-slush or ice-water inside. Direct application of ice-slush to the kidney surface helps its irrigation with cooled water from outside [76,87,104,124,129-132, 155].

The methods mentioned above are quite primitive, rough and inconvenient and, in principle, can not ensure full contact between the ice pieces with the whole external surface of the kidney. Furthermore, direct application of ice to the kidney can lead to multiple external necroses of the kidney [124], after the ice melts the water flows down into the wound. On one hand, because it is a hypotonic liquid, it can break the osmotic balance on the kidney surface and consequently lead to additional sclerosing. On the other hand, the permanent irrigation of the kidney with a large quantity of cold saline solution, except for the great inconvenience of the operating personnel, is very dangerous in respect to the introduction of infection through the wet operating sheets. At the same time the demands for aseptic organ transplantation are extremely high.

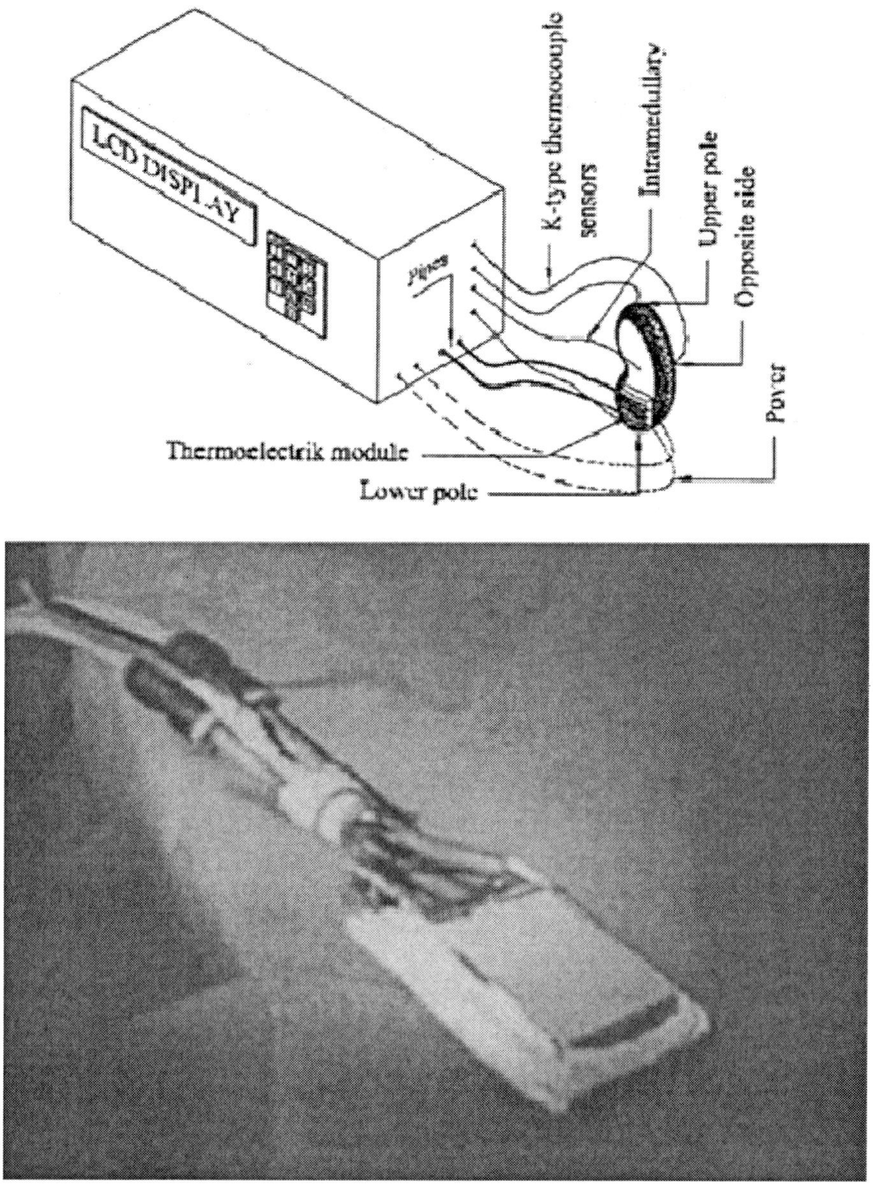

Figure 151. P. Isik's apparatus for the kidney cooling.

Thus, the description of the known technical means for the maintenance of kidney hypothermia during transplantation, in the process of renal blood vessel anastomosing, shows that further improvement is required. Therefore, in most cases the kidney transplantation is actually carried out without any cooling, by sewing of its blood vessels.

A paradox arrises. On the one hand, great means are spent for the permanent duty of the surgeons group to obtaini cadaverous kidneys, or living donors give their organs, then the transplant underwent a long-term conservation by means of an expensive apparatus. Great means are also spent on the urgent transport of a transplant to the recipient, a big quantity of highly qualified and paid surgeons are involved in the fulfillment of the operation. Its cost can sometimes exceed $100,000 [120].

On the other hand, during the transplantation itself, the renal vessels sewing, which can last sometimes 30-60 or more minutes, the kidney is left without any hypothermic protection, gets warm because of contact with surrounding internal organs, surgeon hands, under the beams of operating lamps, and consequently it is subjected to warm ischemic injuries. Therefore is loses, to a marked degree, the previous conservation.

The purpose of the above mentioned apparatus and devices for external cooling of the kidney is not only the cooling of a kidney transplant, but also for the local hypothermia of a "dry" kidney (with a temporarily blockaded blood circulation) by removal of multiple and staghorne stones. Strictly speaking, they were created initially just for that. But even the most perfect apparatus in this field [31,195] require no less than 8-10 minutes in order to cool the human kidney to +20°C. Other devices even spend 15-20 minutes for this [66,87]. This circumstance can not be considered permissible, because the low cooling rate extends the period of disparity between high nutritional requirements of the renal tissue and the limited amount of available energetic resources. Therefore, by these operations, it is very important not only to cool the kidney to a desirable temperature but also to cool it as much as possible rapidly, uniformly, safe, easy and at the same time the manipulations related to cooling should not hinder the execution of the operation's main stages, particularly, throughout the process of blood vessel suturing until renal blood flow restoration.

As a principal cause of the low efficacy of the described devices is the insufficient contact of the heat exchanger with the kidney surface. We concentrated the main part of our efforts in this direction and designed a special original apparatus for local renal hypothermia [158].

The goal of the creation of this apparatus was ensuring a full adjoining of the heat exchanger to the whole external surface of the kidney, achievement of a more sufficient heat diversion from the kidney and acceleration of cooling of a human kidney of any size and configuration, inside as well as outside the organism.

These goals were achieved in that the apparatus is comprised of a Dewar reservoir for refrigerant agent, pump, autonomous refrigerator, control and monitoring system, connecting tubes and heat exchanger, and the latter is made from an elastic material (silicon) as a double wall closed chamber according to the form and size of the kidney.

The apparatus has passed several modifications. The last model (Figure 152, 153) is comprised of a Dewar reservoir 1, capacity (2,5 l)for a refrigerant agent (0,4% chlorhexidin and 15% ethyl alcohol water solution or antiseptic solution Djapa), autonomous refrigerator 2, pump 3 with a productivity of 1 l/min together with the feeding block and accumulator ensuring the capability for work within one hour in case of interruption of central electrofeeding, control system 4 for measuring and regulation of temperature in the reservoir, environment, heat exchanger and cooling organ, degree of filling of reservoir and heat exchanger, link tubes 5 and the heat exchanger 6.

The heat exchanger 6 comprises the external 7 and internal 8 elastic walls, which after the firm uniting along the whole perimeter creates a closed chamber 9 according to the form and size of the kidney. The chamber has wedge form cuts 10 in the middle of the minor curvature and the slits 11 on edges. For comfortable transport the apparatus is gathered in a box with wheels at the bottom.

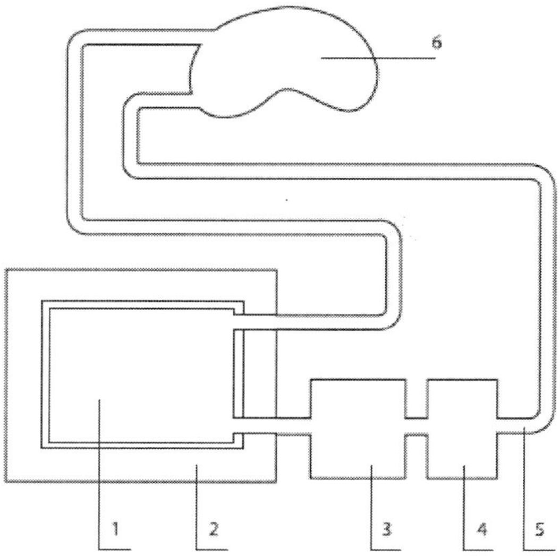

Fig. 1

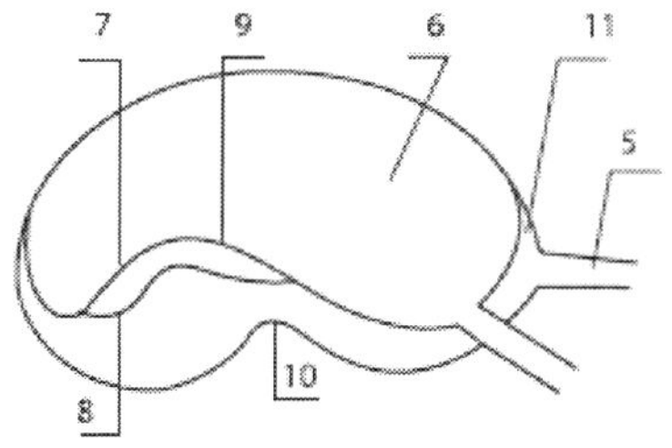

Fig. 2

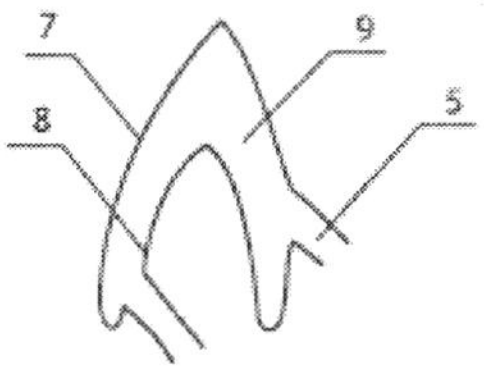

Fig. 3

Figure 152. T. J. Shioshvili's apparatus for local renal hypothermia. Schematic form.

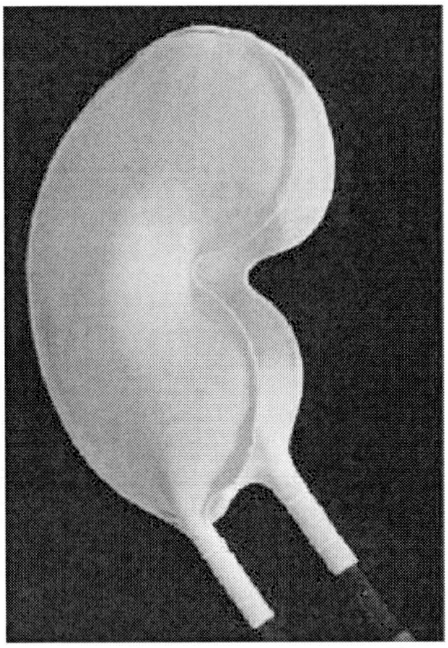

153.,

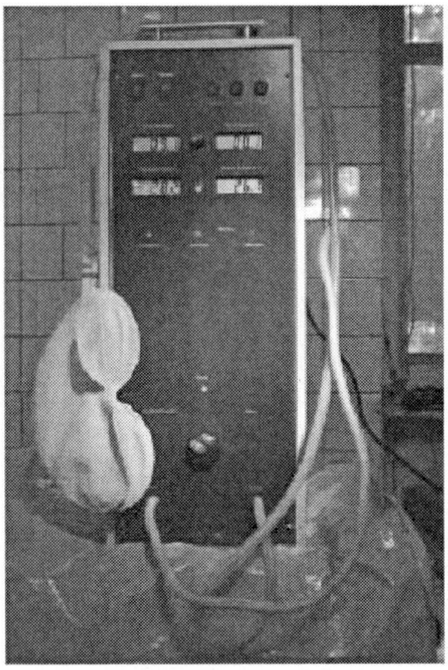

153.,

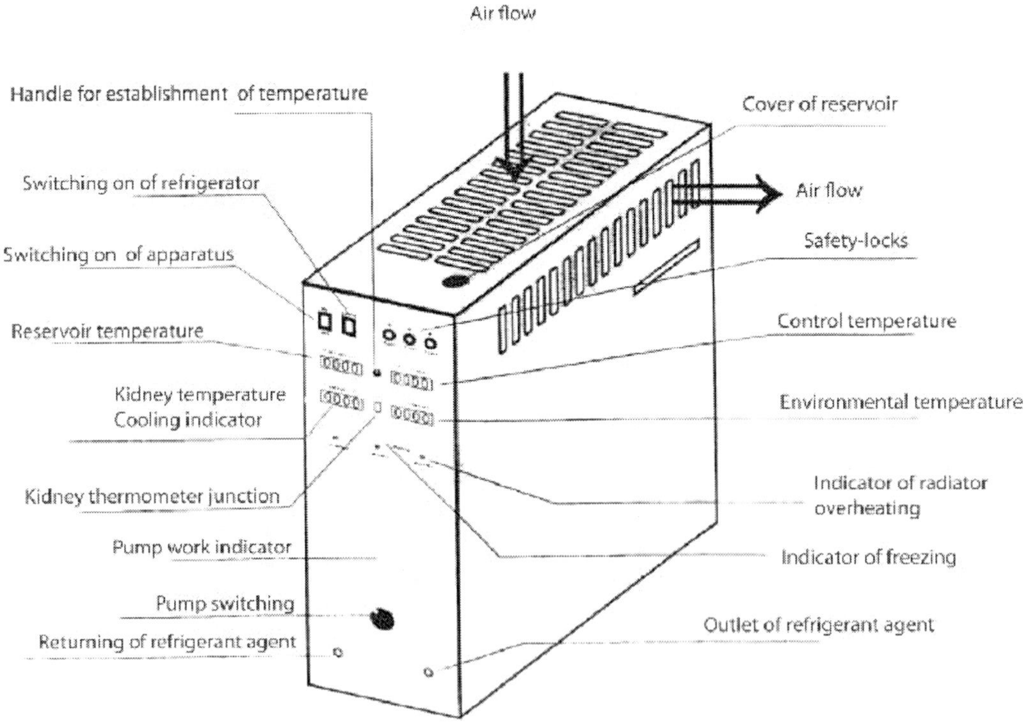

153.,

Figure 153. T. J. Shioshvili's apparatus for local renal hypothermial. Natural picture.
$153._1$ – heat exchanger; $153._2$ – apparatus look in front; $153._3$ – apparatus look from a side.

The control system comprises thermocouples with ranges of measuring from +50 to -50°C which can be seen on liquid crystal displays.

The apparatus works in the following way. 40 minutes before application the refrigerator of the apparatus is switched on. After achievement of the desired temperature of the refrigerant agent in the reservoir (0,5°C) the latter is directed by pump to the external cooling system, the heat exchanger which covers the kidney. Passing through the tube system, the refrigerant agent creates a temperature +1+1.5°C on the internal wall of the heat exchanger. By moderate inflation with liquid, the heat exchanger clings to the entire external surface of the kidney and ensures favorable conditions for its efficient cooling.

The wedge form cuts in the middle of the minor chamber curvature ensure the comfort of manipulations in the field of the kidney gate. The slits on the chamber edges make putting it on the kidney easier.

The heat exchanger is made from silicon with a thickness of 0.4-0.6 mm. The plates of a silicon row are subjected to wringing under a special press-form and polymerization in vacuum. Consequently it was created as a united hermetic chamber which can resist sterilization many times from all methods used in medicine.

Two sizes heat exchanger were made. Because of elasticity they actually embrace all possible versions of size and form of human kidneys.

The described apparatus can be used for two principal purposes: by the operations on the "dry" kidney (removal of stagghorn, multiple stones, partial resection of the kidney); and by auto- and allotransplantation of the kidney and other small organs (testes) for ensuring their hypothermic protection during the operation.

The apparatus can provide rapid and safe cooling and maintenance of stable temperature for the kidney in wide ranges between 37°C and +2°C during an unlimited amount of time.

The apparatus passed the state technical trials in the All-Union Research and Trial Institute for Medical Engineering of the Public Health Ministry of the USSR (Moscow) and clinical testing in 4 clinical institutions of Moscow and 5 of Tbilisi.

The invention is certificated with patents of USSR N340327, USA N3738372, UK N1331002, and Norwey N130751.

The apparatus was demonstrated at the International Exhibitions in Moscow, London, Izmir, Posnan, Prague, Bratislava, Nicosia, Plovdiv, New-Delhi, Barcelona, and Ho Chi Mihn.

At the International Spring Fair in Leipzig (1982) the apparatus was awarded a gold medal.

8.4. Results of a Practical Application of Apparatus for the Local Renal Hypothermia in Experiments and Clinics

The described apparatus for local renal hypothermia was used in two principal directions: 1) Organ auto- and allotransplantations; 2) Nephrotomy and partial resection of a "dry" kidney.

8.4.1. Employment of Apparatus in Organ Transplantations

With these purposes 101 autotransplantations of the kidney in experiments on dogs, 10 kidney and 45 testicle autotransplantations, 6 kidney and 2 testicle allotransplantations from living donors and 6 kidney and 42 testicle allotransplantations from cadavers in clinics were performed.

The kidney autotransplantations on dogs were made in order to investigate the influence of denervation and reinnervation on the kidney in pure experiment, without any immune factors of incompatibility.

The technical aspects of a cooling dog kidney were comprehensively described in chapters 7.3 and 8.3.

From 10 patients subjected to the kidney autotransplantation, 5 suffered before the operation from hydronephrosis, the structure of a significant part of the ureter was determined. In 5 other cases, high level arterial hypertonia was caused with a narrowing of the renal artery.

In all these cases the kidneys were shifted into the iliac fossa with an accompanying correction of the passage of the ureter or renal artery.

By clinical autotransplantation, right after nephrectomy, the kidney was covered with the heat exchanger of a working apparatus for local renal hypothermia, simultaneously the kidney perfusion was begun with an heparinized saline solution for washing away the blood. The kidney was cooled to +20°C in 2,5 minutes. Then the heat exchanger together with the kidney was transported in the iliacal region and a sewing of the renal artery to a. iliaca int. end-to-end and the renal vein to v. iliaca ext. end-to-back was performed. Through this period the heat exchanger was moderately inflated with refrigerant agent and completely isolated the kidney from the surrounding wound tissues and surgeons hands. Only renal magistral blood vessels protruded outside the heat exchanger. Under the constant temperature control, a stable level of renal hypothermia (+20+25°C) was maintained. Furthermore, the actions associated with kidney cooling didn`t hinder the surgeon in vessel anastomosing at all. At the end of the operation a surgical reinnervation of the kidney was performed, as described above.

Case report N1. A 35 year old woman was entered into the clinic with obstructive symptoms in the left kidney. It was found that 2 years earlier she was underwent a gynecologic operation because of fibromyoma. Urological x-ray examinations showed an extended stricture in the left ureter juxtavesical segment and a pyeloectasy. The Boari-plasty operation was performed with a satisfactory, near clinical result. But 2 years later a relapse of ureteral stricture and pyeloectasy occurred, involved in the sclerotic process was almost half of the inferior ureter. The functional state of kidney parenchyma were quite preserved. Therefore its autotransplantation was performed into the iliac fossa with connection of a. renalis to a. iliaca int. end-to-end, v. renalis with v. iliaca ext. end-to-back and antirefluxive ureterocystoneostomy after Leadbetter-Politano. During the operation, first the excision of the injured part of the lower ureter and the preparation of the iliacal blood vessels were performed. Then the wound was prolonged upwards and the left kidney and its blood vessels were separated and cut. The kidney was covered with the heat exchanger of the apparatus for local renal hypothermia [158] and cooled to +20°C in its cortical substance in 3 minutes. This level of hypothermia was maintained during the whole period of blood vessel sewing, which lasted 45 minutes. After the blood recirculation and ureterocystoneostomy, surgical reinnervation of the kidney was performed as described above. The near postoperative period proceeded without complications. The excretory urography between 1 and 20 years later showed a normal functional state of the transplanted kidney (Fig 154).

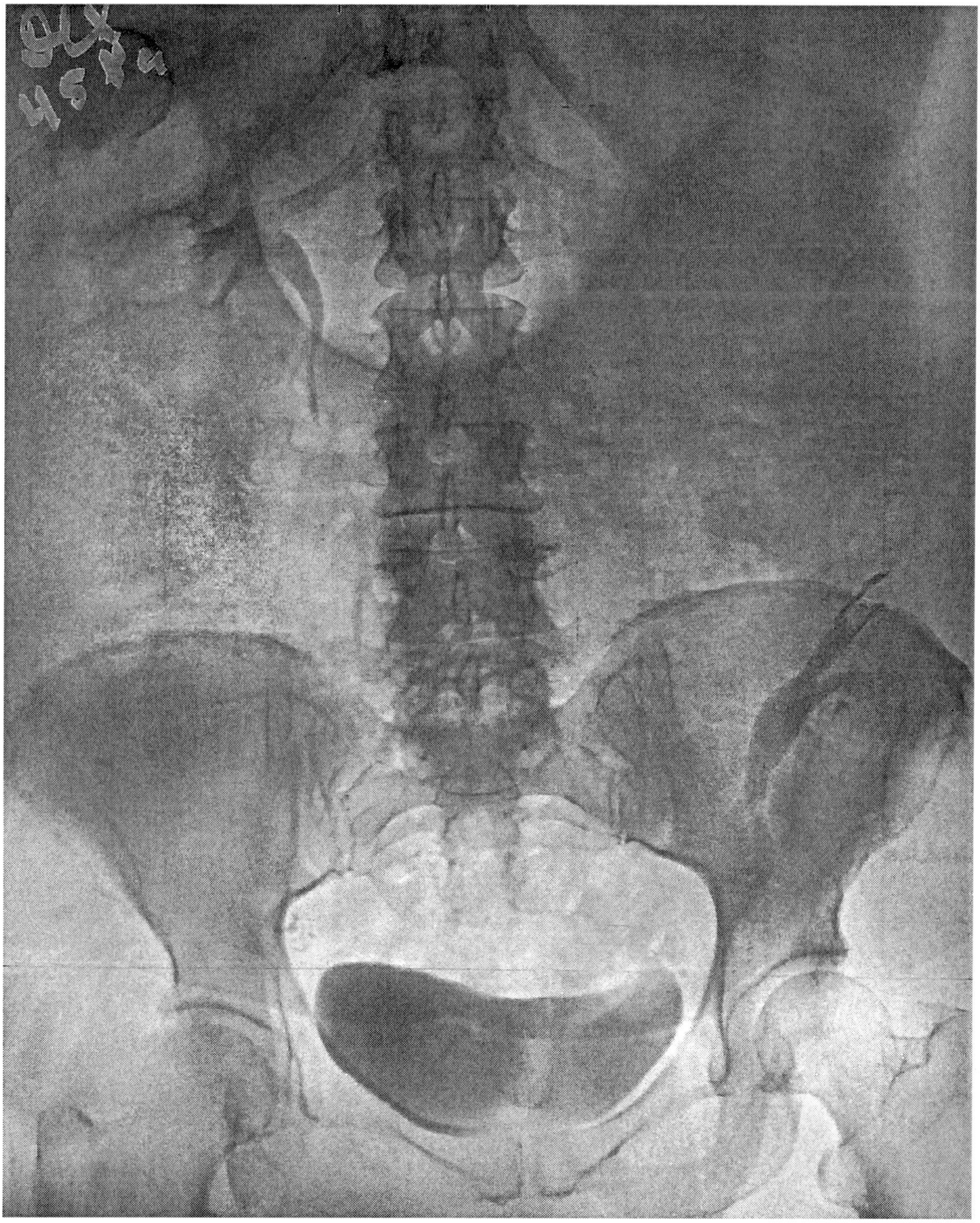

Figure 154. Clinical case. 20 years after the autotransplantation and surgical reinnervation of the left kidney. Excretory and motor functions are normal.

Case report N2. A male (23 years old) was entered in the clinic with a left side pyeloectasia. The excretory urography revealed a stricture in the pyeloureteral segment. A plasty operation was undertaken for its correction, but in the course of operation it was found that that the length of the strictured upper part of the ureter was 15 cm. It made the fulfillment of any kind of orthotopic plastic operation including ureterocalicoanastomosis impossible. Therefore an autotransplantation of the kidney in the iliac fossa was made. The same techniques of hypothermic protection (+20+25°C) during the ischemia (42 minutes) and surgical reinnervation of the kidney were used. The proximal end of intact lower segment of the ureter was anastomosed with the pyelon after the Haynes-Anderssen-Bishop method. The near and remote clinical results were satisfactory.

The apparatus for local renal hypothermia was used further for 6 kidney allotransplantations from living donors in patients with a terminal stage of renal insufficiency. One group of surgeons prepared the iliacal vessels of the recipient, while the others carried out a nephrectomy on the donor. Just after removal, the kidney was placed into the heat exchanger of the apparatus and cooled simultaneously from the outside as well as through perfusion to +20°C within 2,5 minutes. Then the heat exchanger, together with the kidney transplant, were placed in the iliacal region. The renal blood vessels protruding from the heat exchanger chamber were anastomosed with iliacal blood vessels within 35-66 (40.3±3.4) minutes. In 2 cases, the preliminary reconstruction of the branched renal artery extended the anastomosing time for 20 minutes. During this entire period the apparatus ensured the desired level of hypothermia

In 6 other clinical cases of terminal renal insufficiency a cadaverous kidney allotransplant was used. The duration of its preliminary conservation by +2+4°C was 16-33 (23.4±2.3) hours.

In the course of the operation the kidney transplant was displaced from the cooling container into the heat exchanger of the apparatus and both were placed in the iliacal region of the recipient. After preparation, the transplant and recipient blood vessels were anastomosed in a standard way within 32-55 (43.5±3.6) minutes. During this period the apparatus maintained kidney temperature between +2+5°C until the recovery of blood circulation.

It has to be mentioned that the clinical material related to kidney allotransplantation, from living as well as cadaverous donors, was obtained from other clinics (Institude of transplantology and artificial organs, Institute of Urology of Russian Federation, Moscow) clinical trials of the designed apparatus for local renal hypothermia, before our investigations in surgical reinnervation. Therefore these transplantations were made without surgical reinnervation. All other cases of organ transplantations performed in our clinic were accompanied with surgical reinnervation.

The mentioned apparatus was used by 45 orthotopic autotransplantations of testes, because the high sensitivity of the testis to ischemia is well known. The indications for this operation as follows: one side abdominal cryptorchidism in children, bilateral abdominal cryptorchidism in adults, abdominal cryptorchidism in a young man with a sole testis, and replantation of a testis after autohemicastration in young man with mental disturbance.

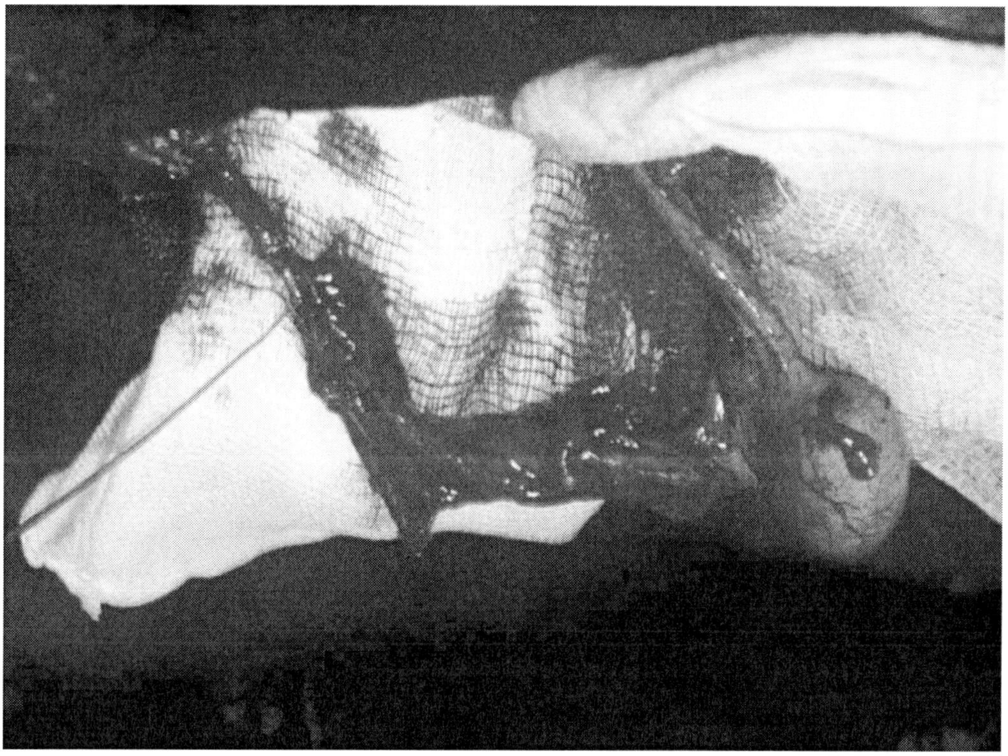

Figure 155. Autotransplanted testis.

The testicle autotransplantation was performed because the short length of testicular vessels made it impracticable to carrying out conventional orchidopexy. Sometimes the deficiency of vasculary pedicle length was 8-12 (10.1±1.1) cm. The testicular vessels were cut higher then the internal inguinal ring and anastomosed end-to-end with the inferior epigastric vessels using microsurgical techniques (Figure 155). The operation lasted 3-3.5 hours on the whole, the duration of testicular ischemia was 45-55 (42.1±1.1) minutes. During this ischemic period the testicules were located in the minor sized heat exchanger. As before, the testicular temperature was maintained firmly at a level of +20+25°C. After recirculation of blood, surgical reinnervation of the testicle was carried out by sewing the perivascular sheets of anastomosed blood vessels. As for ductus deference, it had a sufficient length in reserve for transference of the testicle into the scrotal sack.

The testicle stayed inside the heat exchanger and didn`t hinder manipulations on blood vessels, in spite of the fact that the heat exchanger dimension were relatively more than the testicle.

The peculiarity of testicle replantation consisted in a longer duration of ischemia (5 hours). It was determined by the fact that after trauma the patient first entered another surgical clinic where deep hypothermia of the testicle (with ice external application) began. In our clinic he was operated on urgently. In the following period of testicle ischemia up to blood recirculation, the apparatus maintained its temperature at a level of +10+15°C.

The same apparatus was also used for 44 testicle allotransplantations in patients with primary (hypergonadotropic) hypogonadism. In 2 cases the transplants were obtained from living donors (patient`s fathers), while in 42 other cases cadaverous testicles were used.

By transplantation from a living donor the duration of testicle ischemia was 41 and 49 minutes. Therefore a moderate level of local hypothermia (+20+25°C) for initial protection was used. In cases of cadaverous testicle transplantation the ischemia duration was 4-32 (11.5±2.4) hours on the whole. In 8 cases (16 testicles) a road accident in the winter (in Moscow) had taken place. Therefore the artificial external cooling of the scrotal sack by means of bubbles with melting ice was begun in the ambulance and then continued in the morgue. There the testicles were excised, perfused with heparinized saline solution and placed into a standard transfer container with a temperature of +2+5°C until the transplantation.

In 13 other cases (26 testicles) the patients died in reanimation clinics. After the statement of death, first the external cooling of the scrotal sack with ice bubbles was performed, and then the testicles were excised and placed in a transfer container.

Thus in all cases of allotransplantations of cadaverous testicles, a deep hypothermia (+2+5°C) was used from the very beginning. Furthermore, during the operation, this level of hypothermia was maintained by means of our apparatus until the recovery of blood circulation in the testicles.

The anastomoses of testicular vessels and testicle surgical reinnervation were performed as before, using the inferior epigastric blood vessels and their perivascular sheets.

As for the ductus deference, it was ligated in the proximal segment, because its dimensions and diameter in transplant were incommensurably with that in the recipient. It made their joining, even by means of a microsurgical invagination method, impracticle.

After the operation the patients were treated with immunosuppressive preparations: urbason, cyclosporine A, asathioprin, chorionic gonadotropin, and heparin within 3 months under immunologic monitoring.

8.4.2. Employment of Apparatus for Local Renal Hypothermia in Experiments and by Nephrotomy and Partial Resection of a "Dry" Kidney in the Clinic

The mentioned apparatus [158] was used in experiments on dogs in order to determine the optimal level of hypothermia for protection of the kidney by 2-hour ischemia. After mobilization of the kidney through a transperitoneal approach and blockade of the vascular pedicle, it was placed into the heat exchanger of the apparatus and cooled under the control of a needleform electrothermometer. The cooling of the kidney to +20°C occurred in 1-1.5 (0.8±0.4) minutes, to 10°C-in 2-3 (2.3±0.3) minutes and to 4°C-in 4-5 (4.3±0.2) minutes. After achievement of these levels of temperature the circulation of refrigerant agent, through the heat exchanger was broken temporarily. By an increase of the temperature in the cortical layer of the kidney higher than +25°C, +15°C and +7°C the circulation of refrigerant agent through the system had been repeated for a short time.

138 patients with staghorn (98), multiple (40) stones and 22 patients with small kidney tumors were operated on using local hypothermia (Table 22).

Table 22. Number of patients traced after surgery

Before the operation	during 1 year after the operation	3 years later	5 years later
Nephrolothiasis 138	108	86	77
Kidney-tumor 22	20	17	15

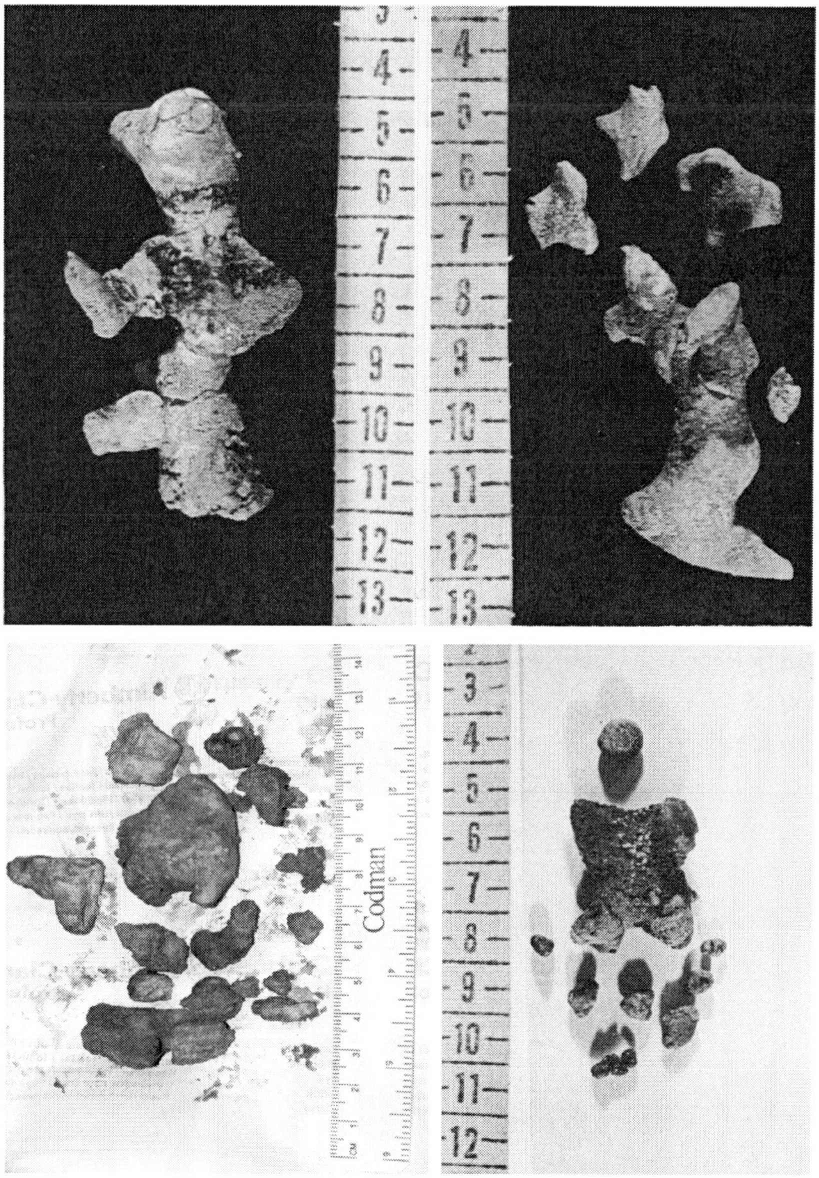

Figure 156. Stones removed from the kidney under the local hypothermia.

The age of patients was 3.5-76 (41.5±3.5) years, among them 90 were males and 70 women. The localization of stones in the right kidney had taken place in 40, in the left one in 70 and, on both sides in 28 cases. Among the 22 oncologic patients, the tumors were in the upper pole of the kidney in 7, in the middle segment in 6 and in the lower pole in 9 cases. Their diameter did not exceed 3 cm.

The method of nephrotomy under local hypothermia was used only in cases when the stones could not be disintegrated by Extracorporal Shock Wave Lithotripsy (ESWL), or removed by means of an ordinary, subcortical pyelotomy or pyelo-calicotomy.

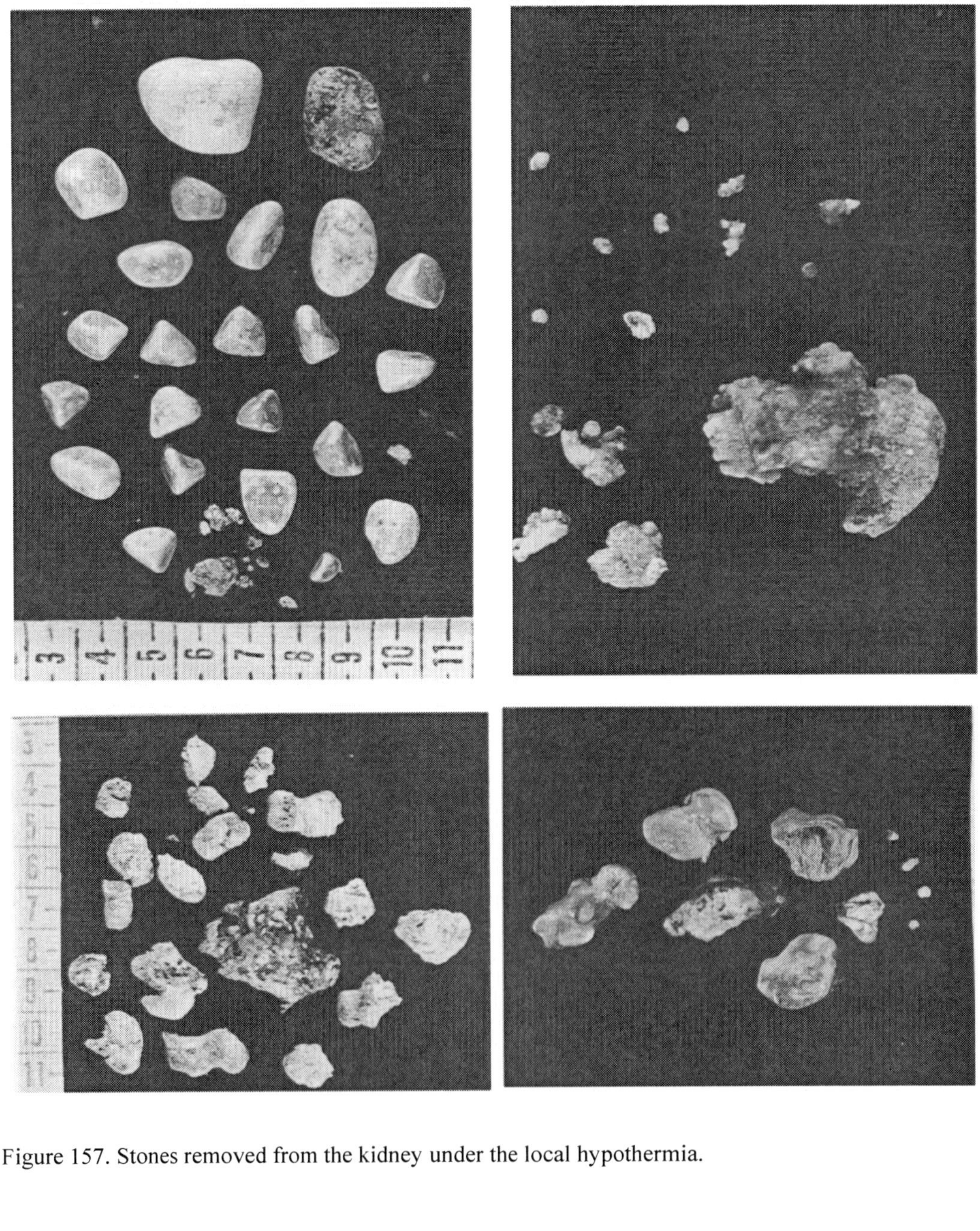

Figure 157. Stones removed from the kidney under the local hypothermia.

Because it is well known from the literature that even 20-minute long normothermic ischemia can cause local necroses in the kidney, and it is impossible to calculate the duration of ischemia necessary for the full removal of staghorn or multiple stones from the kidney exactly, we considered the application of local hypothermia in all cases of a blockade of the renal blood circulation including those of short duration, important (less than 30 minutes). Such tactics permitted us to achieve, from the very beginning, the most economical intensity of metabolism in the "dry" kidney, perform a radical operation in quiet conditions without any hurry and prevent ischemic microinfarctions in the kidney.

Through a lumbotomy or intermusculary approach the kidney was mobilized. Its initial temperature in the cortical substance was 37.0±0.2C. The blood circulation was broken by the method mentioned above [162]. The heat exchanger of the apparatus for local renal hypothermia was introduced to the wound and put on the kidney. Thanks to the circulation of a cold refrigerant agent through the exchanger, the temperature in the cortical substance of the kidney of an adult patient was decreased to +20°C in 2-4 (3.1±0.2) minutes and one of a children in 1-2 (1.4±0.3) minutes. Each cooling ensured the temperature of +20+25°C in the kidney within 20-25 minutes. In the case of more prolonged ischemia the kidney was cooled repeatedly. Once, by 80-minute long ischemia a 4-time switching on of the apparatus was needed.

An exact plan for the large stone removal from the kidney was defined more precisely before the operation. By corresponding localization and size, a radial nephrotomy was preferred (85 cases). By too large stones a Zondeck`s incision was used (11). In the other 42 cases, localization of the stone in one of the poles with accompanying parenchyma atrophy in this place, it was resected together with the stone by a wedge-like incision.

The extraction of stones actually proceeded in a bloodless operating field (Figures 156,157). Then the kidney cavities were intensively bathed with a saline solution for washing off small fragments and sand from the stone.

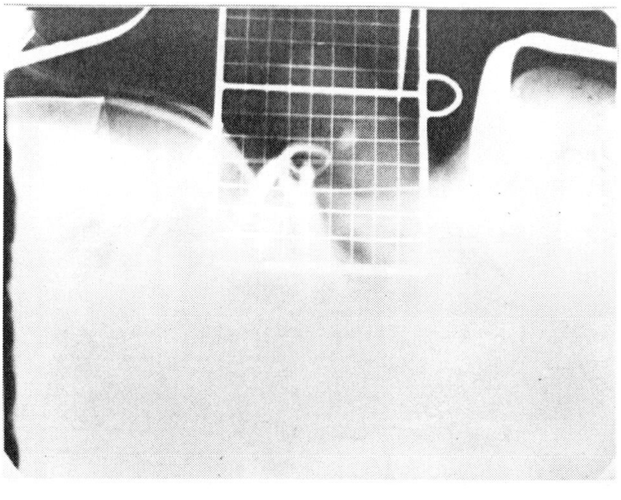

Figure 158. An intraoperative x-ray control examination of the kidney on the background of a metallic net revealed a residual stone.

After that a control x-ray or ultrasonographic examination of the operated kidney was performed. In order to simplity the finding of a residual stone fragment in the kidney, these examinations were performed on the background of a metallic net with 1 cm size checks. It has to be noticed that, thanks to this additional examination, 18 residual stones were revealed and this "false relapse" prevented (Figure 158). On the contrary, in 3 operations performed without such control examination small stones (1 x 1 cm) ("false relapse") were unfortunately left in the lower pole of the kidney. The kidney defects were sewed with П-form sutures.

A segmental resection of the kidney in cases of small tumors (22) was carried out similarly as for the stones. Moreover, it has to be emphasized that the employed wedgelike resection gave more congruent residual kidney surfaces, which simplified the following wound sewing and increased its safety. In contrast with this, a spherical enucleation tumor form, generally used by such operations in other clinics, could not ensure such congruence and a hazard of bleeding would to a marked degree increase.

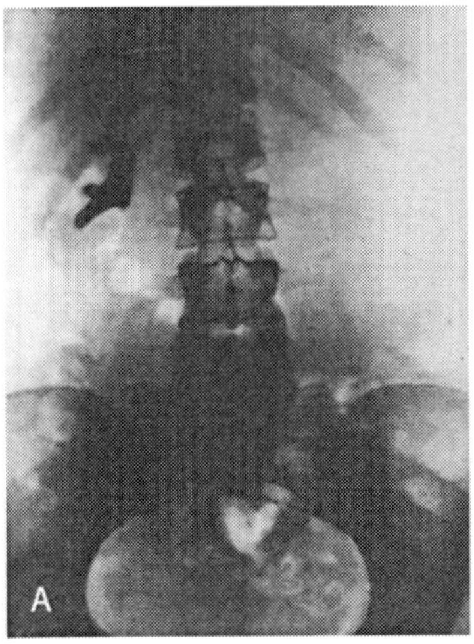

159.$_1$

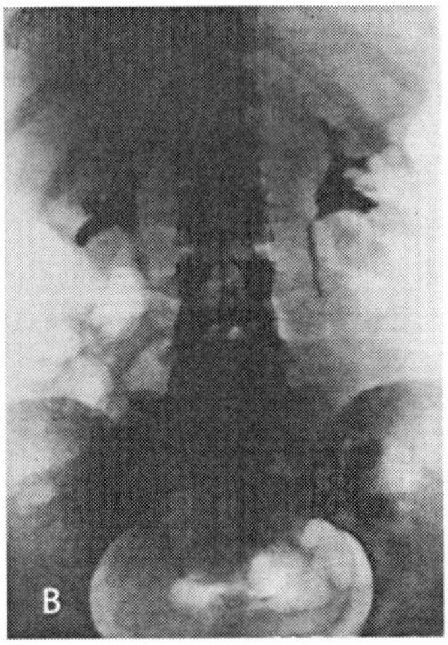

159.$_2$

D

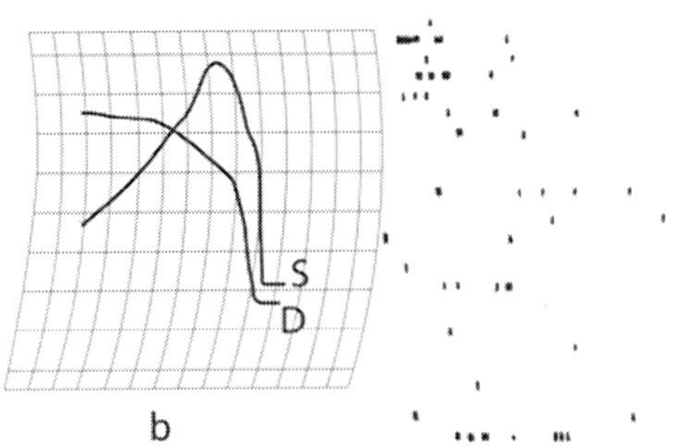

159.$_3$

S

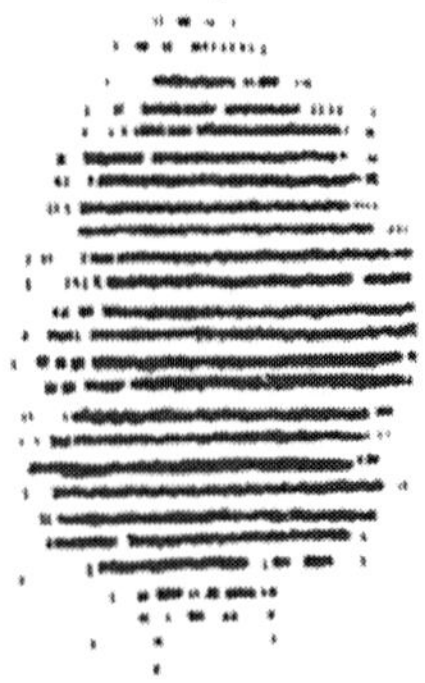

2

159.$_4$

Figure 159. X-ray and radiologic data of a patient with a right-side stag horn nephrolithiasis before the operation. 159.$_1$ – survey X-ray picture of the urinary tract. 159.$_2$ – Excretory urogram; 159.$_3$ – Radiorenogram; 159.$_4$ – Renoscintigram. Indices of damaged right kidney are sharply reduced.

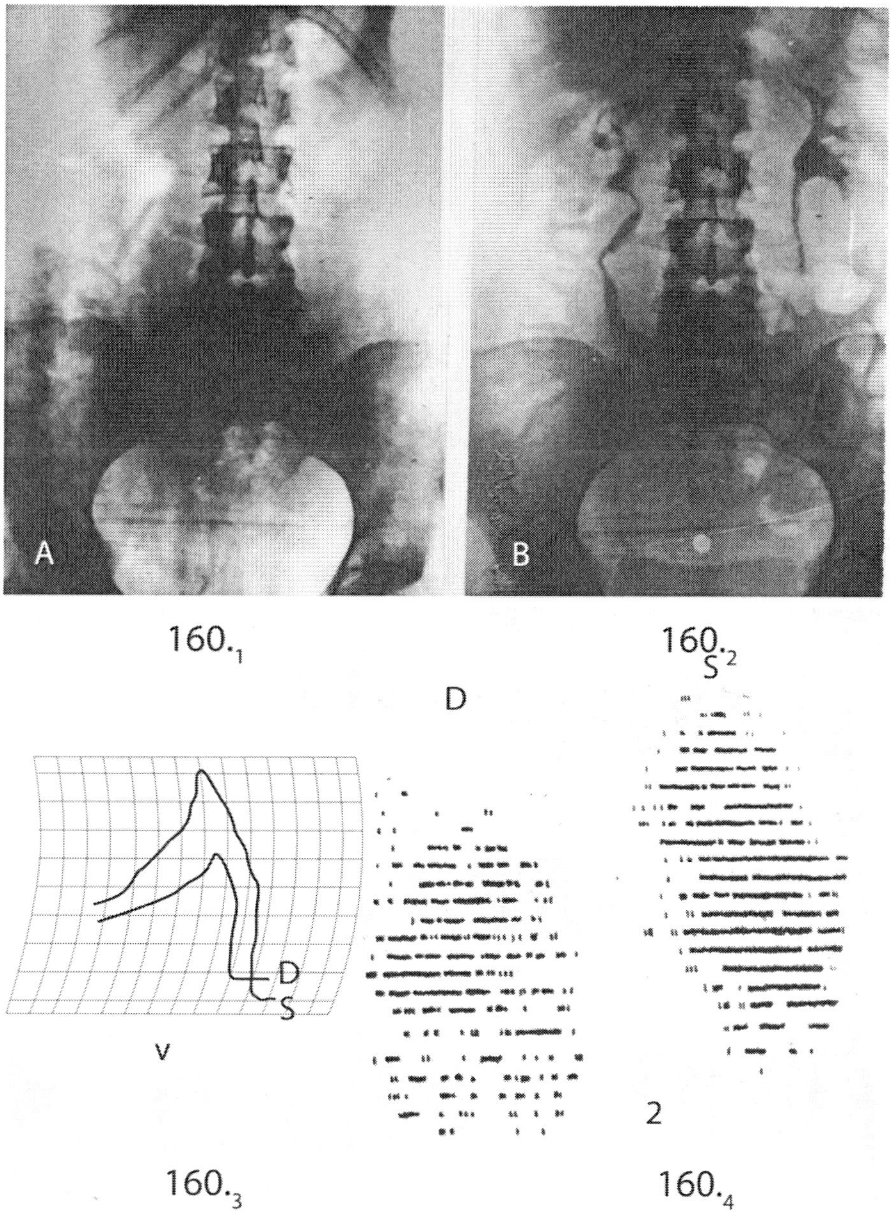

Figure 160. X-ray and rediologic data of the same patient 3 years after the operation on the "dry" kidney under local hypothermia. 160.$_1$ – Survey X-ray picture of the urinary tract; 160.$_2$ – Excretory urogram; 160.$_3$ – Radiorenogram; 160.$_4$ – Renoscintigram. Anatomic and functional indices of the operated (right) kidney are emproved significantly.

The recovery of blood circulation in the kidney in our cases was not accompanied, as a rule, with any significant bleeding from the kidney wound. Very seldom only single additional capsulary sutures were needed. The duration of kidney ischemia on the whole was 12-80 (32.7±4.6) minutes.

In the postoperative period there were no serious complications. In one case a hyperthermic reaction within 1 week of the section nephrotomy had taken place. Significant secondary bleeding was not observed, therefore a compensative blood transfusion was not needed.

Remote clinical results had been traced by 108 petients with nephrolithiasis and 20 with kidney tumors up to 5 years.

From all observed patients with kidney stones 2 patients were dead after 3 years and 1 after 5 years from heart infarction.

The autopsy didn`t show any stone relapse.

Among the observed living patients a true relapse of kidney stones had taken place in 2 cases, 3 years after surgery and a "false relapse" occurred in 3 cases. In the first group, it was determined for general metabolic reasons which could not be sufficiently corrected. In the second group small "false relapse" stones 1 x 1 cm in the lower pole were left, but due to technical reasons, a control intraoperative examination was unfortunately not performed. But these stones within 5 years didn`t show a tendency for growth, neither did functional disorders, except of a moderate leukocyturia in the urine sediment.

In one case, a secondary nephrectomy was made 3 years after the first operation because of advanced nephrosclerosis and unmanageable arterial hypertension.

The excretory urography performed within 3-6 months after the surgery showed a complete restoration or significant improvement of functional condition of the kidneys in 98 cases of 138 (71%), a moderate improvement in 39 cases (28,3%) and a worsening in 1 case (0.7%) (Figures 159.1,2, 160.1,2).

The parallel radiorenographic examinations permitted a more differentiated qualitative and quantitative evaluation of the functional state of the kidneys. Before the surgery the renogram curves were two-phase with decreased amplitude of the vascular segment and a prolonged excretory phase (obturative type) (Figures159.3). The Hirakawa-Corcoran`s renographic index (RI) was 27.3±2.7 ($p<0.001$) (Table 23).

3 months after the operation the renograms became three-phase with increased amplitudes of vascular and secretory segments and a shortening of the semi-excretion period. RI increased by this term to 38.3±2.2 ($p<0.05$) (Table 23).

In the following period, 1, 3 and 5 years later, further improvement of x-ray and renographic indices was observed. Consequently, RI increased which gradually achieved a lower limit of the norm. (Figure 160.1,2,3, Table 23).

Table 23. Changes of Hirakawa-Corcoran`s renographic index in patients operated under local renal hypothermia because of nephrolithiasis

Indices	Before the surgery	3 months after surgery	1 year later	3 years later	5 years later
M±w	27,3±2,7	38,3±2,2	45,0±3,5	48,6±3,0	53,3±3,6
n	138	128	108	86	77
p	<0,001	<0,01	>0,05	>0,05	>0,05

Table 24. Changes of Hirakawa-Corcoran`s RI in patients with segmental resection of tumourous kidneys under local hypothermia

Indices	Before the operation	6 months after surgery	1 year later	3 years later	5 years later
M±m	51,1±2,4	48,4±3,8	54,7±3,2	53,6±4,1	52,7±3,6
n	22	22	22	22	22
p		>0,05	>0,05	>0,05	>0,05

The dynamics of changes in renoscintigrams coincided on the whole with a general tendency to improvement in renograms.

In cases when, before the operation the renoscintigrams were represented with rare touches, after the operation they were gradually succeeded with more frequent touches (Figures 159.4, 160.4).

Clinical results were evaluated as excellent in cases of an absence of stone relapse, full functional restoration of an operated kidney, disappearance or decrease of leukocyturia level, full recovery of patient`s capacity for work; as good in case of absence of a stone relapse, partial improvement of operated kidney functions, residual insignificant leukocyturia, recovery of patient`s capacity for work; as satisfactory in case of kidney functional improvement as compared with preoperative, true or false stone relapse, preservation of a moderate leukocyturia, pain in the back, partial recovery of patient`s capacity for work; and as unsatisfactory when the mentioned indices remained without improvement as compared to preoperative or changed for the worse.

The generalization of existent data shows that the results of surgical treatment of nephrolithiasis were in 71 (51.4%) cases excellent, in 59 (42.8%) good, in 7 (5.1%) satisfactory and in 1 case (0.7%) unsatisfactory.

Among 75 patients previously suffering from arterial hypertonia, after the operation in 60 patients (80%), the arterial blood pressure became normal.

In cases (22) of kidney tumor segmental resection the near as well as remote clinical results, both from general surgical and oncological points of view within 5 years, were without complications. For oncologic reasons all these patients were actively examined during 5 years.

All patients were cancer free within the whole period of this observation.

The preoperative functional state of the injured kidneys after the excretory urography and radiologic examinations, was without serious upsettings.

The same investigations performed 6 months, 1, 3 and 5 years after the operation didn`t reveal any essential disorders. The Hirakawa-Corcoran`s RI remained stable on a normal level between 48.4±3.8 and 52.7±3.6 ($p>0.05$).

8.4.3. Discussion of Clinical Results

The consideration of near and remote clinical data shows that the designed and employed method of intervention on a "dry" kidney under local hypothermia fully corresponded to requirements of modern surgery.

During the operation the surgeons had all the necessary conditions for careful, pedantic and radical execution of an operation without any hurry. The operating field was bloodless which permitted them to manipulate all the time under good visual control. In the case of several nephrotomies, there was an opportunity to leave them open without any bleeding hazard for an effective inspection, bathing and sewing of wounds after the full removal of stones and their sand remnants at the end of the operation was permitted.

The employed method for blood circulation blockade, on the one hand, ensured a bloodless operating field and, on the other hand, prevented an increase of intrarenal pressure. It was confirmed by an outpouring of a small amount of residual blood (5-10 ml) by nephrotomy.

The comfort and efficacy of application of the designed apparatus for local renal hypothermia must be emphasized. Its elastic heat exchanger was introduced to the wound very easily, by conventional lumbotomy as well as by a relatively narrow intermuscular approach, and covered the kidney completely. By moderate filling with refrigerant agent the heat exchanger closely fit to the kidney's whole external surface. It created favorable conditions for the tender, uniform and effective cooling of the kidney. Two sizes of this heat exchanger were actually suitable, one for human adults, and one for the kidneys and testes of children as well as for experimental animals.

This apparatus cooled an adult patient`s kidney to +20°C in 2-4 (3.1±0.2) minutes and a childs kidney in 1-2 (1.4±0.3) minutes, meaning 2-3 times more rapid that other apparatus and devices for the same purpose. Taking into account that during hypothermia the kidney blood circulation was interrupted and its vitality was ensured only at the expense of its own energetic reserves, such essential acceleration of kidney cooling to achieve the most economical level of metabolism can be considered as an important advantage in the prevention of ischemic injury of the kidney.

As for evaluation of the regime used for hypothermia (+20+25°C) and widening of indications to hypothermia in cases of a blockade of the renal blood circulation, the near and remote clinical data show that among 138 operated kidneys, in 71 cases (51,4%) the results were excellent, in 59 (42.8%) were good, in 7 (5.1%) were satisfactory and in 1 (0.7%) was unsatisfactory. In all 22 patients with small kidney tumors, clinical results both from oncologic and functional points of view were excellent.

From 138 operated kidneys 2 true and 3 false stone relapses had taken place. In contrast with this, according to known literary data the frequency of relapse by staghorn and multiple nephrolothiasis is 22-25% [132,134]. Therefore, the decrease of frequency of a true relapse to 2 (1.4%) and general relapse to 5 (3.7%) cases can be considered a satisfactory result.

In my opinion, it can be explained in the following way: 1) the employed temperature regime (+20+25°C) was the best indeed, ensuring sufficient protection from anoxia with a duration up to 2 hours and at the same time caused minimal cold injury in the kidney; 2) a positive role played the widening of indications to the application of local hypothermia and its use in all cases of renal blood circulation blockade, including those of short duration. Such tactics permitted the minimizing of the harmful consequences of anoxia and prevention of ischemic microinfarctions in the kidney, which could be the basis of true stone relapse formation.

As for the 3 false stone relapses in the initial period of our work, they were accidental and their reasons were quite removable.

It also has to be mentioned that normalization of arterial blood pressure in 60 among 75 patients suffering from arterial hypothermia before the operation, occurred. The objective reasons of this phenomenon could be radicalism of intervention, decrease of intrarenal pressure, and elimination or lowering of an inflammatory process in the kidney.

In conclusion, it can be noted that recommendations about the optimal level of hypothermia and the described apparatus can be used in the clinic for auto-and allotransplantations of kidneys and testes. In case of need, this apparatus can ensure a stable, uniform and safe hypothermia up to +2°C.

CONCLUSION

1) The kidney denervation in situ and by autotransplantation is accompanied with degeneration of most of its intraorganic nervous apparatus with principal damage of adrenergic structures and cessation of catecholamins production; single cholinergic nerve fibers are kept.
2) After denervation and autotransplantation of kidneys without surgical reinnervation by 6 months, a germination of single unmyelinized nerve fibers is observed; they do not achieve connection to nephrons and are finished in the connective tissue. Over 2 years they are unable to produce impulsation; all this testifies to their anatomical and functional insufficiency.
3) After denervation and autotransplantation of kidneys without surgical reinnervation by 4-6 months, a firm depression of functional indices occurs, the volume of renal blood circulation, filtration, secretion, reabsorption, excretion, and renographic index. At the same time it is accompanied by lymphoid infiltration, dystrophy, local and diffusive sclerosis and gradual atrophy of the kidney parenchyma. 2 years after the operation the complex functional and morphological examinations of the kidneys allows for a common potential of 60-70% of the standard.
4) After denervation and autotransplantation of the kidneys without surgical reinnervation, upsettings of intraorganic nervous apparatus is inevitably accompanied by typical pathologic, functional and morphologic disorders; these are all reasons to consider them as being determined by the seccation of the adaptive-trophic influence of the renal nervous system because of its insufficient regeneration.
5) After surgical reinnervation of denervated and autotransplanted kidneys by means of sewing of perivascular fascial shreds after Kirpatovsky, within 2 months an intensive regeneration of nerve fibers is observed; by 4-6 months they form terminals in the field of blood vessels, glomerulas, juxtamedullar apparatus, tubules, walls of calices and pyelon. At the same time an anatomical restoration happens at the postganglion part of the kidney nervous apparatus from THXII-LII up to the kidney cortical substance.
6) The regenerated nervous structures of a surgically reinnervated kidney autotransplant are able to achieve normal secretion of specific nervous mediators, catecholamines and acetylcholine with conduction of afferent and efferent impulsation. Neurophysiologic examinations performed 6 months after the operation do not reveal any qualitative deviations in the work of the recovered nervous apparatus of the

kidney. There is a lag of some quantitative indices of biopotentials (for 20-40%), but the value of this lag doesn`t exceed the corresponding one observed by other neuroplastic operations with direct sewing of nerves.

7) After the surgical reinnervation of a denervated as well as autotransplanted kidney, a gradual restoration of their functional data has taken place: the volume of renal blood circulation in 1-2 months, and secretion and reabsorption in 2-4 months. Parallel morphologic examinations show a gradual disappearance of blood stagnation and lymphoid infiltration in the kidney parenchyma (after 1-2 months), and a decrease of dystrophy degree in nephron channels (after 2-4 months). After 4-6 months and further up to 2 years the structure of the surgically reinnervated kidney on macro-, micro- and electron microscopic levels doesn`t differ from the structure of an intact kidney.
8) I. Kirpatovsky`s method of kidney surgical reinnervation ensures restoration of its nervous apparatus of full value, which is able to exert a beneficial and adequate regulative and trophic influence on the organ and keeps its high and stable level of work for a long time. This method can be recommended for wide application in surgery as well as by auto- and allotransplantation of the kidney for achievement of more favorable remote clinical results.
9) The two-hour long normothermic (+37°C) ischemia causes irreversible functional and morphologic changes in the kidney. During the 6 months after the operation the radiorenograms and renoscintigrams correspond to an unfunctioning kidney; necrotic changes and a full suppression of succinatdehydrogenase activity in the kidney parenchyma are revealed.
10) Deep hypothermia (+4+7°C) lessens the harmful consequences of two-hour ischemia, but is accompanied with prolonged disorders of blood circulation and disccordination of metabolic processes in the kidney.
11) The best level of hypothermia for the protection of a kidney by two-hour long ischemia is the temperature zone of +20+25°C. It ensures sufficient resistance to anoxia and minimal circulatory upsettings in the kidney.
12) The improved apparatus for local renal hypothermia examined and approbated in experiments and clinics can be recommended for wide application in surgery for ensuring adequate hypothermia for auto- and allotransplantations of kidneys and testicles, as well as for removal of staghorn, multiple stones and small tumors from the kidney with temporarily blocked blood circulation.

References No. 2

[1] Abbou C.C., Hoznek A., Salomon L., Ben Slama M.R., Chopin D. Is open surgery for partial nephrectomy an obsolete surgical procedure? *Curr. Opin. Urol.*, 1999; 9 (5): 383-389.

[2] Abele R.P., Novick A.C., Ishigami. Comparison of flushing solutions for in situ renal preservation. *Urology,* 1981; 18 (5): 485-489.

[3] Ackermann J.R.W., Barnard C.M. Successful storage of kidneys. *Brit.J.Surg.,* 1966; 53: 525-532.

[4] Alexeenko A.V. Morphologic changes by kidney ischemia in conditions of a local hypothermia. - In book: Materials of the 2nd scient. *Conf. of physicians.* Khabarovsk, 1968, p. 131-132.

[5] Allanson B.R., Gross R.H.M. Ultrastructural changes in renal proximal tubule cells of Tilapia mosambica peters following exposure to low temperature. - *Biologie,* Paris, 1970; III: 611-612.

[6] Andrews P.M., Bates S.B. Improving Euro-Collins flushing solution`s ability to protect kidneys from normothermic ischemia. *Miner. Electrolyte Metab.* 1985; 11 (5): 309-313.

[7] Arshba S.Y., Shioshvili T.J. *The use of a local hypothermia by operations on the "dry" kidney.* - Headline, Tbilisi, 1975, p. 1-4.

[8] Asojan G.A., Kulaev G.K. Some data about the terms of conservation by means of a transorganic gas perfusion. In the book: *Actual questions of organ and tissues transplantation.* Works of the 2nd Moscow Medical Institute, Moscow, 1978; 23: 132-133.

[9] Badenoch A., Darmady E.M. Effects of temporary occlusion of renal artery in rabbits and its relationship to traumatic uremia. - *J.Path.Bact.,* 1947; 59 (1-2): 79-94.

[10] Bagnenko S.F., Maisiuk I.G., Reznik O.N. First experience of use of a double ballon three-lumen catheter for decreasing the time of heat ischemia in asystolic kidney donors in Russia. *Vestn.Khir.im. I.I. Grekova.* 2004; 163 (2): 99-103.

[11] Belzer F.O., Ashby B.S., Duhphy J.E. 24-hour and 72-hour preservation of canine kidneys. - *Lancet,* 1967, 2: 536-539.

[12] Belzer F.O., Ashby B.S. Seventeen hour preservation and transplantation of cadaver kidney. - *Transplantation,* 1968, 6: 863-864.

[13] Belzer F.O. Current methods of kidney storage. - *Cryobiology,* 1969; 5: 444-446.

[14] Belzer F.O., Kounts S.L. Preservation and transplantation of human cadaver kidney: a two-year experience. - *Ann.Surg.,* 1970; 172: 394-403.

[15] Bigelow W.G., Lindsay W.K., Greenwood W. Hypothermia. Its possible role in cardiac surgery: An investigation of factors governing survival in dogs at low body temperatures. - *Ann.Surg.,* 1950; 132 (5): 849-866.

[16] Bilenko M.V., Cherkasova M.B., Judin L.A. A functional investigation of auto- and homotransplanted kidney by means of hippuran J131. In book: *Conference in complex investigation of kidney transplantation problem.* Moscow, 1965, p. 20-21.

[17] Bilenko M.V. Organ conservation. In book: Lectures in transplantology. *Works of P. Lumumba`s People`s Friendship University,* Moscow, 1969, p. 49-59.

[18] Bilenko M.V. Biological aspects of a kidney transplantation: *Medic Doctor dissertation.* Moscow, 1971, -62 p.

[19] Bilenko M.V. Biological aspects of a kidney allotransplantation. Moscow, *Medicine,* 1978, -384 p.

[20] Birkeland S., Vogt A., Krog J., Semb C. Renal circulatory occlusion and local cooling. *J. Appl. Physiol.,* 1959; 14 (2): 227-232.

[21] Birkeland S., Krog J., Vogt A. Renal function following renal ischemia under renal hypothermia. In: *XX Int. Physiol. Congr. Brussels,* 1956, 98-99.

[22] Bogardus G.M., Schlosser R.J. The influence of temperature upon ischemic renal damage. - *Surgery,* 1966; 39: 970-974.

[23] Bogomolow A.M. Local hypothermia in the kidney surgery. Medic Kandid. Dissertation. *Donezk,* 1969, -15 p.

[24] Buchman A.A., Slutzkin I.M. Local hypothermia in operations on the kidney. Urology a. Nephrology, *Moscow,* 1968; 5: 14-17.

[25] Cain H., Fazekas S. Studien über die Folgen einer vorübergehenden experimentällen Nierenischämie. I. Die morphologiachen Veränderugen des akuten Schadens und funktionelle Deutung. - *Virchows Arch.path.Anat.,* 1963; 336: 389-416.

[26] Calne R.Y. Ipotermia sperimentale del rene. - *Minerva Med.,* 1965; 56 (45): 1920-1921.

[27] Carra F., Macchini N., Pedetta S. L`ipotermia profonda selettiva nella preventione del danno ischemico del rene. II. Polikliniko. - *Sez.Chir.*, 1962, (3): 11-46.

[28] Carra F., Macchini N. L`ipotermia selettiva nella preventione del danni renale da ischemia. - *Minerva mod.,* 1965; 56 (45): 1932-1933.

[29] Carrel A. La technique operatoire des anastomoses vasculaires et la transplantation des visceres. - *Lyon Med.,* 1902; 98: 859-864.

[30] Cerilli G.J. Hypothermia in management of acute renal failure. - *Surgery,* 1963; 54 (2): 309-315.

[31] Cockett A.T.K. The kidney and regional hypothermia. - *Surgery,* 1961; 50 (6): 905-910.

[32] Collins G.M., Bravo-Shgarman M.M., Terasaki P.I. Kidney preservation for transplantation. II. A simple technique for 12-hour storage and air transport. - *Transplantation*, 1969; 8: 821-828.

[33] Collins G.M., Hartley L.C.J., Clunie G.I. A kidney preservation for transplantation. 5. Comparison of perfusate for hypothermic storage. - *Med.J.Austral.,* 1971; 22: 1171-1172.

[34] Cunarro J.A., Johnson W.A., Uehling D.T., Updike S.J., Weiner M.W. Metabolic consequences of low-temperature kidney preservation. *J. Lab.Clin.Med.,* 1976; 88 (6): 873-884.

[35] Darmady E.M. Correlation of renal function and structure. - *J.Clin.Path.,* 1965; 18: 493-499.

[36] Debruyne F.M. Surgical prevention in removal of staghorn calculi. - *J.Acta urol.belg.,* 1974; 42 (4): 421-433.

[37] Derkovsky M.M. Apparatus for conseration of transplanting organs. *Cold techniques,* 1969; 11: 37-39.

[38] Djandieri K.M. Examination of biochemical changes in early periods of the kidney regeneration. In the book: *Materials of 1st Conference of georgian urologists,* Tbilisi, 1961, p. 222.

[39] Dottori O., Ekestrom S., Hansson L.O. Local cooling of the kidney using perfusion technique. - *Acta chir. Scand.,* 1962; 124: 180-186.

[40] Dreikorn K., Horst R., Rohl L. 48- to 96-hour preservation of canine kidneys by initial perfusion and hypothermic storage using the Euro-Collins solution. *Eur.Urol.,* 1980; 6 (4): 221-224.

[41] Drobner V.L. Prevention of an acute renal insufficiency by kidney ischemia (Experimental investigation). Medical Candidate Dissertation. *Petrosavodsk,* 1971, -29 p.

[42] Drogaytzev A.D., Gorbatov O.I. Method of local renal hypothermia in experiment. *Journal of experimental surgery and anaesthesiology.* Moscow, 1964; 6: 76-78.

[43] Drogaytzev A.D. Local renal hypothermia. *Medical Candidate Dissertation,* Moscow, 1965, -17 p.

[44] Drogaytzev A.D., Gorbatov O.I. New modification of the renal local perfusion hypothermia. *Journal of experimental surgery and anaesthesiology.* Moscow, 1965; 3: 377-379.

[45] Drogaytzev A.D., Sorokina M.I., Kusmina L.N., Gorbatov O.I. Survival of dogs and dynamics of some biochemical indices after the kidney temporary ischemia. In the book: *Conference in complex problems of kidney transplantation.* Moscow, 1965, p. 49-50.

[46] Duguid W.H., Seright W., Thompson J.D. The effect of hypothermia on the lesion of experimental renal ischemia. -*Brit.J.Surg.,* 1958; 46: 273-281.

[47] Eilert H.B., Eggert D.E., Derlacki D.I. *Kidney Graft storage after surface cooling. Arch.Surg.*, 1971; 102: 197-198.

[48] Eisendrath D.N., Strauss D.C. The effect on the kidney of temporary compression of its vessels. - *J.A.M.A.,* 1910; 55 (27): 2286-2290.

[49] Enfendgiev M. About a nephrolythotomy. *Urology* (Moscow), 1961; 2: 11-16.

[50] Farcon E.M. In vivo hypothermic perfusion during renal surgery. *Urology,* 1974; 3 (4): 414-420.

[51] Fisher E.R., Copeland C., Fisher B. Correlation of ultrastructure and function following hypothermic preservation of canine kidney. - *Lab.Invest.,* 1967; 17: 99-119.

[52] Fraley E.E., Malt R.A. Intracellular defect produced by renal ischemia. - *Surgery,* 1967; 62: 221-226.

[53] Gayer G. Electron histochemistry. Moscow, *MIR.* 1974. - 488 p.

[54] Gill J.S., Abreu S.C., Dasai M.M. Laparoscopic ice slush renal hypothermia for partial nephrectomy: the initial experience. *J.Urol.* 2003; 170 (1): 52-56.

[55] Glosman O.S., Golzova T.G., Zikeeva A.I. Influence of hypothermia in the development of experimental nephrocalcinose in rats. *Arch. Pathol. Moscow,* 1961, 4: 37-42.
[56] Gorjunov V.G. Kidney local hypothermia and its clinical application. *Medic Candidate Dissertation.* Moscow, 1969, - 20 p.
[57] Gow J.G., Ross J.C., Hill C.A. *Partial nephrectomy.* - Lancet, 1959; II: 759-761.
[58] Gritzman U.J., Levitzkaya L.A., Goldina B.G. Experimental basis of kidney conservation at 0°C temperature. In the book: *Current problems of operational surgery. Moscow,* 1968, p. 66-67.
[59] Hamilton P.B., Phillips R.A., Hiller A. Duration of renal ischemia required to produce uremia. - *Amer.J.Physiol.,* 1948; 152: 517-522.
[60] Hanley H.G., Joekes A.M., Wickham J.E.A. Renal hypothermia in complicated nephrolithotomy. - *J.Urol.,* 1968; 99 (5): 517-520.
[61] Hardy J.D. High ureteral injuries. Management by autotransplantation of the kidney. - *J.A.M.A.,* 1963; 184 (2): 97-101.
[62] Hardy J.D., Eraslan S. Autotransplantation of the kidney for high ureteral injury. - *J.Urol.,* 1963; 90 (5): 563-574.
[63] Hendren T.H., Hardin C.A. Low molecular dextran effect on temporary renal ischemia. - *Arch.Surg.,* 1964; 68 (2): 206-208.
[64] Herrell S.D., Jahoda A.E., Husain A.N., Albala D.M. The laparoscopic cooling sheath: novel device for hypothermic preservation of kidney during temporary renal artery occlusion. *J. Endourol.,* 1998; 12 (2): 155-161.
[65] Ishikawa M., Sugimura X. Hypoxia due to occlusion of renal blood vessels. - *Urol. Int.,* 1961; 12: 228-245.
[66] Isik H. A new microcontroller supervised thermoelectric renal hypothermia system. *J.Med.Syst.,* 2005; 29 (5): 441-447.
[67] Isselhard W., Denecke H., Witte J., Berger M., Fischer J.H. Renal function after hypothermic kidney ischemia with orthograde and retrograde O2 persulflation in situ. *Res.Exp.Med.* (Berl.), 1972; 157 (3): 231-234.
[68] Isselhard W., Witte J., Denecke H., Berger M., Fischer J.H. Kidney function following hypothermic aerobic ischemia in situ. *Pflugers Arch.;* 1972: Suppl. 332: R 26.
[69] Jones W.R., Politano V.A. The effects of renal artery occlusion on renal function under normothermia and regional hypothermia. - *J.Urol.,* 1963; 89 (4): 535-540.
[70] Kalandadze N.I., Schioschwili T.J. Histomorphologie und Aktivität der Suksinatdehydrogenase der Niere nach experimenteller Ischämie bei verschiedenen Temperaturen. - *Z.Urol.Nephrol.,* 1973; 66 (7): 497-502.
[71] Kallerhoff M., Holscher M., Kehrer G., Klass G., Bretschneider H.J. Effects of preservation conditions and temperature on tissue acidification in canine kidneys. *Transplantation,* 1985; 39 (5): 485-489.
[72] Kallerhoff M., Blech M., Kehrer G., Kleinert H., Langheinrich M., Sickmann W., Helmchem U., Bretschneider H.J. Kidney function parameters following ischemia stress using the Euro-Collins Solution or the Bretschneider cardioplegic HTK Solution. *Urologe A,* 1987; 26 (2): 96-103.
[73] Kallerhoff M., Blech M., Isemer F.E., Kehrer g., Kleinert H., Langheinrich M., Helmchen U., Bretschneider H.J. Metabolic, energetic and structural changes in

protected and unprotected kidneys at temperatures of 1 degree C and 25 degrees C. *Urol. Res.*, 1988; 16 (1): 57-62.

[74] Koletsky S., Persky L., Stueber P. Regional renal hypothermia. - *Surgery,* 1958; 44 (1): 77-83.

[75] Kovacs S., Persky L., Stueber P. The protective value of hypothermia in renal anoxia: evaluation by selective cooling of the kidney. - *Anaeth. Analg.,* 1959; 38: 157-161.

[76] Krendel B.M. Extracorporal surgery and autotransplantation of the kidney. Survery of foreign literature. *Urology and Nephrology,* Moscow, 1977; 5: 80-89.

[77] Lande S.I., Subramaniam F.V., Tiedemann R.N. 24 hour venous-arterial perfusions of awake dogs with a simple membrane oxygenator. - *Tr.Amer.Soc.Artif.Int. Organs,* 1969; 15: 181-186.

[78] Landman J., Rehman J., Sundaram C.P., Bhavani S., Monga M., Pattaras J.G., Gokden N., Humphrey P.A., Clavman R.V. Renal hypothermia achieved by retrograde intracavitary saline perfusion. *J. Endourol.,* 2002; 16 (7): 445-449.

[79] Landman J., Venkatesh R., Lee D. Renal hypothermia achieved by retrograde endoscopic cold saline perfusion: technique and initial clinical application. *Journal of Urology.* 2003; 61: 1023-1025.

[80] Larionov V.G. Autotransplantation of conservated kidneys. *Medical Candidate Dissertation.* Smolensk, 1965, -16 p.

[81] Levy M.N. Oxygen consumption and blood flow in the hypothermic perfused kidney. - *Amer.J.Physiol.,* 1959; 147: 111-114.

[82] Lieberthal W., Rennke H.G., Sandock K.M., Valeri C.R., Levinsky N.G. Ischemia in the isolated erythrocyte-perfused rat kidney. Protective effect of hypothermia. *Ren. Physiol. Biochem,* 1988; 11 (1-2): 60-69.

[83] Lillehei R.C. In vitro preservation of whole organs by hypothermia and hyperbaric oxygenation. - *Cryobiology,* 1964; 1: 181-193.

[84] Lilli R. Pathohistologic techniques and practical histochemistry. Moscow, *Mir,* 1969, -645 p.

[85] Lopatkin N.A., Lopuchin J.M., Pytel J.A. About the transplantation of a cadaverous kidney. *Urology a. Nephrology. Moscow,* 1967; 5: 34-48.

[86] Lopatkin N.A., Maso E.B., Krendel B.M. Extracorporary surgery of the kidney in the treatment of a vasorenal hypertonia. *Urology a. Nephrology, Moscow,* 1977; 5: 31-35.

[87] Lopatkin N.A., Maso E.B., Gorjunov V.G. Local hypothermia in operations because of nephrolithiasis. *Urology a. Nephrology, Moscow,* 1968; 5: 17-23.

[88] Lopatkin N.A., Lopuchin J.M., Kuchinsky I.N. Homotransplantation of a cadaverous kidney in the clinics. In the book: *Actual problems of organ transplantation. Moscow,* 1969, p. 185-214.

[89] Lopuchin J.M., Shifrin E.G., Cheknev B.M. Organ conservation in conditions of hypothermia and hyperbaric oxygenation. In the book: *Actual problems of organ transplantation. Moscow.,* 1969, p. 168-182.

[90] Lopuchin J.M. Current state of organ transplantation problem. Moscow, *Znanie,* 1971, -79 p.

[91] Lopuchin J.M., Kogan E.M., Karaganov J.D. Ultrastructural grounds of liver, kidney and heart vitality. Moscow, *Medicine,* 1977, -255 p.

[92] Lovelock J.E. Denaturation of lipid-protein complexes as a cause of damage by freezing. - *Proc.Roy.Soc., B.,* 1957; 147: 427-433.

[93] Lowenstein L.M., Paddock J.K. Brush border membrane injury and regeneration following renal ischemia. *Int.J.Biochem,* 1980; 12 (1-2): 235-236.

[94] Maathuis M.H., Manekeller S., van der Plaats A., Leuvenink H.G., Hart N.A., Lier A.B., Rakhorst G., Ploeg R.J., Minor T. Improved kidney graft function after preservation using a novel hypothermic machine perfusion device. *Ann. Surg.,* 2007; 246 (6): 982-991.

[95] Macksood A.I., Szilagyi D.E., Smith R.F. The maintenance by cold perfusion of the viability of the devascularised canine kidney. - *Surg.Forum,* 1961; 12: 190-191.

[96] Majno G., La Gaftuta M., Thompson T.E. Cellular death and necrosis: chemical, physical and morphological changes in rat liver. - *Virch.Arch.Path.Anat.,* 1960; 333: 421-425.

[97] Makarenko V.S. Survival of animals and changes of blood some biochemical data by acute circulatory disorders in the kidney. In the book: Materials of 1st Congress of the Belorussian physiological cociety, *Minsk,* 1962, p. 123-125.

[98] Makarenko V.S. Functional state of kidneys after one-side kidney ischemia. *Journ. Public Health of Belorussia,* 1965; 3: 30-31.

[99] Makarenko V.S. Recovery of kidney function after its acute ischemia. In the book: Some questions of morphology and physiology, *Minsk,* 1966, p. 46-48.

[100] Manax W.G., Block J.H., Longerbeam J.K., Gillehei R.C. Successful 24 hour in vitro preservation of canine kidneys by the combined use of hyperbaric oxygenation and hypothermia. *Surgery,* 1964; 56: 275-282.

[101] Manax W.G., Bloch J.H., Largiaber F. Organ perfusion before transplantation with particular reference to the kidney. - *Surgery,* 1965, 54: 528-534.

[102] Marberger M., Takaha M., Lorenz J., Gunter F., Fischer D., Orestano F. Short time in situ preservation of the ischemic kidney by a simple initial hypothermic perfusion with various cold solutions. An animal experimental study. *Urologe A.*, 1975, 14 (4): 199-204.

[103] Marberger M., Piroth D., Gunter R., Alken P., Scheiblich H. The impact of in situ ballon occlusion of the renal artery and hypothermic perfusion on renal blood flow. *Urol. Res.,* 1978; 6 (1): 49-55.

[104] Marberger M., Eisenberger F. Regional hypothermia of the kidney: surface or transarterial perfusion cooling? A function study. *J. Urol.,* 1980; 124: 179-183.

[105] Marshall E.K., Crane M.M. The influence of temporary closure of the renal artery on the amount and composition of urine. - *Amer. J. physiol.,* 1923; 64 (2): 387-403.

[106] Martines G., Motta G., Musacci G.F. Rilievi ultrastrutturali nella ipotermia renale profonda. (Nota technical preliminarie). - *Minerva chir.,* 1967; 22 (3): 115-117.

[107] McAnulty J.F., Huang X.Q. Nonesterified fatty acid content of rabbit kidney cortex slices after warm ischemia and low temperature preservation. *Cryobiology,* 1996; 33 (1): 70-81.

[108] McAnulty J.F., Huang. X.Q. The efficacy of antioxidants administered during low temperature storage of warm ischemic kidney tissue slices. *Cryobiology,* 1997; 34 (4): 406-415.

[109] Merill J.P., Murray J.E., Harrison J.H. Successful homotransplantation of the human kidney between identical twins. *J.A.M.A.,* 1956, 160 (4): 277-282.

[110] Metzner P.J., Boyce W.H. Simplified renal hypothermia: an adjunct to conservative renal surgery. - *Brit J. Urol.,* 1972; 44: 76-85.

[111] Mikeladze A.L., Shioshvili T.J. Electron microscopic investigation of kidneys by ischemia and hypothermia. In the book: Materials of iInternational Conference in electron microscopy. *Varna,* 1971, p. 128.

[112] Mikeladze A.L., Arshba S.J., Shioshvili T.J. Electron microscopical investigation of kidneys after their experimental ischemia in various temperature conditions. *Cytology, Leningrad,* 1972; 14 (5): 579-584.

[113] Mikeladze A.L., Shioshvili T.J. Kidney ultrastructure by ischemia and hypothermia, Tbilisi, *Mezniereba,* 1975, -122 p.

[114] Minor T., Schumacher H.B., Wideman Y.R.F. Comparison of renal oxygen consumption and blood flow with cooling and rewarming. - *Surgery,* 1967; 61: 256-259.

[115] Mitchell R.M., Woodruff M.F. The effects of local hypothermia in increasing tolerance of the kidney to ischemia. - *Transplant.Bull.,* 1957; 4: 15.

[116] Mitchell R.M. Renal cooling and ischemia. - *Brit J. Surg.,* 1959; 46: 593-597.

[117] Molkoff J.N., Golikova S.D., Kirjanoff V.K. Transplantation of vitally important organs. In the book: Materials of 7th Allunion Conference in organ a. tissue transplantation. *Rostov,* 1976; 1: 38-38.

[118] Molotkoff V.G., Larionov V.G. Pathologic anatomy changes in dog kidneys after autotransplantation of the conservated right kidney. In the book: Works of Smolensk Medical Institute, *Smolensk,* 1963; 16: 119-137.

[119] Momose S., Hirata K., Baba M. Renal ischemia and hypothermia. - *Urol.intern.,* 1961; 12 (4-5): 161-163.

[120] Moor F. History of organ transplantation. Moscow, *Mir,* 1973, - 312 p.

[121] Navarro A.P., Sohrabi S., Colechin E., Griffiths C., Talbot D., Soomro N.A. Evaluation of the ischemic protection efficacy of a laparoscopic renal cooling device using renal transplantation viability assessment criteria in a porcine model. *J.Urol,* 2008; 179 (3); 1184-1189.

[122] Neely W.A., Turner P.H.D. The effect of arterial, venous and arteriovenous occlusion on renal blood flow. - *Surg.Gynec.Obst.,* 1959; 108: 669-672.

[123] Nekrasova I.A. Influence of a short-time ischemia on the kidney and a protective role of the local hypothermia in operations with blockaded kidney blood circulation. Medical Candidate Dissertation. *Donetzk,* 1971, -17 p.

[124] Newman H. Renal hypothermia produced by direct application of ice. - *J.Urol.,* 1963; 89 (3): 319-324.

[125] Oblomova U.F. Recovery processes in pigeon kidneys after one-side nephrectomy. Medical Candidate Dissertation. *Samarkand,* 1967, -16 p.

[126] Oganesjan A.S. Influence of a cold on the kidney diuresis and filtration. News of Armenian Academy of Sciences, Biology a. Agricultural Sciences, *Erevan,* 1956; 9 (9): 33-38.

[127] Opitz E., Rotter W., Hilscher W. Uber die 'Wiederbelebungszeit" der Rattenniere. - *Verh.Gtsch.Ges.Path.,* 1953; 37: 336-342.

[128] Osipovich V.V. Some mechanisms of kidney vicarious hypertrophy. *Medical Candidate Dissertation.* Novosibirsk, 1965, -11 p.

[129] Ovnatanjan K.T., Sernjak P.S., Bogomolov A.M., Suslov V.V. Local hypothermia in kidney staghorne and multiple stone surgery. *Experimental surgery a. anaesthesiology, Moscow,* 1965; 6: 50-53.

[130] Ovnatanjan K.T., Bogomolov A.M., Suslov V.V. 50 operations on the "dry" kidney after local hypothermia. *Clinical surgery, Moscow,* 1967; 1: 1-6.

[131] Ovnatanjan K.T., Suslov V.V., Bogomolov A.M. Surgery of a cooled kidney. I. Grekov`s Herald of surgery, *Moscow,* 1969; 2: 53-59.

[132] Ovnatanjan K.T., Suslov V.V., Bogomolov A.M., Gluchova K.Z. Local hypothermia in urological practice. Kiev, *Zdorovja,* 1969, -156 p.

[133] Paddock J.K., Lada W., Lowenstein L.M. Regeneration of the renal brush border after renal ischemia in rats. *Am. J. Physiol.,* 1981; 241 (1): 28-33.

[134] Palivoda N.I. Clinic and treatment of kidney staghorn stones. Medical Candidate Dissertation. *Minsk,* 1968, -19 p.

[135] Palmer J.M., Guernsey J.M., Connolly J.E. An experimental study of selective renal hypothermia. - *Amer.J.Surg.,* 1963; 106 (8): 224-232.

[136] Pegg D.E., Green C.J. Renal preservation by hypothermic perfusion. I. The importance of pressure control. - *Cryobiology,* 1973; 10 (1): 56-66.

[137] Peirce E.C., Mathewson W.T. Design and fabrication of blood oxygenator for circulatory assist devices. - In: *Artificial program conference.* Washington, 1969; p. 405-416.

[138] Petrovsky B.V., Solovjev G.M., Govallo V.I. *Kidney transplantation.* Moscow, Medicine, 1969. - 240 p.

[139] Pichlmaier H. Praktische Ergebnisse bei der Nierenverplanzung. - *Therap.Ber.,* 1969; 19: 631-638.

[140] Prather G.C. Method of hemostasis during nephrostomy. - *J.Urol.,* 1934; 32 (6): 578-599.

[141] Proctor E., Mathews G., Archibald J. Acute orthotopic transplantation of hearts stored for 72 hours. - *Thorax,* 1971; 26: 99-102.

[142] Rojdestvensky V.I. Influence of a temporary breaking of renal blood circulation on the kidney function. Works of P. *Lesgaft Scientific Institute, Leningrad,* 1927; 12 (2): 97-117.

[143] Rossotto P., Motta G., Azzena G.F. Stidio metabolico sull azione protettiva della ipotermi profonda nell anossia renale. - *Minerva med.,* 1966; 57 (88): 3687-3690.

[144] Rothauge C.F., Voss H., Bettge S. Nierenfunktion und Nierendurchblutung in Hypothermie. - *Bull soc.int. Chir.,* 1960; 19 (4): 393-397.

[145] Ruffo A., Rossotto R., Motta G. Histopatologie dell ipotermie d`organo. - *Minerva med.,* 1965; 56 (45): 1872-1887.

[146] Ruffo A., Rossotto R., Motta G. Ipotermia selettiva del rene. - *Minerva med.,* 1965; 56 (45): 1921-I-1931.

[147] Ruffo A., Rossotto R., Motta G. L`hypothermia d`organe et ses applications en urologie. - *Presse med.,* 1965; 73 (6): 293-294.

[148] Ruffo A., Rossotto R., Motta G. Rilievi ultrastrutturali nella ipotermia renale profonda. - *Minerva med.,* 1966; 57 (88): 3697-3722.

[149] Schioschwili T.J. Locale Hypothermie bei Operationen an der "trockenen" Niere. - *Z.Urol.Nephrol.,* 1971; 64 (7): 503-507.

[150] Schioschwili T.J. Apparat für die locale Hypothermie der Niere. - *Z.Urol.Nephrol.,* 1973; 66 (7): 493-496.

[151] Schirmer H.K.A. The effect of intermitten and prolonged renal artery occlusion upon respiration and anaerobic glycolysis of dog kidney. - *L.Urol.,* 1965; 94 (5): 511-513.

[152] Schloerb P.R., Waldorf R.D., Welsh J.S. The protective effect of kidney hypothermia on total renal ischemia. - *Surg.Forum,* 1957; 8: 633-635.

[153] Semb C. Renal tuberculosis and its treatment by partial resection of the kidney. - *Acta Chir.Scand.,* 1949; 98 (3-6): 457-475.

[154] Semb C. Partial resection of the kidney: anatomical, physiological and clinical aspects. - *Ann.Roy.Coll. Surg. Eng.,* 1956; 19: 137-155.

[155] Semb C. Local cooling of the kidney for protection against operative trauma. - *Acta Chir.Scand.,* 1959; Suppl. 245: 368-372.

[156] Semb C., Krog J., Johanser K. Renal metabolism and blood flow during local hypothermia, studied by means of renal perfusion in situ. - *Acta Chir. Scand.,* 1960; 253: 196-202.

[157] Semb C., Hoeg K., Vogt A. Die Teilresektion der Niere und die Nierenfunktion. - *Urologie,* 1963 (3): 131-140.

[158] Shioshvili T.J. Apparatus for local renal hypothermia. USSR Author`s certificate N 340327, 1972; USA Patent N 3738372, 1972; UK Patent N 1331002, 1973; Norway Patent N 130751, 1974.

[159] Shioshvili T.J. Electron microscopical investigation of god kidneys after a temporary ischemia in various temperature regimes. In the book: *Materials of the 8th Allunion Conference in electron microscopy.* Moscow, 1971; 3: p. 61-61.

[160] Shioshvili T.J. Local hypothermia in operations on a "dry" kidney. *Medical Candidate Dissertation,* Tbilisi, 1972, - 23 p.

[161] Shioshvili T.J. Indications and contrarindications to use of the local renal hypothermia in clinics. In the book: *Questions of clinical a. experimental urology.* Tbilisi, 1972; 8: 32-36.

[162] Shioshvili T.J. Temporary blockade of the blood circulation in operations on the kidney. In the book: *Questions of clinical a. experimental urology,* Tbilisi, 1973, 9: 34-35.

[163] Shioshvili T.J. Radiologic evaluation of functional changes in kidneys after various degrees of a local hypothermia by ischemia. *Journ.experim. surgery a. anaesthesiology,* Moscow, 1974; 3: 81-83.

[164] Shioshvili T.J. Results of the clinical use of a "dry" kidney`s hypothermia. *Eur. Urol.,* 1977; 3: 154-158.

[165] Shioshvili T.J. *Local hypothermia by operations on the "dry" kidney.* Tbilisi, Sabtchota Sakartvelo (Sovjet Georgia), 1978, - 148 p.

[166] Shumakov V.I., Stengold E.S., Onishenko N.A., Matveeva G.A. Dying energetics in isolated organs. *Journ. Experim. Surgery a. Anaesthesiology,* Moscow, 1974; 1: 54-59.

[167] Shumakov V.I., Stengold E.S., Onishenko N.A. Conservation of the kidney in experiments and clinics. *Surgery,* Moscow, 1972; 2: 95-102.

[168] Shumakov V.I., Zubarev V.A., Stengold E.S. Techniques and method for a kidney conservation. *Medical techniques,* Moscow, 1972; 3: 6-9.

[169] Shumakov V.I., Onishenko N.A. Pathohenesis of an injurying influence of hypothermia on isolated organs. In the book: *Actual questions of organ conservation.* Moscow, 1978; 1: 41-59.

[170] Shumakov V.I., Stengold E.S., Onishenko N.A. *Organ conservation,* Moscow, Medicine, 1975, - 252 p.

[171] Siegel M.B., Lowenstein L.M., Levinsky H.G. Choline uptake into renal phospholipids following renal ischemia in rats. *Circ. Res.,* 1979; 44 (1): 62-67.

[172] Starzl T.E. *Experience in renal transplantation* . - Philadelphia-London, 1964. - 246 p.

[173] Stewart H.H. The surgery of the kidney in the treatment of renal stone. - *Brit.J.Urol.,* 1960; 32: 392-415.

[174] Stoll H., Carlson C.B. The anuria following temporary anemia of the kidney. - *Amer.J.physiol.,* 1923; 67: 153-158.

[175] Stubbs A.J. Antrophic nephrolithotomy in the solitary kidney. *J. Urol.,* 1978; 119: 457-460.

[176] Stueber P.J., Kovacs S., Koletsky S. Regional hypothermia in acute renal ischemia. - *J.Urol.,* 1958; 79 (5): 793-800.

[177] Thoenes W. Mikromorphologie des Nephron nach temporaren Ischemie., - *In. V.Int.* Congr. Electron Mikroscopy. - Philadelphia, 1962; 2: 2-4.

[178] Thoenes W. Mikromorphologie des Nephron nach temporaren Ischemie. - *Stuttgart: G.Thieme,* 1964. - 199 S.

[179] Toledo-Pereyra L.H., Najarian J.S. Pulsative flow and viability of isolated perfused kidneys. - *Transplantation,* 1973; 16 (1): 63-64.

[180] Tovstoles K.F., Shevtzoff I.P., Banjkovsky N.S. Use of a "dry" operating field and local hypothermia in the surgery of kidney staghorn stones. In the book: *Materials of 1st Conference of Caucasian Republics,* Sukhumi, 1977, p. 194-195.

[181] Tziskarishvili L.D. *About the vitality of a kidney in case of ligation of its vascular pedicle,* Tbilisi, Grusmedgis, 1952, - 21 p.

[182] Tziskarishvili L.D. Ligation of kidney main vessels by its TBC injury. In the book: *Works of the 1st Conference of Azerbaijanian urologists.* Baku, 1958; p. 215-219.

[183] Van Slyke D.D., Phyllips R.A., Hamilton P.B. Effect of shock on the kidney. *Tr. Ass. Amer. Physicans*, 1944; 58: 119-127.

[184] Venkatachalam M.A., Bernard D.B., Donohoe J.F., Levinsky N.G. *Ischemic damage and repair in the rat proximal tubule: differences among the S1, S2 and S3 segments. Kidney Int.,* 1978; 14 (1): 31-49.

[185] Venkatachalam M.A., Jones D.B., Rennke H.G., Sandstrom D., Patel Y. Mechanism of proximal tubule brush border loss and regeneration following mild renal ischemia. *Lab. Invest.,* 1981; 45 (4): 355-365.

[186] Veroux G., Basile M., Benigno A. L`uso dell ipotermia selettiva nella preventione del danno renale da ischemia acuta. Studio dell attivite fosfatasica. - *Minerva med.,* 1966; 57 (83): 3722-3725.

[187] Vesirov M.D. Investigation of a kidney acute ischemia in experiment. *Medic. Candidate Dissertation. Makhatchkala,* 1968, - 20 p.

[188] Vineberg S.S. Kidney stones. Moscow, *Medicine,* 1971, - 199 p.

[189] Viville C., Schueller D., de Petriconi R. Contact renal refrigeration with continuous control of the intrarenal temperature in surgery for staghorn calculi. *J.Urol.* (Paris), 1983; 89 (5): 345-349.

[190] Wakabayashi Y., Narita M., Kim C.J. Renal hypothermia using ice slush for retroperitoneal laparoscopic partial nephrectomy. *Urology,* 2004; 63: 773-775.

[191] Ward J.P. Determination of the optimal temperature for regional renal hypothermia during temporary renal ischemia. *Brir. J.Urol.,* 1975; 47: 17-24.

[192] Webb L. Inhibitors of ferments and metabolism. Moscow, *Mir,* 1966, - 362 p.

[193] Weiss L., Armstrong J.A. Structural changes in mammalian cells associated with cooling to -79°C. - *J.Biophys. Biochem.Cytol.,* 1960; 7: 673-678.

[194] Wickham J.E.A., Hanley H.G., Joekes A.M. Regional renal hypothermia. - *Brit.J.Urol.,* 1967; 39 (6): 727-743.

[195] Wickham J.E.A. A simple method for regional renal hypothermia. - *J.Urol.,* 1968; 99 (3): 246-247.

[196] Wickham J.E.A., Coe N., Ward J.P. One hundred cases of nephrolithotomy under hypothermia. - *J.Urol.,* 1974; 112 (6): 702-705.

[197] Wilson G.S.M. Clinical experience in renal hypothermia. - *J.Urol.,* 1963; 89 (5): 666-669.

[198] Yoho A., Stueber P.J., Koletsky S. Further experiences with occlusion of the renal pedicle. - *J.Urol.,* 1961; 86 (2): 185-188.

[199] Zimmerman H. Experimentelle histologische, histochemische und funktionelle Untersuchungen zur Frage der Nierenschädigung nach temporärer Ischämie. - *Beitr. path.Anat.*, 1957; 117 (1): 65-84.

[200] Zufarov K.A., Gontmacher V.M. Atlas. Electron microscopy of the kidney. *Medicine,* Tashkent, 1969; - 102 p.

INDEX

A

B

E

F

G

H

I

K

L

M

N

O

P

Q

R

S

T

U

V

W